# BURN TRAUMA

TRAUMA MANAGEMENT
Volume IV

*Series Editors*

F. William Blaisdell, M.D.
Professor and Chairman
Department of Surgery
University of California, Davis
Sacramento, California

Donald D. Trunkey, M.D.
Professor and Chairman
Department of Surgery
The Oregon Health Sciences University
Portland, Oregon

# BURN TRAUMA

**Robert H. Demling, M.D.**
Professor of Surgery
Harvard Medical School
Director, Longwood Area Trauma/Burn Center
Boston, Massachusetts

**Cheryl LaLonde**
Burn Technician and
Senior Research Associate, Department of Surgery
Brigham and Women's and Beth Israel Hospitals
Boston, Massachusetts

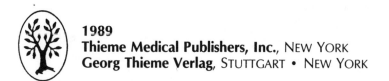

**1989**
**Thieme Medical Publishers, Inc.**, NEW YORK
**Georg Thieme Verlag**, STUTTGART • NEW YORK

Thieme Medical Publishers, Inc.
381 Park Avenue South
New York, New York 10016

BURN TRAUMA
Robert H. Demling, Cheryl LaLonde

**Library of Congress Cataloging-in-Publication Data**

Demling, Robert H.
Burn trauma / Robert H. Demling, Cheryl LaLonde.
p.   cm. -- (Trauma management : v. 4)
Includes index.
ISBN 0-86577-281-9
1. Burns and scalds.   I. LaLonde, Cheryl.   II. Title.
III. Series.
[DNLM: 1. Burns.   2. Burns--therapy.   3. Multiple Trauma.   WO 700
T776 v. 4]
RD96.4.D46 1989
617.1'1-dc20
DNLM/DLC
for Library of Congress                                              89-4566
                                                                        CIP

Copyright © 1989 by Thieme Medical Publishers, Inc. This book, including all parts thereof, is legally protected by copyright. Any use, exploitation or commercialization outside the narrow limits set by copyright legislation, without the publisher's consent, is illegal and liable to prosecution. This applies in particular to photostat reproduction, copying, mimeographing or duplication of any kind, translating, preparation of microfilms, and electronic data processing and storage.

*Important note:* Medicine is an ever-changing science. Research and clinical experience are continually broadening our knowledge, in particular our knowledge of proper treatment and drug therapy. Insofar as this book mentions any dosage or applications, readers may rest assured that the authors, editors, and publishers have made every effort to ensure that such references are strictly in accordance with the state of knowledge at the time of production of the book. Nevertheless, every user is requested to carefully examine the manufacturers' leaflets accompanying each drug to check on his own responsibility whether the dosage schedules recommended therein or the contraindications stated by the manufacturers differ from the statements made in the present book. Such examination is particularly important with drugs that are either rarely used or have been newly released on the market.

Some of the product names, patents, and registered designs referred to in this book are in fact registered trademarks or proprietary names even though specific reference to this fact is not always made in the text. Therefore, the appearance of a name without designation as proprietary is not to be construed as a representation by the publisher that it is in the public domain.

Printed in the United States of America.

5   4   3   2   1

TMP ISBN 0-86577-281-9
GTV ISBN 3-13-736301-2

# Dedication

This book is dedicated to: my mother; my wife, Pat; and my children, Jill and Kate, whose continued support and understanding have made this book possible, and to the burn care team whose dedication to patient care is the primary moving force behind new advances in the burn field.

R.H.D.

# Contents

| | |
|---|---|
| Preface | ix |

## Section 1—Resuscitation Phase (0 to 36 Hours)     1

| | |
|---|---|
| 1. Airway and Pulmonary Abnormalities | 3 |
| 2. Restoration and Maintenance of Hemodynamic Stability | 24 |
| 3. Management of the Burn Wound | 42 |
| 4. Transfer to Burn Facility | 66 |

## Section 2—Postresuscitation Phase (2 to 6 Days)     69

| | |
|---|---|
| 5. Pulmonary Abnormalities | 71 |
| 6. Maintaining Hemodynamic Stability | 84 |
| 7. Daily Care of the Burn Wound | 101 |
| 8. Early Wound Excision and Grafting | 118 |

## Section 3—Inflammation-Infection Phase (7 Days to Wound Closure)     147

| | |
|---|---|
| 9. Pulmonary Abnormalities | 149 |
| 10. Hemodynamic and Metabolic Support | 168 |
| 11. Management of the Burn Wound | 179 |
| 12. Infection and Sepsis | 193 |

## Section 4—Rehabilitation and Wound Remodeling Phase     207

| | |
|---|---|
| 13. Rehabilitation and Wound Remodeling | 209 |
| 14. Treatment | 213 |

## Section 5—Electrical Burns 221

15. High Tension Electrical Burns 223
16. Low Tension Oral Burns 240
17. Lightning 242

## Section 6—Management of Burns in the Multiple Trauma Patient 245

18. Management of Burns in the Multiple Trauma Patient 247

## Section 7—Reference Section 257

19. Respiratory Function 259
20. Hemodynamics and Perfusion 272
21. Nutritional Support 290
22. Topical Antibiotics 299

Index 305

Color Plates 309

# Preface

The burn patient undergoes a number of dramatic physiologic and metabolic changes over the course of the injury state. These changes are so marked that the physician may have the feeling of treating a different patient every several days as the process evolves. It is essential to have a clear understanding of the pathophysiologic differences and the necessary treatment modifications needed over time following the burn. To help clarify this process, the burn injury is divided into the following phases, which will be discussed in separate sections, and in addition, we have covered the specific areas of electrical injury and burns in the presence of other trauma:

1. Resuscitation phase (0 to 36 hours)
2. Postresuscitation phase (2 to 6 days)
3. Inflammation, infection phase (7 days to wound closure)
4. Rehabilitation and wound remodeling phase (admission to 1 year postburn)
5. Electrical burns
6. Combined trauma and burns
7. Reference section (appendix respiratory function)

A reference section on general critical care management has been added to complement the information presented in the four phases, since the major burn patient becomes a very complex critical care patient. The final outcome of the patient is based as much on provision of critical care as it is on skillful management of the wound.

## EPIDEMIOLOGY

It is estimated that each year 1% of the population of the United States has a burn injury. There are more than 2 million burns annually, of which one fourth will require medical care and produce significant, at least temporary, disability. Approximately 100,000 burn patients required hospital admission and more than 10,000 persons die of burn-related causes annually in the United States. The most common age groups involved are the toddler (2 to 4 years), for whom scalds are the most common cause, and the young adult (17 to 25 years), usually male, for whom the most common cause is a flammable liquid. Structural fires account for less than 5% of hospital admissions but are responsible for more than 45% of burn-related deaths. The National Fire Prevention and Control Administration estimates that there are 2,600,000 reported fires and 30,000,000 unreported fires annually. Half of these are believed to be started by children. These fires result in 7500 deaths and 310,000 serious injuries and an annual economic loss of nearly $14 billion dollars, which includes property and personal injury losses. More than two thirds of fire deaths occur in residential rather than work-related fires. Hotel and other multiple victim fires account for less than 5% of total fire-related deaths. Males between the ages of 18 and 25 years are at highest risk. Heating unit failures account for the highest percentage of home fires, followed by cooking accidents. Cigarette smoking accidents rank as the number one cause of fatal fires, being responsible for more than 2000 deaths per year. Most fire-related deaths have a smoke inhalation injury as a major contributor to the fatality. Although the incidence of burns does not appear to be decreasing substantially, fire-related deaths have decreased by 20% in recent years, due in part to mandatory smoke alarms in multifamily dwellings. Scalds are the leading cause of burn injury in children, especially under 5 years of age. The severity of injury is related to the water temperature and the time of exposure. For a third degree burn, the relationship of temperature to time is:

| | |
|---|---|
| 120°F | 10 minutes |
| 130°F | 30 seconds |
| 140°F | 10 seconds |
| 150°F | 2 seconds |

The area of the body most commonly involved is the upper extremity (70%), with the next most common area being head and neck (50%). Injuries to these areas, of course, can result in significant long-term morbidity, both from impaired function and altered appearance. Although progress in prevention has been limited, there have been major recent advances in the care of burn patients. Probit analysis methods have revealed an improved survival rate among patients in burn centers. In 1964, combination second- and third-degree burns that involved 50% of the total body surface in persons 10 to 30 years of age led to a mortality rate of about 50%. In 1974, the mortality rate among the same patients was about 30%. In 1984, a number of burn centers reported mortality rates of less than 10% for this degree of injury. Even a few years ago, burns that affected 70 to 80% of total body skin led to a mortality rate of 90% among this same age group. Many centers now report that many more of these patients are surviving. One major reason for the impressive recent progress in this field has been the expansion of the use of specialized centers for burns. There are now 150 burn units (1700 specialized burn-care beds) in the United States, compared with only a dozen just 20 years ago. About 21,000 patients with burns (approximately one third of all patients hospitalized for burns) are treated yearly in these centers. The centers have made possible not only improved care, but the multidisciplinary research responsible for the advances to be described.

Robert H. Demling, M.D.

# SECTION 1
# Resuscitation Phase (0 To 36 Hours)

Cardiopulmonary instability characterizes this period. Life-threatening airway and breathing problems are of major concern at this time, with carbon monoxide, upper airway edema, and the immediate effect of smoke inhalation injury being the most common problems. The initial phase is also characterized by hypovolemia as plasma volume is lost into the burn tissue. The burn itself, except for initial assessment as to severity and depth, and the need for escharotomies in selected cases, is of less immediate concern. Wound management becomes a higher priority component in later phases. The adequacy of initial treatment of pulmonary and circulatory abnormalities sets the stage for subsequent management. Any early management error will lead to a dramatic increase in morbidity and mortality during the subsequent injury phases.

# 1

# Airway and Pulmonary Abnormalities

Abnormalities of ventilation and oxygenation are a common finding in the immediate postburn period. There are six fairly distinct critical disease processes that must be recognized and aggressively managed. The first four are associated with the inhalation injury complex and are presented in the approximate order in which symptoms will develop. The symptom complex, diagnosis, and treatment of each disease process will be discussed.

A respiratory reference section is provided in Chapter 19 to assist in the monitoring and support of lung function during all phases of lung injury.

## GENERAL SECTIONS

- Smoke Inhalation Injury Complex
    - Hypoxia from Low Fraction of Inspired Oxygen
    - Carbon Monoxide and Cyanide Toxicity
    - Upper Airways Obstruction from Tissue Edema (Internal and External)
    - Chemical Burn to Upper and Lower Airways
- Lung Changes from Skin Burn
- Impaired Chest Wall Compliance
- Common Pitfalls in Pulmonary Support
- Summary Section

## SMOKE INHALATION INJURY COMPLEX

Pulmonary insufficiency caused by the inhalation of heat and smoke is the major cause of mortality in the fire-injured person, accounting for more than 50% of fire-related deaths. The magnitude of the problem has been much better appreciated in recent years. The use of many new synthetics in home furnishings and clothing have resulted in a much more complex form of injury, due to the extremely toxic combustion products of these advances in technology. A closed space fire can result in a severe hypoxic insult as well as lung damage from the inhalation of toxic fumes. The exposure time, the concentration of fumes, the elements released, and the degree of concomitant body burn are critical variables. These factors cause a very complex injury with morbidity and mortality risks, especially when combined with a body burn. Improved knowledge of the pathophysiology combined with an aggressive treatment plan has made it possible to improve the outcome (Fig. 1–1).

## Hypoxia from Low Fraction of Inspired Oxygen

The inspired air in a fire has a decreased oxygen tension ($PO_2$) in view of oxygen utilization during combustion. The fraction of inspired oxygen ($FiO_2$) will frequently reach 0.1 leading to an alveolar $PO_2$ ($PAO_2$) of 50 to 60 mmHg and in turn an arterial

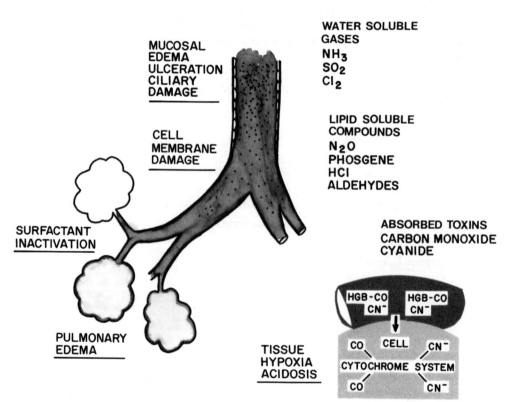

**Figure 1–1.** Chemical injury to the lung.

oxygen tension (PaO$_2$) of less than 40 mmHg. The hypoxic insult can lead to severe organ dysfunction, in particular brain, as a result of both ischemia and subsequent reperfusion injury. A brief neurologic study using the Glasgow coma scale is a part of the initial evaluation. Treatment is the immediate administration of high-flow oxygen. A persistent neurologic dysfunction after reversal of carbon monoxide toxicity and hypovolemia may well reflect the initial hypoxic insult.

## Carbon Monoxide and Cyanide Toxicity

Carbon monoxide toxicity is one of the leading causes of death in fires. While oxygen is being used during combustion, carbon monoxide is being released, since it is a basic by-product of combustion. Carbon monoxide is rapidly transported across the alveolar membrane and preferentially binds with the hemoglobin molecule in place of oxygen. In addition, carbon monoxide shifts the hemoglobin-oxygen curve to the left, thereby impairing oxygen unloading at the tissue level. The result is a major impairment in oxygen delivery, since 98% of oxygen is carried to the tissues on hemoglobin. With prolonged exposure, carbon monoxide can also saturate the cell, binding to cytochrome oxidase, thereby further impairing mitochondrial function and adenosine triphosphate (ATP) production. Production of hydrocyanide, the gaseous form of cyanide, is a well-recognized cause of morbidity and mortality, especially with burning of synthetics such as polyurethane. Although cyanide can be absorbed through the gastrointestinal tract or skin, it is most dangerous when aerosolized and inhaled because of its rapid absorption through this large surface area. The hydrocyanide then binds to the cytochrome system, thereby inhibiting cell metabolism and ATP production. All cells, in particular the liver, have a detoxifying process for hydrocyanide with the enzyme rhodenase converting hydrocyanide to thiocyanate, which is then excreted in the urine. This protective system can be overcome by a large amount of cyanide, especially if the patient is also hypovolemic, thereby impairing cyanide metabolism and clearance.

### *Symptoms*

Symptoms of carbon monoxide toxicity are usually not present until carboxyhemoglobin exceeds 15%, i.e., 15% of the hemoglobin is bound to carbon monoxide rather than oxygen (Table 1–1). Symptoms are those of decreased tissue oxygenation, with initial manifestations being neurologic due to the impairment in cerebral oxygenation. Major myocardial dysfunction can also develop, with evidence of myocardial ischemia or even infarction, especially with preexisting coronary artery disease. In addition, the neurologic dysfunction caused by carbon monoxide exposure can lead to a progressive and permanent cerebral dysfunction. Frequently, a patient will awaken transiently after severe inhalation injury only to have progressive neurologic deterioration 24 to 48 hours later. This process is believed to be due to the prolonged brain hypoxia from both the carbon monoxide and the low environmental oxygen tension. Cyanide toxicity presents in a very similar fashion to carbon monoxide, with severe metabolic acidosis and obtundation in severe cases. Diagnosis, however, is more difficult because cyanide levels are not always readily available or very reliable.

**Table 1-1** Carbon Monoxide Toxicity

| Diagnosis | | |
|---|---|---|
| Increased carboxyhemoglobin level (may be normal if treatment initiated before arrival) | Low oxygen saturation relative to $PaO_2$ | Unexplained metabolic acidosis |

**Carbon Monoxide Intoxication**

| CARBOXYHEMOGLOBIN LEVEL (%) | SYMPTOMS |
|---|---|
| 0–5 | Normal value |
| 15–20 | Headache, confusion |
| 20–40 | Disorientation, fatigue, nausea, visual changes |
| 40–60 | Hallucination, combativeness, coma, shock state |
| $\geq 60$ | Mortality >50% |

## Diagnosis

Carbon monoxide toxicity is measured using the carboxyhemoglobin level. The persistence of a metabolic acidosis in the patient with adequate volume resuscitation and cardiac output suggests persistent carbon monoxide (or cyanide) impairment of oxygen utilization and delivery. However, hypovolemia and other cell poisons cannot be excluded. $PaO_2$ will remain relatively normal, since the chemical alteration of hemoglobin or of the cytochrome system by carbon monoxide will not affect the amount of oxygen dissolved in arterial plasma. However, the measured oxygen saturation of hemoglobin will be markedly decreased relative to the $PO_2$.

*Oxygen saturation will be less than that expected from the measured $PaO_2$.*

Therefore, if there is a discrepancy between the measured $PaO_2$ and measured oxygen saturation, carbon monoxide toxicity is present until proved otherwise. A high carboxyhemoglobin also indicates a significant smoke exposure, and therefore a chemical burn to the airways is likely to be present. A low carboxyhemoglobin does not always indicate a minimal smoke exposure because administration of oxygen at the scene of the fire can displace some of the carbon monoxide before arrival at the emergency room. Blood cyanide levels can be measured to make the diagnosis of cyanide toxicity. Normal levels, e.g., in smokers, is less than 0.1 mg/L. A lethal level is considered to be about 1 mg/L.

## Treatment

Treatment of carbon monoxide toxicity consists of the early displacement of carbon monoxide from hemoglobin by administration of 90 to 100% oxygen. The half-life of carboxyhemoglobin in the patient when breathing 20% oxygen is about 120 to 200 minutes, whereas the half-life when breathing 90 to 100% high-flow oxygen is 30 minutes, i.e., the concentration of carboxyhemoglobin is reduced by approximately 50% every 30 minutes if an oxygen concentration of 90 to 100% is used.

*Oxygen administration is required for all major burns until carbon monoxide toxicity can be ruled out or until carboxyhemoglobin levels return to normal.*

Hyperbaric oxygen (2 to 3 atm) produces an even more rapid displacement and is most useful in cases of prolonged exposure, when carbon monoxide is also present in the mitochondria, since the carbon monoxide is more difficult to displace from the cytochrome system. The drawback of hyperbaric oxygen use is the inability to "get to the patient" during this crucial period of hemodynamic and pulmonary instability. Hyperbaric oxygen is best used in cases in which the patient has severe neurologic compromise with high carboxyhemoglobin, more than 50%, but no major burns or severe pulmonary injury and is not responding to high-flow oxygen with clearance of symptoms. However, the vast majority of cases can be successfully managed by simply using 90 to 100% oxygen.

Endotracheal intubation and use of 90 to 100% oxygen with mechanical ventilator assist is indicated for those patients with impaired neurologic function and a high carboxyhemoglobin. This patient group not only needs a more aggressive attempt at displacing the carboxyhemoglobin using positive pressure at a high $FiO_2$, but is also at a high risk for aspiration, as any neurologically impaired patient would be.

Cyanide management remains controversial. In general, cardiopulmonary support is usually sufficient treatment, since the liver via the enzyme rhodenase will clear the cyanide from the circulation. Sodium nitrite is used (300 mg intravenously over 5 to 10 minutes) in severe cases, especially those in which the diagnosis is made by blood levels. Methemoglobin is produced by the nitrite, which, in turn, binds the cyanide. However, methemoglobin does not transport oxygen and a tissue hypoxia can develop, which is similar to the original cyanide effect. Ordinarily, thiosulfate is also given, which, in turn, binds the cyanide to form thiocyanate. One must be reasonably sure of the diagnosis of cyanide toxicity before giving sodium nitrite.

**Table 1-2** Treatment of Carbon Monoxide and Cyanide Toxicity

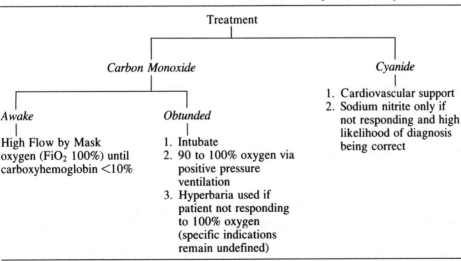

## Upper Airways Obstruction from Tissue Edema (Internal and External)

Direct heat injury caused by the inhalation of air heated to a temperature of 150°C or higher ordinarily results in burns to the face, oropharynx, and upper airway (above the vocal cords). Even superheated air is rapidly cooled before reaching the lower respiratory tract because of the tremendous heat-exchanging efficiency of the oropharynx and nasopharynx.

Heat produces an immediate injury to the airway mucosa, resulting in edema, erythema, and ulceration. Although these mucosal changes may be anatomically present shortly after the burn, physiologic alterations will not be present until the edema is sufficient to produce clinical evidence of impaired upper airway patency. This may not occur for 12 to 18 hours. The presence of a body burn magnifies the injury to airways in direct proportion to the size and depth of the skin burn. The massive fluid requirements necessary to treat the skin burn are in part responsible, as are mediators released from the burned skin.

Another compounding injury is any face or neck burn that will accentuate the problem by producing marked anatomic distortion and, in the case of the deep neck burn, external compression on the larynx. A particularly dangerous injury is the third degree facial burn in which minimal external edema is present. The lack of external edema is due to the nonelastic third degree burn, which does not allow expansion. Intraoral edema in this case is usually massive but unrecognized unless looked for. A more superficial burn causes massive external edema but may produce much less mucosal edema and airway compromise. The effect of deep face burns on airway maintenance are:

1. Airway obstruction by intraoral and laryngeal edema
2. Anatomic distortion by face and neck edema, which increases the difficulty of endotracheal intubation
3. Oral edema decreasing clearance of intraoral secretions
4. Impaired protection of the airway from aspiration

The local edema process usually resolves in 4 to 5 days.

### *Symptoms*

Symptoms of obstruction, namely, stridor, dyspnea, increased work of breathing, and eventually cyanosis, do not develop until a critical narrowing of the airway is present. Upper airway noise indicative of increased turbulent airflow often precedes obstruction. It is difficult to distinguish noise from a narrowed airway from that caused by increased oral and nasal secretions due to smoke irritation. The airway edema and the external burn edema process have a parallel time course so that by the time symptoms of airway edema develop, external and internal anatomic distortion will be extensive.

### *Diagnosis*

A history must be obtained regarding the nature of the burn. This information may not always be available from the Emergency Medical Service transport team if the patient has been transferred from another emergency room rather than the scene and if the patient cannot provide the information. Inspection of the oropharynx looking for soot or evidence of a heat injury should be done with every burn victim. A number of techniques have been used to assess further the degree of injury and determine the need for endotracheal intubation. Spirometry and the measurement of flow-volume curves will detect early airway changes but requires a cooperative patient without severe facial burns to obtain reliable data. Xenon lung scan is an extremely sensitive method for detecting any airways dysfunction. The method is not readily available and is not widely used. Quantitation of injury is a problem with this method. Fiberoptic bronchoscopy or laryngoscopy will determine whether physical evidence of pharyngeal or laryngeal mucosal injury is present, namely, erythema and edema (Color plate 1, page 311). *Laryngoscopy is the most rapid and least complicated diagnostic tool.* Unfortunately, unless serial studies are performed, none of these tests can accurately predict the severity of subsequent airway compromise, since the edema is progressive during the first 18 to 24 hours.

## Treatment

Maintaining an adequate airway is essential for successful early management. There are four standard criteria (the four Ps) for the need for endotracheal intubation:

1. Maintain airway *p*atency
2. *p*rotect against aspiration
3. *p*ulmonary toilet to decrease mucous plugging and infection risks
4. Need for *p*ositive-*p*ressure ventilation

The upper airways injury can meet at least the first two indications and frequently the third if patient fatigue begins to develop because increased work of breathing will result from the airway compromise.

Intubation of the trachea is not without its own complications because the cough mechanism is impaired, especially in the patient with good respiratory mechanics. In addition, intubation increases the risk of nosocomial infection. A judgment decision must be made in the initial assessment as to whether the airway can be managed safely without an endotracheal tube. *When in doubt, it is safer to intubate.* There are many other indications in the burn patient besides airway edema for the need for intubation, which will be discussed later in this chapter.

Three major categories of patients, who are at risk for upper airways compromise, are described.

**Heat and Smoke Exposure Plus Extensive Face, Neck Burns.** A patient with a significant inhalation injury and deep facial burns is managed by early endotracheal intubation. Management without intubation is allowed only if closely monitored for any signs of obstruction of upper airways, and *only* if intubation can be safely and rapidly performed when needed. However, increasing anatomic distortion caused by face and neck burns usually makes a later intubation very difficult. Therefore intubation is best performed on admission, since one cannot wait until the inevitable massive face and neck edema develops to make this decision. Those not intubated need to be placed in an intensive care unit environment with the head elevated and with experienced personnel ready to intervene if necessary. An important principle to follow in these patients is to: *Make the decision to intubate in the first 4 to 8 hours based on progression of symptoms, and the clear understanding that the edema process will get worse over the next 12 to 18 hours.*

**Burn Alone: No Inhalation.** Patients with very deep second or third degree burns to the face, particularly lips and neck, also frequently require early intubation, especially in the presence of other burns. Neck compression from burn edema and inability to handle secretions make respiratory distress a likely event and make a delayed intubation very difficult. Emergency tracheotomies are difficult, at best, to perform in these patients and lead to airways infection. The resolution of edema will require 4 to 5 days. The intubated patient can now be anesthetized over the next several days if burn excision is needed.

Patients with small second degree facial burns from flashes of flame or hot liquids without a smoke exposure or intraoral burns are at less risk for airway compromise. Elevation of the head of the bed while maintaining a controlled fluid resuscitation is the appropriate management. The airway can usually be maintained without a tube and the edema will resolve in 2 to 3 days.

**Heat and Smoke Inhalation: No Facial Burns.** The criteria for early intubation in this group is based on the findings on initial laryngoscopy or bronchoscopy as well as the respiratory function of the patient. If the airway cannot be adequately managed by

**Table 1-3** Initial Assessment of Airway (to Intubate or Not to Intubate)

Stridor Retraction
Respiratory Distress
$PaO_2 < 60$    $PaCO_2 > 55$
Deep Burns: Face, Neck

*Present*
1. Intubate now!
2. Use adequate sized tube
3. Humidified oxygen
4. Transport to intensive care unit-burn center
5. Elevate head

*Absent*
Look for Signs of Airway Injury
1. Oropharyngeal erythema
2. Hoarseness, changing pulmonary status

*Present*
Perform Laryngoscopy

*Absent*
Follow Closely if History of Smoke Exposure (Remember Deterioration of Blood Gases Is a Late Finding)

Upper Airway Edema Present
1. Intubate now!
2. Use adequate sized tube
3. Humidified oxygen
4. Transport to intensive care unit-burn center

Modest Erythema but No Significant Edema
1. Follow closely, symptoms often delayed
2. Consider fiberoptic bronchoscopy if history of smoke exposure

positioning or ventilation by aggressive pulmonary toilet, immediate intubation is indicated. The lack of significant external anatomic distortion usually allows for a safer intubation, if delayed, than in the presence of a face or neck burn.

## Chemical Burn to Upper and Lower Airways

This aspect of inhalation injury is often an extension of the upper airways injury just described but is generally much more serious than that produced by heat alone. Toxic gases contained in smoke as well as carbon particles coated with irritating aldehydes and organic acids can result in injury to both upper and lower airways (Table 1–4). The location of injury will depend on the duration of exposure, the size of the particles, and the solubility of the gases.

Breath holding and laryngospasm, as a result of airway irritation, are protective mechanisms against excessive exposure in the conscious patient. The unconscious patient, however, loses this protection, resulting in a more severe injury to the lower airways. Information as to status of consciousness at the scene should be sought in the history.

Water-soluble gases found in smoke from burning plastics or rubber, such as ammonia, sulfur dioxide, and chlorine, react with water in the mucous membranes to produce strong acids and alkalies that lead to irritation, bronchospasm and mucous membrane ulceration, and edema. Severe impairment of the ciliary mechanism of the mucosa occurs, leading to impairment of the removal of particles and mucus. Lipid-soluble compounds, such as nitrous oxide, phosgene, hydrogen chloride, and various toxic aldehydes, are transported to the lower airways on carbon particles that, in turn, adhere to the mucosa. All these agents produce cell membrane damage. There is also marked early increases in bronchial blood flow, which accentuates the edema formation.

Alveolar edema is not a major component of the early disease state and therefore not responsible for the early impaired gas exchange. Several clinical studies have verified that

**Table 1-4** Toxic Elements in Housefire Smoke

| Gas | Source | Effect |
| --- | --- | --- |
| Carbon monoxide | Any organic matter | Tissue hypoxia |
| Carbon dioxide | Any organic matter | Narcosis |
| Nitrogen dioxide | Wall paper, wood | Bronchial irritation<br>Dizziness<br>Pulmonary edema |
| Hydrogen chloride (phosgene) | Plastics (polyvinylchloride) | Severe mucosal irritation |
| Hydrogen cyanide | Wool, silk, nylons (polyurethane) | Headache<br>Respiratory failure<br>Coma |
| Benzene | Petroleum plastics | Mucosal irritation<br>Coma |
| Aldehydes | Wood, cotton, paper | Severe mucosal damage<br>Extensive lung damage |
| Ammonia | Nylon | Mucosal irritation |

lung water is significantly increased only after massive inhalation injuries in which damage has extended to the very small airways. In this circumstance, the source of the water remains undefined. The increased airways fluid from mucosal irritation looks and acts physiologically like any increase in alveolar water. Alveolar flooding in these severe cases may well be due to retrograde flow of bronchorrhea. The airways are, of course, perfused by the bronchial vessels in which permeability has been altered. There is no clear evidence that there is an alteration in the integrity of the pulmonary microcirculation with a moderate smoke inhalation injury with the exception of certain toxins, such as some hydrocarbons that are absorbed through the airways and recirculate to the lung. A body burn markedly potentiates the inhalation-induced lung dysfunction caused by chemical injury. Mortality rate for patients with severe inhalation injury alone is 5 to 8%. Mortality rate of the combination of a major burn and smoke inhalation far exceeds that of either injury alone.

## Symptoms

Symptoms may well be absent on admission, with the true magnitude of the degree of injury only becoming evident after 24 to 48 hours. Early symptoms usually consist of bronchospasm manifested as wheezing and bronchorrhea. An intense initial bronchorrhea caused by the irritation of the airway mucosa in combination with increased oral and nasal secretions can give the appearance of fulminant pulmonary edema. The source of these secretions, however, is not the pulmonary circulation in the vast majority of cases. Injury at the alveolar level is usually fatal. The presence of soot in the lung secretions is certainly evidence of smoke exposure but is not a necessary finding. Early bronchospasm and bronchiolar edema initiated by the irritant gases causes a marked decrease in lung compliance and increased work of breathing. Impaired clearance of secretions will accentuate the problem. The resulting ventilation-perfusion (V/Q) mismatch will create impaired gas exchange with an increasing alveolar-arterial oxygen gradient and minute ventilation. In summary, the symptom complex is as follows:

> Bronchorrhea, wheezing
> Coughing, dyspnea
> Increase work of breathing
> Impaired gas exchange

## Diagnosis

Diagnostic aids are history of closed space exposure, physical findings (soot, presence of symptoms), increased carboxyhemoglobin, direct visualization of injury (laryngoscopy, fiberoptic bronchoscopy), and indirect visualization, V/Q xenon scan).

A *history* of confinement in a closed space during the burning process is a good indicator of potential lung damage. However, single breath exposures to toxic chemicals are sufficient to produce major airways damage. An absence of a history, especially by transferring medical personnel, often means a lack of detailed information about the circumstances of injury. The true story often takes hours or days to determine. *Physical findings* on admission that suggest smoke exposure include a facial burn, soot in the sputum, dyspnea, coughing, wheezing, and bronchorrhea. If present, these findings are helpful. However, many patients demonstrate minimal symptoms early after injury and only when airways edema develops do symptoms become evident. An elevated *carboxyhemoglobin* level indicates an exposure to the elements in smoke. Often, considerable displacement of the carbon monoxide has occurred before arrival due to standard institution of oxygen at the scene.

*Laryngoscopy* will demonstrate the presence of mucosal irritation at and above the cords and provide information about the need for endotracheal intubation. Absence of upper airways changes almost always means absence of lower airways injury. Visualization of the upper and lower airways by *fiberoptic bronchoscopy* can provide information on the anatomic extent of injury but initial findings have not been found to prognosticate accurately the magnitude of injury to allow anticipation of the subsequent course.

*V/Q xenon scan* will indicate whether small airways constriction is present because of an impairment in normal alveolar xenon clearance. However, this test is no longer commonly used, since direct visualization is the preferred approach.

## Treatment

Initial treatment of a chemical burn consists of an aggressive approach to upper airway maintenance and pulmonary support, which includes maintenance of small airways patency and removal of soot and the mucopurulent secretions (Fig. 1–2). Careful well-monitored fluid resuscitation is necessary to avoid accentuation of the process. Undervolume resuscitation will aggravate the pulmonary dysfunction as much as will overresuscitation. The addition of positive end-expiratory pressure (PEEP) is frequently necessary to maintain small airway patency and an adequate functional residual capacity by assisting in holding the edematous airway open until edema resolution. Early endotracheal intubation and PEEP have been reported to decrease pulmonary deaths after severe burns and smoke inhalation. Positive-pressure support should precede evidence of severe respiratory compromise, since prevention of airway closure is much more readily accomplished than is the reopening of collapsed airways. A large enough tube, i.e., at least a 7 mm internal diameter, should be used in adults because very thick secretions develop as a result of the lung injury. If the initial tube is too small, it will be very dangerous to change once massive facial and airway edema develops. Although the nasotracheal route may be more comfortable to the patient, the size of the tube may need to be compromised and lead to later problems for secretion clearance. The continued use of additional humidified oxygen to maintain adequate oxygen delivery as well as to assist in the clearance of secretions is indicated. Elevation of the patient's head and chest 20 to 30° is also helpful.

Bronchospasm is a frequent component of the chemical injury. However, diagnosis can be complicated by rhonchi and upper airways noises, caused by increased secretions. A helpful clue to determining the magnitude of increased airways resistance is the difference between dynamic and static compliance. The difference between the two reflects increased resistance to airflow, which will, of course, also include the endotracheal tube. Bronchospasm can be treated with bronchodilators, either parenteral or via aerosol. The $beta_2$ sympathomimetic agents, metaproterenol (Allupent) or isoetharine (Bronkosol), are effective bronchodilators. Intravenous aminophylline, although a good bronchodilator, is frequently limited in its use because of the tachycardia seen in the early postburn period (Table 1–5).

## TREATMENT

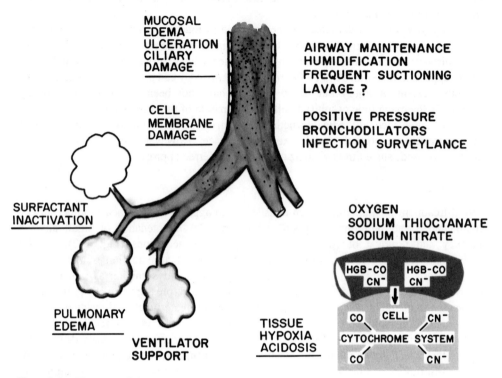

**Figure 1–2.** Treatment of chemical burn in the lung.

Beginning about 18 to 24 hours after a burn, increasing airway resistance is often due to bronchiolar edema and airway plugging rather than bronchospasm. The impaired gas exchange often responds to further increases in PEEP in addition to bronchodilators. PEEP in excess of 10 cm $H_2O$, will produce some impairment in cardiac output if hypovolemia is also present. Prophylactic antibiotics are not indicated. The injured airways mucosa will frequently become colonized with bacteria, especially if an endotracheal tube is present. Prophylactic antibiotics will only select for the more resistant organisms. It is now well-demonstrated that corticosteroids in the presence of a body burn increase rather than decrease the smoke inhalation morbidity and mortality. Steroids are therefore contraindicated in the presence of a burn. With inhalation injury in the absence of a burn, no benefit has been demonstrated.

Close monitoring of the adequacy of gas exchange is necessary, particularly during the early evolution of the inhalation injury. An indwelling arterial line or a pulse oximeter is required. The pulse oximeter indicates arterial oxygen saturation using a photosensor that detects the color of the blood flowing beneath the probe.

Table 1-5  Bronchodilator Therapy

| Drug | Actions | Side Effects | Indications | Dosage |
|---|---|---|---|---|
| Aminophylline | Relaxation of airway and pulmonary vascular smooth muscle. Improves diaphragm function. Some positive inotropic, chronotropic activity. Mild diuretic effect. Renal clearance with active metabolites | Nausea, vomiting, central nervous system stimulation can be seen with therapeutic doses, as can tachycardia and other arrhythmias. Response potentiated with renal insufficiency | Control of bronchospasm acute and chronic | Intravenous 5 mg/kg initially followed by infusion. 0.2–0.75 mg/kg/hr. Therapeutic plasma concentration 10 to 20 $\mu$g/ml |
| Isoetharine (Bronkosol) | Stimulation of $\beta$-adrenergic receptors, $\beta_2 > \beta_1$. No $\alpha$ stimulation. Smooth muscle relaxant for airways and vessels. Rapid onset of action. Metabolized by liver, lung; renal excretion | Nausea, vomiting, central nervous system stimulation. May see some cardiac stimulation at higher doses. Rare paradoxical bronchoconstriction | Control of acute bronchospasm when only modest cardiac stimulation can be tolerated to help clear thick secretions | Via aerosol 0.25 to 1 ml of 1% isoetharine diluted 1:3 with saline. Duration about 4 hr |
| Epinephrine | Relaxation of bronchial smooth muscle via $\beta_2$ stimulation. Also decreases airway edema by constricting bronchial arterioles. Immediate onset of action. Metabolized in liver and nerve endings. Renal excretion | Cardiac stimulation both $\beta$ and $\alpha$ central nervous system stimulation. Tachyphylaxis can develop rapidly | Control of acute bronchospasm, especially with allergy-induced reactions | Intramuscular, subcutaneous 0.2 to 0.5 mg every 20 minutes. Via aerosol, 0.1 to 1.0% solution |
| Terbutaline | Stimulation of $\beta$ receptors, $\beta_1 > \beta_2$. No $\alpha$ effect. Relaxation of airway and vessel smooth muscle. Immediate onset. Longer acting than most other agents. Metabolized in liver with renal excretion | Cardiac stimulation usually only at high doses. Fewer gastrointestinal side effects | Control of acute and chronic bronchospasm. Longer action and more potent than isoetharine as a bronchodilator to help clear thick secretions | Subcutaneous 0.25 to 0.5 mg every 4 hours. Orally, 2.5 to 5 mg every 6 to 8 hours |

**Table 1-6** Assess for Lower Airways Injury (to Ventilate or Not to Ventilate With Positive Pressure)

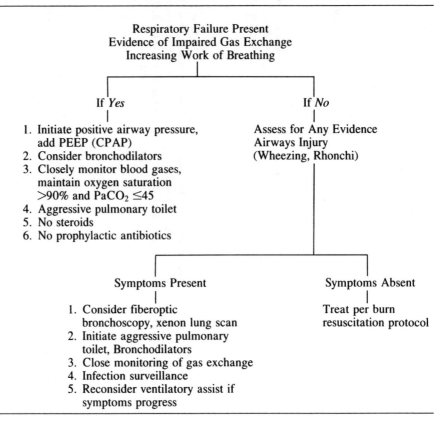

## LUNG CHANGES FROM SKIN BURN

The increase in pulmonary complications seen after burns even in the absence of inhalation injury has in the past been attributed to an increase in lung protein permeability. Recent evidence would indicate that this is not the case. Although there are biochemical changes in lung tissue, particularly increased lipid peroxidation reflecting oxygen radical injury, there is no measurable lung microvascular protein leak, at least not in man. A number of human studies have verified no increase in lung water during the resuscitation phase despite massive soft tissue edema.

Lung changes as a result of the body burn, however, do include a transient increase in pulmonary artery pressure and a modest, but significant, decrease in $PaO_2$. Ventilatory changes include an increase in closing volume and an increase in airways resistance, indicating small airways pathologic changes. A number of bronchoconstrictor and vasoactive mediators are released from burn tissue, as indicated in the following diagram:

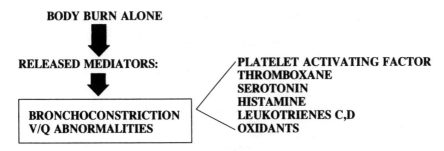

The mediator-induced process is relatively modest in degree in the absence of a concomitant smoke inhalation injury. The two injuries together, however, may dramatically compound the degree of injury produced by either alone. The *findings of skin burn alone* are:

    Mild pulmonary hypertension
    Modest decrease in $PaO_2$
    Decreased compliance
    Increased closing volume

*Treatment is supportive, but pharmacologic manipulation of mediators is on the horizon.*

## IMPAIRED CHEST WALL COMPLIANCE

Respiratory excursion can be markedly impaired by a burn to the chest wall. The process is most evident with a circumferential third degree burn. The loss of elasticity in the chest wall due to the burn tissue will markedly increase the work of breathing required to maintain functional residual capacity and an adequate tidal volume. As more subeschar edema develops, compressing the chest wall, the end-expiratory intrathoracic volume begins to decrease. Edema from a second degree burn is also sufficient to alter lung mechanics. The loose aureolar tissue in the axilla and lateral chest wall will sequester large amounts of edema fluid, leading to a very heavy tense chest wall. Full-thickness burns produce a more severe limitation because tissue expansion is markedly impaired and intrathoracic volume becomes compressed. The result is a significant V/Q mismatch, atelectasis, and hypoventilation. Maximum respiratory effort is frequently required just to maintain adequate gas exchange. Any process that compromises the necessary increase in inspiratory force and muscle activity, such as hypoxia, hypovolemia, pain, or sedation, will accentuate the severity of lung dysfunction.

    Symptoms may not be clearly evident until edema formation peaks at about 10 to 12 hours. The first clinical evidence of the chest wall restrictive defected is often labored breathing followed by a rapid respiratory deterioration, particularly in the patient who is not receiving ventilator support. Clearance of secretions can be impaired due to the inability to generate a hyperinflation. In the combined chest burn and inhalation injury, it is very difficult to distinguish the degree of impairment in total lung compliance due to the increased airway edema and bronchospasm compared with that due to the impaired chest wall. The increasing airway pressure required to expand the stiff chest wall will lead to

Table 1-7  Pathophysiology of Chest Wall Compliance

Chest Wall Burn Plus Edema
↓
Restrictive Chest Wall Defect
↓
1. Decreasing total lung compliance
2. Increased work of breathing
3. Decreasing functional residual capacity = atelectasis
4. Impaired cough mechanism
   Resulting in
1. Hypoventilation: Impaired gas exchange
2. If mechanical ventilation is used, watch for:
   Increasing airway pressure
   Accentuation of V/Q mismatch
   Impaired venous return
   Decreased cardiac output

---

impaired hemodynamic function as the high pressure is transmitted to the mediastinum, impairing venous return. The hemodynamic instability is very difficult to treat simply by volume loading because any resulting increase in central venous pressure will dramatically increase the rate of fluid and protein loss into the burn tissue, accentuating the chest wall edema.

## Diagnosis

A high index of suspicion coupled with an understanding of the mechanism of injury is essential. A decreasing compliance as reflected by clinical evidence of increased work in the absence of an inhalation injury indicates the problem is the chest wall burn. It is more difficult to sort out the process when an inhalation injury is also present.

## Treatment

The three main treatment principles are:

1. Recognize the problem
2. Control the tissue edema process (elevation of upper body if hemodynamically stable)
3. Surgically decompress the chest wall constriction

As soon as the patient is hemodynamically stable, the head and chest should be elevated 30° to decrease chest wall edema. Fluid resuscitation should be well controlled, especially in the immediate postburn period to avoid both under- and overresuscitation. If symptoms develop that are compatible with chest wall restriction in a third degree burn, an escharotomy is required (Fig. 1–3). *The burn does not have to be circumferential to produce a restrictive defect.* A longitudinal incision should be placed in the midaxillary lines then connected across the lower chest wall. Bleeding is usually easily controlled, if the incisions stay within the margins of the third degree burn, since the dermal vessels are already heat thrombosed. The incision must extend into the subeschar area to allow adequate chest wall expansion. If a charred chest is present on admission, reflecting

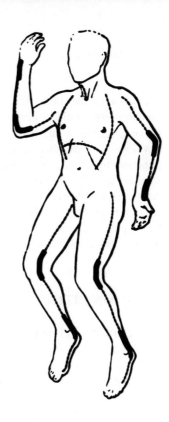

**Figure 1–3.** Escharotomy incisions are shown for deep extremity and chest wall burns.

**Table 1-8** Treatment of Chest Wall Burn

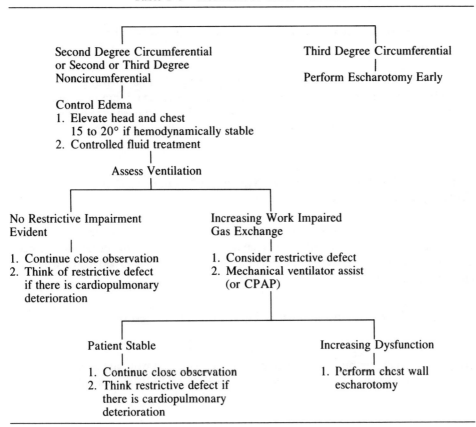

19

extension of the burn into fat and possibly fascia (i.e., a fourth degree burn), an escharotomy should be performed on admission. An extremely deep burn tissue results in tissue contraction due to desiccation, making the chest wall tight even before edema develops. Use of microcrystalline collagen to pack the incision sites can help control punctate bleeding. Larger vessels usually require suture ligatures or cautery. Escharotomies are usually not required in a second degree burn unless the burn is very deep or the edema is so massive that the burned skin is tight. Even with an escharotomy, the restrictive process can be of such magnitude that hypoventilation is clearly evident. In these patients, endotracheal intubation and positive-pressure ventilation should be initiated before obvious pulmonary deterioration.

## COMMON PITFALLS IN PULMONARY SUPPORT

### Using Initial Arterial Oxygen Tension to Reflect Adequacy of Oxygenation

In the presence of carbon monoxide, the $PaO_2$ can no longer be used to reflect oxygen-hemoglobin saturation. Avoid the error of decreasing the $FiO_2$ when the $PaO_2$ is above 100 torr before the status of the carboxyhemoglobin level is known.

### Using a Small Nasotracheal Tube in the Presence of Smoke Inhalation

The concerns with smoke inhalation are an immediate problem of airway patency and an additional major problem of pulmonary toilet. A tube less than 7 mm in an adult is too small for adequate suctioning and thick secretions will compromise ventilation at a time when it is not safe to change the tube due to face, neck, and airway edema.

### Endotracheal Intubation Without Addition of Some Positive End-Expiratory Pressure

A chest wall burn, generalized edema, inhalation injury, use of narcotics, all decrease functional residual capacity and all are common in the burn patient. PEEP applied early can help avoid atelectasis and airway collapse. Begin with 5 cm $H_2O$ and increase up to 10 cm $H_2O$, if needed.

### Fluid Restricting a Patient with a Burn Plus an Inhalation Injury

Hypovolemia will not protect the inhalation-injured lung and will only augment the V/Q mismatch because less of the lung is perfused, especially if PEEP is required.

## Avoiding Colloid Because of Concern About Adult Respiratory Distress Syndrome

The lung does not develop a protein leak initially after a major burn unless a massive inhalation injury is present. If colloid is needed for improved hemodynamic stability, it should be given. There is no evidence to indicate that protein has a deleterious effect on the lung after smoke inhalation.

## Underestimating the Effect of the Chest Wall on Ventilation

Patient positioning, to minimize chest and face edema, and escharotomy are often not done until severe pulmonary dysfunction has already developed. Prevention remains far more effective than treatment of respiratory failure.

# SUMMARY OF DIAGNOSIS AND TREATMENT OF EARLY PULMONARY ABNORMALITIES: SMOKE INHALATION INJURY COMPLEX

## Clinical Presentation

I. Hypoxia, Carbon Dioxide, Cyanide (Immediate Onset)
   Lethargy, Disorientation, Obtundation
   No Cyanosis
   Auscultation and Radiographs Normal
II. Heat Component of Smoke (Onset 12 to 24 Hours)
   Dyspnea, Tachypnea, Possible Cyanosis
   Auscultation; Stridor, Upper Airway Noise
   Radiographs; Normal Chest
III. Chemical Component of Smoke (Onset Delayed)
   Dyspnea, Tachypnea, Cyanosis, Tachycardia
   Auscultation; Diffuse Wheezing and Rhonchi
   Radiographs: Usually Normal Until Severe Atelectasis, Alveolar Edema, or Bronchopneumonia Is Evident

## Diagnosis

History: Closed Space Containment, Impaired Consciousness at Scene, Toxic Chemicals Known to Be Released

Clinical Findings: Facial Burn, Soot in Sputum, Cough
Wheezing: Often Asymptomatic on Admission

Chest Radiograph: Usually Normal on Admission

Carboxyhemoglobin: If Increased Indicates Smoke Inhalation
If Absent May Mean Displacement Has Already Occurred

Oxygen Saturation: Lower than Predicted by $PaO_2$ Means Increased Carboxyhemoglobin

Laryngoscopy: Indicates Upper Airways Injury Is Present
Difficult to Quantitate Degree of Injury

Bronchoscopy: Indicates Presence or Absence and Level of Injury but Cannot Accurately Prognosticate

V/Q Xenon: Indicates Small Airways Involvement but Cannot Accurately Prognosticate

## Decreased Chest Wall Compliance

Cause: Deep Burns to Chest Wall as Well as Tissue Edema Impairing Tissue Elasticity

Clinical Presentation: Decreased Dynamic and Static Compliance
Decreased Functional Residual Capacity
Increased Work of Breathing

Diagnosis: High Index of Suspicion
Recognition of Pathophysiology

# TREATMENT SUMMARY (0 TO 24 HOURS)

## Airway-Pulmonary Abnormalities

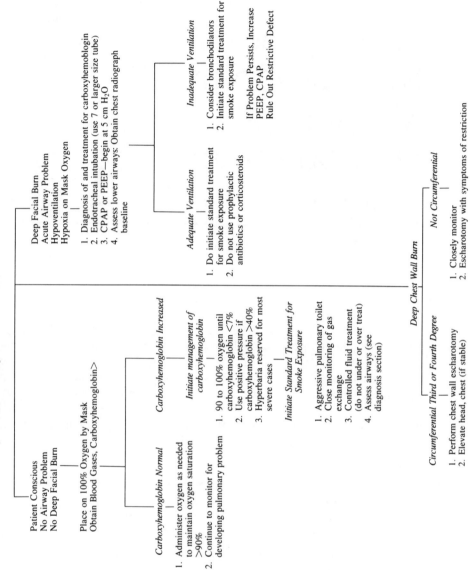

# 2

# Restoration and Maintenance of Hemodynamic Stability

Massive fluid shifts occur during this period that can lead to a severe impairment in oxygen delivery to tissues. An understanding of these early fluid shifts is necessary in order to avoid hemodynamic instability and initiate the appropriate treatment modalities. Appropriate monitoring is also necessary. The basic concepts of the pathophysiology and treatment of burn shock will be described. Important reference information relative to fluid balance, pharmacologic support of the circulation, coagulation, and acid-base abnormalities common during this period can be found in the reference section.

**GENERAL SECTIONS**
- Pathophysiology of Burn Shock
    - Burn Edema
    - Changes in Nonburn Tissue (Nonburn Edema)
    - Systemic Hemodynamic Changes
    - Hematologic Changes
- Practical Approach to Treatment
    - Choice of Resuscitation Fluid
    - Intravenous Access
    - Rate of Infusion
    - What to Monitor
    - Indications for Inotropic Support
    - Common Pitfalls in Initial Fluid Resuscitation
    - Treatment Summary

# PATHOPHYSIOLOGY OF BURN SHOCK

The postburn vascular changes in volume shifts involve four processes: (1) a loss of intravascular volume into the interstitium, both in burn and nonburned tissues; (2) an increase in burn tissue osmotic pressure leading to further edema in burn tissue; (3) a generalized impairment in cell membrane function resulting in nonburn cell swelling from an extracellular to intracellular water shift; and (4) a shift of intravascular water into interstitium in nonburn tissues due to hypoproteinemia.

## Burn Edema

Massive fluid and protein shifts occur in the burn tissue itself as a result of alterations in vascular permeability and in the burn tissue interstitium. The specific pathophysiology of the edema process is described in this chapter instead of the chapter on burn wound because of the relationship to resuscitation. The most pronounced shift occurs in the first several hours as a result of the increased protein permeability and the apparent increase in burn tissue osmotic pressure.

### *Increased Vascular Permeability*

Direct thermal injury to tissues results in striking changes in the microcirculation. There is clearly an increase in protein permeability in the injured microcirculation, leading to marked loss of intravascular water and protein. The protein is carried across the vascular endothelial membrane along with the large fluid shift, the latter being dictated by the balance of osmotic and hydrostatic pressure.

Despite a fairly uniform description of the pathologic changes, there remains some controversy over the mechanism of injury producing these changes. One controversy revolves around the significance of direct vessel injury versus that produced as a result of vasoactive substances released from the burn. The concept of a mediator-induced injury is of considerable importance, since this would allow for possibly modulating the degree of burn edema by mediator inhibition. Vasoactive mediators, such as vasodilator prostaglandins, histamine, bradykinin, and oxygen radicals can produce edema by either a direct increase in vascular permeability or indirectly by an increase in microvascular hydrostatic pressure superimposed on an already altered membrane (Fig. 2–1). The marked impairment in the vascular permeability in burn tissue leads to a loss of the gradient between plasma and interstitial protein content for even very large macromolecules. This fact plus the dependence of edema on maintenance of perfusion and hydrostatic pressure means that the rate rather than the type of resuscitation fluid controls the burn edema process.

To summarize, the *mechanisms of increase in vascular permeability* are:

1. Direct heat-induced endothelial cell injury
2. Mediator-induced, endothelial cell injury, oxygen radicals, histamine, prostaglandins

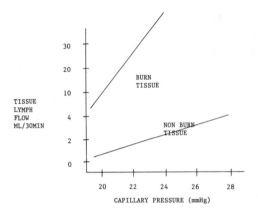

**Figure 2–1.** Relationship between capillary hydrostatic pressure and fluid loss across the capillary.

## *Increased Burn Tissue Osmolarity*

The rate of the initial fluid loss from the microcirculation into the interstitium of the burn tissue has been found by a number of investigators to be in excess of that due simply to an increase in vascular permeability. An increase in burn tissue osmotic pressure estimated at 200 to 300 mgHg has been hypothesized to explain the rapid water shift (and with it protein) into the burned tissues. An early 10 to 15 mEq/L increase in burn tissue sodium content over that of plasma is noted. This increase, believed to be due to sodium binding to the injured collagen, appears to be responsible for the initial imbalance of osmotic pressures. One milliosmol generates an osmotic pressure of 19 mmHg. This loss of extracellular sodium must be recognized and replaced.

## *Rate of Edema Formation*

The fluid and protein shifts are the greatest in the first several hours due to the combined effect of increased permeability and an imbalance of osmotic forces. The *complications of burn edema are:*

1. Hypovolemia
2. Hypoproteinemia
3. Decreased tissue oxygen tension
4. Increased tissue pressure

Edema formation in a small wound is maximum at about 6 hours after injury, since blood volume and vascular pressures to the wound are maintained. The degree of systemic hypovolemia caused by fluid loss into a large burn surface will retard the rate of edema formation, with the quantity of subsequent edema dependent on the adequacy of the fluid resuscitation.

Severe hypoproteinemia will occur as a result of the protein loss into the wound. The major protein losses occur in the first 6 to 8 hours postburn during the peak of the fluid loss, after decreasing plasma proteins to less than 50% of normal. The protein-rich interstitial edema fluid appears to form a gel after about 12 hours, leading to obstruction of local lymphatic vessels and impairing edema clearance. The gel is due to leaking of clotting proteins into the interstitium leading to fibrin deposition. Tissue oxygen tension decreases with edema process as the distance between viable cells and the closest capillary increases. This process will have the most deleterious impact on the marginally viable cells. Resolution of edema depends on restoration of lymphatic patency, which may take a number of days to weeks. Therefore, edema in deeper burns resolves more slowly than superficial burns.

## Changes in Nonburn Tissue (Nonburn Edema)

Generalized nonburn tissue edema is also a characteristic finding after a major burn. Edema formation in nonburned tissues is clearly evident in patients with burns exceeding 30% of the total body surface. The process is not due simply to an increase in vascular permeability, since permeability is only transiently altered in nonburned tissues. A number of studies have verified that much of the vascular to extravascular fluid shift in nonburn tissue is caused by the burn-induced plasma hypoproteinemia. The cause is not just due to a decrease in plasma osmotic pressure, since the plasma to interstitial colloid osmotic pressure gradient can be maintained relatively constant as a result of a concomitant decrease in interstitial protein content. The edema appears to be due, at least in part, to an alteration in the microvascular interstitium itself by the low protein content decreasing the resistance to fluid accumulation. The nonburn edema formation can be attenuated by maintaining a normal protein content. However, plasma protein content is almost impossible to maintain during the first 8 hours due to the early rapid losses after a major burn. Total fluid requirements can be substantially decreased if nonburn edema is controlled by the addition of protein and nonprotein colloids to the crystalloid infusion after a large burn.

There is also a generalized alteration in the cell membranes of nonburned tissue, in particular muscle, in the presence of a shock state. A decrease in cell membrane potential occurs, leading to a shift of sodium and water from the extracellular space into the intracellular space. The significance of this process is dependent on the degree of shock and can be minimized by early restoration of tissue perfusion.

## Systemic Hemodynamic Changes

Decreased oxygen delivery to tissues is the primary problem during this period. Cardiovascular instability arises from the microvascular and cell membrane alterations just described. The rate of loss of plasma volume is the greatest during the first 4 to 6 hours, decreasing substantially by 18 to 24 hours. The degree of hypovolemia is relative to burn size (see rule of nines in Chapter 3). A persistent low-flow state, however, will result in a further increase in the volume deficit as extracellular fluid shifts into the intracellular space.

Cardiac output is initially depressed, owing primarily to hypovolemia. Afterload is also increased due to a marked increase in systemic vascular resistance from vasoactive mediators, such as catecholamines. Systemic hypertension is seen in about 10% of burn patients due to this mediator response. A decrease in cardiac contractility from a circulating myocardial depressant factor has also been reported, but the factor has yet to be identified. A decrease in cardiac contractility is most evident in third degree burns in excess of 40% total body surface and is probably due to myocardial edema rather than a

**28** Burn Trauma

circulating factor. Positive-pressure ventilation frequently required in the early postburn period may further decrease perfusion. Cardiac output is usually restored toward normal well before restoration of a normal plasma volume as a result of the increased heart rate typical of the early postburn period.

Central venous pressure and pulmonary artery wedge pressure usually remain low even when cardiac output and perfusion are adequate, for vasculature in a burn patient can be perceived as a large garden hose in which holes are punched in a proximal segment (burn) of the hose. Changes in upstream pressure lead to a change in the rate of leak through the holes, whereas downstream pressure and flow remains relatively constant. An overzealous attempt at restoring blood volume over and above that necessary for adequate perfusion can markedly accentuate edema-related complications, because fluid and protein losses in burn tissue are markedly aggravated by any increase in venous pressure.

Blood volume in severe burns can remain decreased for days in view of the ongoing fluid and protein losses. Even with massive fluid replacement, blood hematocrit greater than 50 often occurs in the early postburn period.

Normal blood volume can be more effectively restored once the leak begins to slow, at about 24 to 36 hours.

## Hematologic Changes

There is frequently evidence of hemolysis, particularly after deep third degree burns or any prolonged exposure to a heat source, with increased free plasma hemoglobin and hemoglobinuria. Increased red cell lipid peroxidation is evident and fragmented red cells are often seen on smear. Many of these injured red cells will have a markedly shortened life span, leading to a decreasing hematocrit. Red cell hematopoesis is also markedly impaired and remains so until the burn wound is closed. A leukocytosis is also characteristic during this early phase. In addition, a marked consumption of platelets, fibrinogen, and plasminogen is seen in the burn wound as well as a marked depletion of

**Table 2-1** Hematologic Changes

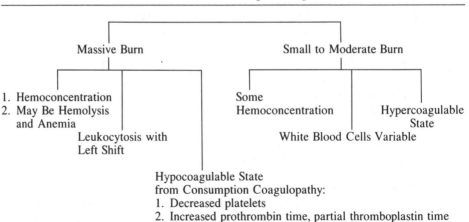

hemostatic components. A hypercoagulable state can be seen in the initial period in moderate burn injuries. A hypocoagulable state, resulting from a depletion of clotting factors, is frequently seen with massive burns. A decrease in the fibrinogen half-life in these patients indicates ongoing intravascular clotting. Thrombocytopenia will be evident in this latter group as well. This is most likely the result of the tremendous stimulus to clotting from the large area of injured collagen.

## PRACTICAL APPROACH TO TREATMENT

The key decisions to be made are:

>What type of fluid to use
>What type of vascular access
>How much to give
>What parameters to monitor
>When are inotropes required

### Choice of Resuscitation Fluid

In general, fluids that contain salt at least in quantities isotonic with plasma are appropriate for use in resuscitation if given in sufficient amounts. Restoration of the sodium loss, is essential. Fluids should be free of glucose (exception being small children), since glucose intolerance is characteristically present due to high circulating levels of stress hormones. The oral route can be used for small burns but intestinal ileus occurs after deep burns in excess of 20% total body surface. A number of salt-containing intravenous fluids are used, including colloids to minimize edema in nonburned tissues and maintain a better blood volume. The specific properties of these fluids are described in Table 2–3.

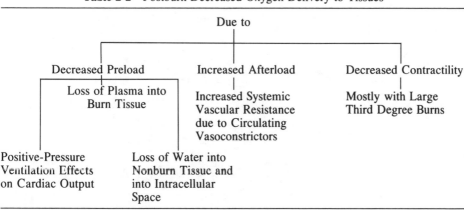

Table 2-2 Postburn Decreased Oxygen Delivery to Tissues

Table 2-3  Preload Expanding Properties of Standard Fluids

| Fluid | Osmolarity (mOms/L) | Colloid Osmotic Pressure (mmHg) | pH | Distribution Space | Approximate Ratio: Volume Infused to Produce 1 CC of Plasma Expansion |
|---|---|---|---|---|---|
| 5% dextrose | 250 | 0 | 4 | Total body water | 8:1 |
| Normal saline | 308 | 0 | 5 | Extracellular | 3:1 |
| Ringer's lactate solution | 270 | 0 | 6.5 | Extracellular | 3:1 |
| Hypertonic lactated saline (250 mEq Na$^+$/L) | 450 | 0 | 6-7 | Extracellular expansion by fluid shifts from cells | <3:1* |
| Plasma | 280-300 | 20-28 | 7 | Intravascular | 1:1 |
| 6% albumin | 250 | 20-24 | 6-7 | Intravascular | 1:1 |
| 6% dextran 70 | 300-303 | 20-40† | 4-7 | Intravascular expansion by extracellular fluid shift | <1:1 |
| 10% dextran 40 | 317-324 | 40-60† | 4-7 | Intravascular expansion by extracellular fluid shift | <1:1 |
| 6% Hetastarch | 310 | Approximately 26 | 6.5 | Intravascular | 1:1 |

\* Depends on tonicity of fluid and plasma osmolarity.
† Rate must be sufficient to maintain plasma concentration of >2 g/dl: Usually 2 cc/kg/hr or more required (colloid distribution space assumes normal permeability characteristics).

## Crystalloid (Isotonic, Hypertonic)

Crystalloid, in particular lactated Ringer's solution, is the most popular resuscitation fluid in the United States. Isotonic crystalloid, if given in large enough amounts, can restore cardiac output toward normal in most patients, the exception being extremes of age and massive burns. Lactated Ringer's solution is preferred to normal saline because it more closely matches extracellular fluid. Since isotonic salt solutions generate no differential in osmotic pressure between plasma and interstitial spaces, the entire extracellular space must be expanded to replace intravascular losses. The amount of isotonic crystalloid required in the first 24 hours is initially estimated on the calculated deficit in sodium lost from the extracellular space. This has been estimated to be 0.5 to 0.6 mEq/% body burn/kg body weight, which equates to 4 ml/kg/% body burn of lactated Ringer's solution. The quantity of crystalloid needed is also dependent on the parameters used to monitor resuscitation.

Since sodium appears to be the key element in crystalloid infusion, solutions with increased sodium concentration have a theoretical advantage in that less water is infused. The hypertonic salt solutions used clinically have a milliosmolar content of 400 to 600 (280 to 300 mOsm is isotonic), thereby transiently generating potential osmotic pressures of several thousand millimeters of mercury in excess of normal until an iso-osmolar state is produced. This equilibrium occurs as the extracellular space is expanded by basically borrowing intracellular water. The current practice is to use a solution with a sodium content of approximately 240 mEq/L by adding two ampules of sodium lactate to each liter of normal saline. Current recommendations are that serum sodium levels should not be allowed to exceed 160 mEq/L during its use. A more isotonic solution should be instituted once a hyperosmolar state develops. Free water cannot be given during infusion because this will simply lead to a more isotonic solution and, in turn, no decrease in total administered fluid. Complications of the use of this solution relate primarily to those of the hyperosmolar state that occurs if too much salt is given. Increased water retention is likely to occur with institution of hypotonic solutions beginning on day 2 postburn.

## Colloids (Protein, Nonprotein)

Since nonburned tissue appears to regain normal permeability very shortly after injury and since hypoproteinemia may accentuate the nonburn edema, protein restoration beginning at about 8 to 12 hours seems appropriate if edema in noninjured tissue and total fluid requirements are to be minimized.

Fresh frozen plasma contains all the protein fractions that produce both the oncotic and nononcotic properties, but disease transmission is a major complication. It is therefore now strongly recommended not to use fresh frozen plasma or human plasma fractions as simply a volume expander. This product should be reserved for correction of documented clotting abnormalities. A 6% albumin solution replaces only the albumin losses. The amount of 6% protein solution to be infused remains undefined. Many investigators have arbitrarily used between 0.5 and 1 ml/kg/% total body surface during the first 24 hours. The amount depends on the magnitude of injury and the degree of hemodynamic instability. The protein should be infused at a constant rate over time rather than pulsed, since the latter approach will transiently increase pressure and increase the rate of edema formation.

Nonprotein colloids are advantageous if colloids are required early to maintain hemodynamic stability because the more expensive protein is lost into the burn. A standard 6% solution of dextran 70 exerts an oncotic pressure more than twice that generated by a 6% albumin solution. This makes the compound advantageous as a volume expander. Dextran 40 (40,000) in a 10% solution is an even more potent volume expander due to the generation of a colloid osmotic pressure six to eight times that of a comparable weight of protein, if infused at a rate of about 2 ml/kg/hr. Dextran 70 (6% or 60 g/L) should not be given in excess of 2 g/kg body weight and dextran 40 (10% or 100 g/L) over 1.5 g/kg over any 24-hour period to prevent a platelet deficit, which will impair clotting. The use of the hapten Promit, a dextran of 1000 molecular weight, before dextran solution essentially eliminates the concern of an allergic reaction to the dextran molecule. Hetastarch, a 6% starch solution, has colloid properties similar to those of a 6% protein solution, generating an oncotic pressure comparable to that of protein. The molecules are much larger than those of most dextrans and vascular clearance is therefore much slower. As with dextran, these products in large volumes, i.e., exceeding several liters, can lead to clotting abnormalities and the potential for immune dysfunction from reticuloendothelial blockade.

*Blood*

Because there is no real early red cell deficit with a burn alone, unless severe hemolysis occurs, blood replacement is usually not needed during this period. Occasionally, however, blood can be a very useful volume expander to restore cardiac output if perfusion is not adequately maintained by other fluids, especially if the patient has lost red cells, e.g., from escharotomies or from hemolysis, in the early postburn period.

## Intravenous Access

A peripheral vein catheter through nonburn tissue is the route preferred for fluid administration. A central line or pulmonary artery line is only occasionally needed to monitor the patient during the initial resuscitation period and is removed as soon as it is no longer needed. The possibilities for *intravenous access are:*

First choice:  Peripheral vein; nonburn area
Second choice:  Central vein; nonburn area
Third choice:  Peripheral vein; burn area
Worst choice:  Central vein; burn area

Monitoring lines are required primarily for the elderly patient or the patient with severe heart disease. An extremely high complication rate has been reported with central catheters in burn patients as a result of infection and embolic episodes related to a hypercoagulable state. An intravenous catheter should not be placed through burn tissue unless no other possible route exists, because of the high infection rate. Central line sites when not totally dedicated to total parenteral nutrition should be rotated every 3 days to minimize the risks of catheter sepsis infection.

# Rate of Infusion

Rate of fluid administration is dependent on the rate of loss, the latter being assessed by the perfusion monitors. An initial rate can be estimated using the size of the burn (combined second and third degree) relative to body surface area and body weight:

24 hour volume = 4cc × % total body surface × body weight
(one half in first 8 hours)

However, the amount of fluid required is that necessary to maintain perfusion and a formula is only an initial guide. If shock is present on admission, a bolus of fluid should be given (colloid is more effective than crystalloid). After perfusion is restored, fluid, usually isotonic crystalloid, should be infused at a relatively constant rate over several hours, making small changes to fine tune perfusion. Boluses, once shock is corrected, are disadvantageous because these simply transiently increase pressure and increase the rate of loss into the burn. The bolus approach is more appropriate for the trauma patient without a large leak where blood volume can be restored and then the infusion rate decreased. Fluid requirements in the first 6 to 8 hours will exceed those in the subsequent 18 hours, since the largest fluid shifts occur early. Approximately half of the first 24-hour requirements will need to be given in the first 8 hours. Once a fluid infusion rate is reached in the first 8 hours, which produces adequate perfusion, only modest hourly rate changes should be made in order to avoid large fluctuation in hemodynamic stability. Beginning at 8 to 10 hours, an attempt should be made to decrease the rate gradually and find that amount and mix of fluids that is the least amount necessary to maintain adequate perfusion.

# What to Monitor

No one monitor of perfusion in the burn patient can be considered to be a completely reliable indicator of tissue oxygenation (perfusion) and therefore several standard hemodynamic monitors and laboratory tests should be utilized. The correct and incorrect parameters to follow will be presented.

## Physiologic Measurements
**Baseline Body Weight.** The baseline weight is used to help estimate the initial fluid infusion rate (via formula). The preburn weight (if available) should be used for assessing nutrition needs and drug dosage.

**Arterial Pressure.** The increased sympathetic tone characteristic of this early period makes arterial pressure an insensitive measure of volume status; however, a minimal level of perfusion pressure (more than 90 mean) must be maintained and therefore blood pressure monitoring is necessary. The specific blood pressure required to maintain adequate organ perfusion and tissue oxygenation in each patient will only become evident as one carefully observes the response to fluid infusion.

An *arterial line* may be required if:

1. Patient is hemodynamically unstable

2. Extremities are burned so that sphingomanometric pressure cannot be obtained,
3. If frequent blood gases are required to monitor not only arterial oxygen tension but pH and arterial carbon dioxide tension.

The arterial catheter should be placed through nonburned skin and should be removed as soon as possible.

A *pulse oximeter* can provide continuous information of percent of oxygen-hemoglobin saturation and is noninvasive.

**Pulse Rate.** Tachycardia is inevitable early postburn due to hypovolemia and catechol release from tissue trauma and pain. The degree of tachycardia can be very useful for determining adequacy of volume replacement. The exception would be the elderly or the patient with preexisting heart disease in which the heart rate cannot increase in proportion to the stimulus. In most patients:

Pulse less than 120 usually indicates adequate volume
Pulse more than 130 usually indicates more fluid is needed

This guideline assumes that the pulse rate response corresponds to the other monitors of perfusion being used.

**Electrocardiographic Monitoring.** Arrhythmias are not common in the young patient as long as oxygenation is adequate, but they become a major concern in the patient older than 45 years as a result of the burn stress response. Rhythm changes may be the first clues of hypoxia and electrolyte or acid-base abnormalities and therefore, continuous electrocardiographic monitoring is required during this period.

**Urine Output.** The status of renal blood flow is usually an accurate reflection of the adequacy of systemic perfusion during this early phase of injury. A urine output of 0.5 to 1 ml/kg/hr normally reflects adequate renal blood flow, assuming there are no factors, such as alcohol, hyperglycemia, or mannitol, that alter the relationship between renal blood flow and urine output. In these cases, a "good" urine output may be seen in the presence of systemic hypoperfusion. A value less than 0.5 ml/kg/hr usually indicates renal hypoperfusion unless an acute renal insult has also occurred. A value more than 1.0 ml/kg/hr usually means too much fluid is being given and therefore excess edema is being produced. A value of 0.5 ml/kg/hr is usually adequate, assuming other perfusion parameters also reflect adequate perfusion. Because of the need for continuous assessment of renal blood flow, an indwelling urinary catheter is necessary for burns in excess of 30% total body surface or in smaller burns with other complicating factors.

**Intake-Output.** What goes in and what comes out should be carefully tabulated. Intake will far exceed output during this phase as edema develops.

**Blood Gases.** The method and importance of monitoring arterial oxygen and carbon dioxide tension has been described in detail in Section 7. The measurement of pH and acid-base balance are also extremely useful for the assessment of tissue oxygenation. A base deficit during this phase usually reflects impaired tissue oxygenation due to hypovolemia or carbon monoxide toxicity (also cyanide). If an arterial line cannot be placed safely, *a pulse oximeter* can be used for assessment of arterial oxygen tension and the measurement of venous pH and carbon dioxide tension can be used. Venous blood will have a higher (2 to 5 mmHg) carbon dioxide tension and a lower pH (0.05 to 0.08) than arterial blood but trends can be followed.

**Body Temperature.** The burn patient is very prone to hypothermia during this early period, especially with infusion of cool fluids. A decrease in temperature will lead to further hemodynamic instability and impaired perfusion. The external environment must be altered to allow for maintenance of a normal temperature for this period (which is 37 to 37.5°C). At a later phase, a higher core temperature will be required.

**Central Venous Pressure (CVP).** The central venous pressure in the large burn at this stage is usually low, 0 to 5 cm $H_2O$, even with adequate fluid resuscitation. This fact is understandable if one remembers that the burn-injured circulation is acting like a sieve. The rate of fluid loss is markedly accentuated by any increase in capillary pressure. Therefore it can be very dangerous to use an arbitrary value of central venous pressure as an endpoint of resuscitation. Too much or too little fluid can be infused based on an arbitrary value. There will be a poor correlation between right atrial pressure and the left ventricular end-diastolic volume if cardiac disease is present.

**Pulmonary Artery Wedge Pressure.** The majority of young patients, even with massive burns, do not require the use of these measurements for initial resuscitation. In this population, the risks of a pulmonary artery line may well exceed its benefits in assessing adequacy of perfusion. As with central venous pressure, pulmonary artery wedge is usually normal to low, 6 to 10 mmHg, early after burn even when adequate perfusion is present. Hypoperfusion is almost always due to hypovolemia. Well-recognized exceptions are: (1) impaired left ventricular function due to impaired left ventricular filling, e.g., high mean airway pressure, pneumothorax; or (2) marked increase in afterload due to a high level of circulating vasoconstrictors. A selected group of patients can benefit from this measurement. These include:

1. Elderly or patients with preexistent heart disease with large burn or smoke inhalation
2. Young patient with massive burn who is not maintaining perfusion despite fluid intake well in excess of predicted

**Cardiac Output, Mixed Venous Oxygen Tension.** The primary objective of fluid management is to maintain adequate tissue oxygen delivery. The direct measurement of cardiac output (cardiac index) can assist in the determination of oxygen delivery. A cardiac index in excess of 2.5 L/min/m$^2$ would be considered normal for a noninjured person. However, after injury, the number itself does not define the adequacy of oxygen delivery relative to needs because injured tissue needs exceed those of normal tissue. The value for mixed venous oxygen tension ($PvO_2$) however, can greatly assist in this determination. With access to mixed venous blood, monitoring of $PvO_2$ can be achieved. As with wedge pressure, this value is not required in most young patients, being reserved for elderly patients or those with other injuries such as inhalation.

$PvO_2$ >35 mmHg: oxygen delivery adequate
$PvO_2$ 30–35 mmHg: oxygen delivery marginal
$PvO_2$ <30 mmHg: oxygen delivery inadequate

*Laboratory Measurements*
**Hemoglobin and Hematocrit.** Baseline hematocrit and hemoglobin is useful to monitor, although changes in the values may not accurately reflect changes in blood volume due to the selective loss of the plasma component of blood. Hemoconcentration

**Table 2-4** Hematocrit Changes After Large Burn

| Finding | Cause |
|---|---|
| Hematocrit increased | Plasma volume decreases while circulating red blood cell volume remains relatively constant |
| Hematocrit normal | Normalization of blood volume has occurred<br>Decrease in both plasma and red blood cell volume, the latter from, e.g., hemolysis |
| Hematocrit decreased | Hemolysis from prolonged heat exposure, with only plasma volume replacement<br>Major loss of blood from nonburn injury with only plasma volume replacement<br>Preexisting anemia<br>Hypervolemia (unlikely) |

invariably occurs after large burns and normalization of blood volume is almost impossible until 24 to 48 hours. Blood loss, for example, from escharotomies, line placement, internal bleeding, and fractures, can easily be underestimated because the rate of plasma loss may exceed the rate of whole blood loss maintaining a normal hematocrit despite severe volume depletion. A declining hematocrit during this period in the absence of hemolysis, however, clearly indicates that there is a source of blood loss someplace.

**White Blood Cell.** Initial white blood cell count may be high, normal, or low, depending on the magnitude of the stress response and white cell sequestration into the burn. The absolute value is not a particularly useful parameter during this period.

**Electrolytes.** Since the initial losses are primarily plasma, the $Na^+$, $Cl^-$, $K^+$ values remain relatively constant despite hypovolemia and vary mainly as a result of the type of resuscitation fluid used. $K^+$ will increase if severe hemolysis has occurred or renal impairment is present. The $HCO^-_3$ content will vary, depending on the status of perfusion and acid-base balance.

**Creatinine and Blood Urea Nitrogen.** Baseline values are helpful to rule out intrinsic renal disease, which will impair the reliability of urine output as an index of perfusion.

**Plasma Proteins.** A marked decrease in plasma proteins occurs early postburn, with the major decrease occurring in the first 4 to 6 hours. Not much can be done about this level until about 10 to 12 hours postburn because of the rapid fluid and protein shift. Plasma albumin should be maintained above 2.5 g/dl.

**Plasma Myoglobin.** The plasma value of myoglobin is obtained with very deep burns, especially electrical burns. Myoglobin released from deeply injured muscle will affect renal function. A higher urine output should be maintained.

**Prothrombin Time, Partial Thromboplastin Time, and Platelets.** An initial value during this period is useful for determining whether clotting factors will be needed. It is not common to have to replace clotting factors and platelets during the first 36-hour period unless a prolonged shock state has initiated disseminated intravascular coagulation or preexisting liver or hematologic disease was present.

## Indications for Inotropic Support

Inotropic support to supplement fluids is indicated if adequate perfusion cannot be maintained without excessive fluid administration. As opposed to the nonburn patient, it is very difficult to "fill the tank" and increase preload to values above normal levels in the major burn patient if this is needed to increase cardiac output. This maneuver may simply lead to a marked accentuation in tissue edema, which in turn can further impair perfusion. Poor ventricular function is most commonly seen in the elderly burn patient or the patient with smoke inhalation requiring increasing positive pressure. Since improved renal blood flow is a major goal, low-dose dopamine (1 to 3 µg/kg/min) is often very useful. The dopamine effect at this range is primarily that of an isolated improvement in renal blood flow. Middle range dopamine (5 to 10 µg/kg/min) or dobutamine will increase contractility and improve cardiac output. Dobutamine produces less tachycardia and essentially no vasoconstrictor effect. Digoxin is not recommended in the immediate postburn period because the rapid fluid shifts can lead to digitalis toxicity and this agent is, in general, a less potent inotrope compared with dopamine or dobutamine. Vasodilators may be beneficial in selected cases of severe increases in systemic vascular resistance or systemic hypertension that is impairing cardiac output by the increase in afterload.

## Common Pitfalls in Initial Fluid Resuscitation

### Initial Underresuscitation

The largest fluid shifts occur in the first several hours postburn. If there has been a significant delay in initiation of fluid infusion and a shock state is present, initial crystalloid infusion based on a formula will often be inadequate. More volume is needed. A volume expander such as a nonprotein colloid or protein solution or hypertonic saline can be very useful along with isotonic crystalloid to correct the shock state.

### Initial Overresuscitation

Aggressive fluid infusion is now frequently initiated in most emergency rooms with placement of large lines. The practice of "wide open" fluid infusion during early assessment and transport regardless of hemodynamic response is to be avoided. The excess fluid cannot be compensated for by decreasing infusion rate in subsequent hours because the extra fluid is already out of the vascular space.

### Striving for Ideal Numbers

It is quite possible to achieve ideal numbers (pulse less than 120, blood pressure more than 100, urine output 0.5 to 1 cc/kg/hr) in a young patient with a moderate-sized uncomplicated burn. Attempts at pushing fluids beyond reasonable amounts to achieve "ideal numbers" in the massive burn (more than 60% total body surface), especially in the presence of inhalation injury or in the elderly, will only accentate edema-induced complications. Adequate perfusion is not the same as "ideal numbers." An intelligent treatment plan considering developing pulmonary and chest wall edema-induced complications must be devised.

## Consideration of Fluid Alone for Treatment of Impaired Perfusion

Hypovolemia from burn-induced fluid and protein shifts is the predominant cause of hypoperfusion, and fluid infusion is the treatment. However, two other processes must be considered. The first is impaired cardiac output due to an increasing mean airway pressure, particularly from a noncompliant chest wall burn. Ventilator adjustments, chest wall escharotomy, elevation of the head of the bed to decrease chest edema, and the use of an agent, such as low-dose dopamine, to assist fluids can be very helpful in maintaining perfusion. Secondly, cardiac depression from a deep body burn is well described, particularly in the elderly. Supplementation of fluids both crystalloid and colloid with a beta agonist can help reverse a downward course reflected by continually increasing fluid requirements and decreasing perfusion.

## Use of Urine Output Alone as Monitor for Volume Restoration

Although usually a reliable indicator of renal perfusion, factors such as high plasma alcohol or glucose levels will often lead to an inappropriately high urine output relative to the status of tissue perfusion. The value of the urine output must be considered to be unreliable under these circumstances.

## Failure to Secure Intravenous Lines

As edema develops, tape unravels and the intravenous catheter slips out of the vein into the surrounding tissue. Not only does this lead to transient hypovolemia, but finding a new site when edema is present can be extremely difficult. A solution is to secure the intravenous line with sutures.

# TREATMENT SUMMARY

## Monitoring Guidelines

1. Blood pressure—only reliable as volume indicator if low
2. Pulse: young patient—pulse less than 120, reasonable perfusion; pulse more than 130, needs more fluid
   Elderly or with heart disease—pulse not accurate reflection of perfusion
3. Urine output—0.5 to 1 cc/kg/hr (nonglycosuric; no alcohol) is adequate
   Exception: Myoglobin or hemoglobinuria
   >1 cc/kg/hr, excessive, decrease fluids (assuming valid reassessment)
4. Electrocardiogram—particularly important for patient more than 45 years old
5. Temperature—To avoid hypothermia (large burn)
   —To avoid hyperthermia (small to moderate second degree burn)

6. Blood gases—High risk of hypoxemia, hypercapnia due to direct pulmonary complications of burn and of treatment
   pH, acid-base—Base deficit very useful indicator of tissue oxygenation
7. Pulmonary artery wedge pressure—For high-risk patient (elderly) inhalation, cardiac output, mixed venous oxygen pressure, if cardiopulmonary stability cannot be achieved
8. Complete blood count—Hemoglobin not reliable indicator of status of red blood cell mass due to selective plasma loss
9. White blood cell—Initial value, usually increased, reflecting stress response, not infection
10. Electrolytes—only initial abnormality may be hyper- or hypokalemia. $HCO_3^-$ value dependent on acid-base balance
11. Blood urea nitrogen, creatinine—Anticipate normal values initially; changes more evident in subsequent days
12. Plasma proteins—Anticipate decrease of about 50% from normal; albumin usually less than 3 g/dl
13. Prothrombin time, partial thromboplastin time, platelets—moderate burn: usually near normal. Massive burn (more than 50% total body surface): abnormal due to consumption

# TREATMENT SUMMARY (0 TO 24 HOURS)

## Maintenance of Hemodynamic Stability

*All Patients* with Burns More than 20% Total Body Surface
Large Bore Peripheral Intravenous Lines
Begin Lactated Ringers Solution; Estimate Initital Rate According to Percent Total Body Surface and Weight
Monitor: Pulse, Blood Pressure, Urine, Electrocardiography, Temperature, Electrolytes, Complete Blood Count
Maintain: Blood Pressure >90 Systolic, Urine 0.5 to 1 cc/kg/hr, Pulse <130, Temperature 36° to 38°

Modify Protocol with

Massive Burns, Inhalation Injury, Elderly, Shock

*Monitoring*

1. Add arterial line if blood pressure cannot be adequately monitored, if unstable, or for access to blood gases
2. Pulse oximeter (ideal for oxygen saturation)
3. Pulmonary artery catheter
   if preexistent heart disease is severe
   if hemodynamic instability persists
   if inotrope needed
4. Monitor cardiac output, wedge, mixed venous oxygen tension
5. Add blood urea nitrogen, creatinine, coagulation panel, plasma proteins

*Fluid Infusion to Include*

1. Colloid or
2. Hypertonic lactated saline (for first 8 to 10 hours)

*Consider*

1. Inotrope if fluid alone not adequate (low-dose dopamine first choice)
2. Vasodilator if severe systemic hypertension present (sodium nitroprusside is best initial choice)

# SUMMARY

## Specific Resuscitation Guidelines

**Patient <40 Years Old and <50% Total Body Surface No Smoke Inhalation**

1. Can give isotonic crystalloid for 24 hours as primary fluid
2. Begin replacing protein deficit at 12 to 18 hours (1 to 2 cc/kg/hr)

**Patient <40 Years Old and >60% Total Body Surface With or Without Smoke Inhalation**

1. Use isotonic crystalloid as primary fluid
2. Add colloid from beginning (2 cc/kg/hr)
3. Consider hypertonic saline early
4. May need to add renal dose dopamine

**Patient >40 or <5 Years Old With Large Burn**

1. Isotonic crystalloid primary fluid
2. Add colloid from beginning (nonprotein or protein) to maintain stability
3. Consider careful use of hypertonic saline
4. May need to add inotropic support

**Patient with Burn and Severe Smoke Inhalation**

1. Will usually need combination of crystalloid and colloid to maintain hemodynamic stability, especially with increasing need for positive pressure
2. Consider low-dose dopamine if urine output poor despite large volume infusion

**Patients Not Responding to Fluid Alone**

1. Look for pulmonary problem, increased airway pressure
2. Consider inotrope β agonist first choice
3. Consider use of blood as volume expander

**Patients in Shock**

1. Give colloid (5% albumin, dextran) along with crystalloid until shock corrected
2. Then use crystalloid as primary fluid

# 3

# Management of the Burn Wound

Recognition of the magnitude of burn injury that is dictated by depth, size, and the prior health of the host is of crucial importance in the overall care plan. Decisions as to wound management are based on this assessment. In addition, it is important to understand that the wound itself in this early period can rapidly evolve toward a deeper injury. The type of early care provided will have a major impact on subsequent morbidity and mortality.

Sections relating to basic pathophysiology and recognition of injury will be discussed along with treatment principles.

## GENERAL SECTIONS

Pathophysiology of Early Burn Wound Changes
    Anatomy and Function of the Skin
    Depth of Burn Injury
    Severity of Injury
Practical Approach to Treatment
    Neutralize the Source of Burn Injury
    Avoid Excess Heat Loss
    Determining the Extent of Injury
    Cleaning and Debriding the Wound
    Infection Control
    Management of Specific Burn Areas
    Impaired Distal Perfusion and Need for Escharotomy
    Pitfalls in Early Wound Management
    Treatment Summary

## PATHOPHYSIOLOGY OF EARLY BURN WOUND CHANGES

### Anatomy and Function of the Skin

The skin is the largest organ of the body, ranging from 0.25 $m^2$ in the newborn to more than 2 $m^2$ in the adult. It consists of two layers, epidermis and dermis, or corium (Fig. 3-1). The outermost layer of the epidermis is composed of dead, cornified cells that act as

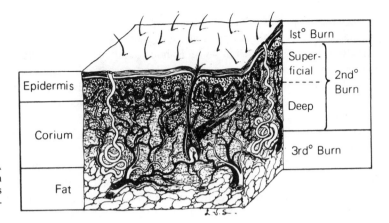

**Figure 3–1.** A schema showing depth of burns. Corium is another term for dermis.

a tough protective barrier against the environment. The second, thicker layer, the corium (0.06 to 0.12 mm), is composed chiefly of fibrous connective tissue. The dermis contains the blood vessels and nerves to the skin and the epithelial appendages of specialized function. The nerve endings that mediate pain are found in the dermis. Partial thickness injuries are extremely painful because the nerve endings are exposed. Full-thickness burns are usually anesthetic due to heat destruction of the nerves.

The skin is also the barrier that prevents loss of body fluids through evaporation and loss of body heat. Sweat glands help maintain body temperature by controlling the amount of heat lost by evaporation. Increased loss of water and heat through burned skin are major problems early postburn. In addition, the skin is the primary protective barrier against invasive infection, preventing penetration of microorganisms into the subdermal tissues. Loss of this function results in increased risk of invasive infection. Another protection that the skin provides is adaptation to changes in the physical environment initiated by the sensory nerve endings in the dermis, which detect the sensations of touch, pressure, pain, cold, and heat. Loss of this function will lead to long-term impairment.

In summary, the *functions of the skin are:*

1. Maintenance of normal body temperature
2. Barrier to evaporative water loss
3. Barrier to invasive infection
4. Metabolic activity (vitamin D synthesis)
5. Protection against environment, using sensation of touch, pressure, pain

## Depth of Burn Injury

Traditionally, burn depth has been classified in degrees of injury based on the amount of epidermis and dermis injured. At present, depth is estimated by *physical appearance, pain,* and *skin texture or pliability*. A number of noninvasive diagnostic techniques have been used and are being evaluated; however, none at the present time have replaced the accuracy of clinical assessment based on experience. A *first degree* burn involves only the thinner outer epidermis layer and is characterized by erythema and mild discomfort. Tissue damage is minimal and protective functions of the skin are intact. Pain, the chief symptom, usually resolves in 48 to 72 hours, and healing takes place uneventfully. The pain is believed to be in large part due to local vasodilator prostaglandin production. In 5 to 10 days, the damaged epithelium peels off in small scales, leaving no residual scarring. The most common causes of first degree burns are overexposure to sunlight or brief scalding by hot liquids of less than 120°F (Table 3-1). *Second degree* burns are defined as those in which the entire epidermis and variable portions of the dermis layer are heat destroyed.

A *superficial second degree* burn involves heat injury to the upper third of the dermis (Color plate 2, page 311). The microvessels perfusing this area are injured and permeability is increased, resulting in the leakage of large amounts of plasma into the interstitium. This fluid, in turn, lifts off the thin heat-destroyed epidermis, causing blister formation. The blisters will continue to increase in size in the postburn period as cell and protein breakdown occurs, releasing osmotically active particles into the blister fluid, which subsequently attract additional water (1 mOsm of solute generates 19 mmHg pressure). A light pink, wet-appearing very painful wound is also seen if blisters are disrupted. Frequently, the epidermis does not lift off the dermis for 12 to 24 hours and what appears initially to be a first degree is actually a second degree burn. Despite loss of the entire basal layer of the epidermis, a burn of this depth will heal in 7 to 14 days due to repopulation by the epithelial cells that are also present in hair follicles, sweat glands, and other skin appendages, anchored deep in the dermis. Minimal scarring is expected to occur, if the burn does not increase in depth, since the wound inflammation that stimulates excessive collagen deposition is short-lived due to the rapid wound closure.

A *deep dermal* or deep second degree burn extends well into the dermal layer and fewer viable epidermal cells remain. Therefore reepithelialization is extremely slow, sometimes requiring months. In these patients, blister formation does not characteristically occur because the dead tissue layer is sufficiently thick and adherent to underlying viable dermis that is not readily lifted off the surface by the edema. The exception would be the very young or very old patient with a very thin dermis. The wound surface is usually red in appearance with white areas in deeper parts. There is only modest plasma surface leakage because of the severe impairment in blood supply (Color plate 3, page 312).

**Table 3-1** Common Characteristics of Burn Injury

| Cause | Depth (Degree) | Pain | Appearance |
|---|---|---|---|
| Hot liquids | | | |
|   Short exposure | Second | Severe | Wet, pink blisters |
|   Long exposure | Second, third | Minimal | Wet, dark red |
| Flames | | | |
|   Flash exposure | Second | Severe | Wet, pink blisters |
|   Direct contact | Third | Minimal | Dry, white, waxy or brown, black leathery |
| Chemicals | | | |
|   Acid, alkali | Second Converts to third | Severe | Light brown to light gray |

Because the remaining blood supply is marginal, there is a high probability of deepening of the tissue damage with time.

The appearance of the deep dermal burn changes dramatically over the next several days as the area of dermal necrosis along with surface coagulated protein turns the wound a white to yellow color. The amount of surface coagulum is accentuated with the use of a topical antibiotic, making the deep second degree burn difficult to differentiate from a third degree burn after 24 to 48 hours. The continued presence of pain can assist in the diagnosis because pain is usually absent in a full-thickness injury. Fluid losses and the metabolic effects of deep dermal burns are basically the same as that seen with the third degree burn. Dense scarring is usually seen if the wound is allowed to heal primarily rather than excised and skin grafted.

A full-thickness or *third degree* burn is defined as destruction of the entire epidermis and dermis, leaving no residual epidermal cells to repopulate. This would will therefore not reepithelialize and whatever area of the wound is not closed by wound contraction will require skin grafting. A characteristic appearance of the now avascular burn tissue on first appearance is a waxy white color typical of any avascular tissue. If the burn extends into the fat or with prolonged contact with a flame source, a leathery brown or black appearance can be seen along with coagulated veins, characterizing charred tissue (Color plate 4, page 312). A short exposure to a very high temperature, such as direct contact with a flame, is the usual cause of a third degree burn. However, prolonged contact with hot liquids as seen with intentional scalding, with only a modest increase in temperature, e.g., 130°F water, can result in a third degree burn. This type of prolonged contact with hot liquids will also lead to hemolysis of red cells as well as release of myoglobin from underlying muscle, resulting in a red pigment deposition in the wound. The appearance of the wound can be mistaken for viable dermis after a flame burn. Therefore *a dark red appearance in a scald burn may represent a full-thickness injury.*

The immersion scald wound will frequently evolve into a deeper burn than initially anticipated. Full-thickness flame burns usually lead to immediate occlusion of the injured capillaries by thrombosis, as with electrocautery. The lack of any painful sensation is due to the heat destruction of the nerve endings. Chemical burns have a much different appearance, even when full thickness, having a light grey to brown discoloration. Pain in chemical burns is usually extreme because the burning process continues for minutes to hours.

The exact depth of many burns cannot be clearly defined on first appearance. The major difficulty is distinguishing a very deep dermal from a full-thickness (third degree) burn that extends just through the dermis (Color plate 5, page 313). This burn is termed an indeterminate burn, since an accurate diagnosis of depth cannot be made initially.

A *zone of ischemia* is present, beneath the heat destroyed outer tissue and the clearly viable tissue, well beneath the surface. The tissue in between is heat injured but still viable. The vasculature to this area has been injured. Some vessels are thrombosed and other vessels are patent but prone to thrombosis because of endothelial cell damage. The marginally viable tissue can be readily converted to nonviable tissue by any further decrease in blood flow caused by local mediator release or infection. A deep second degree or healable burn can therefore progress to a third degree burn. Vasoactive mediators, such as thromboxane and products of oxygen radical release, appear to be involved in the progressive ischemia and attempts at blocking these mediators has met with some success both in the laboratory and in man. Avoidance of any process that will lead to further local ischemia, such as tissue desiccation or hypovolemia, must be avoided. Tissue oxygen tension also decreases with the burn edema process as the distance between viable cells and the closest capillary increases. This process will have the most deleterious impact on the marginally viable cells. Prevention of wound conversion is of major importance in the resuscitation period.

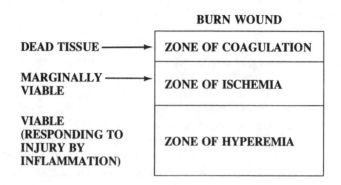

## Severity of Injury

The size of the burn is defined in terms of percent of total body surface area. A useful initial guide is the use of the "rule of nines," in which the body is divided into areas with 9% of total body surface. The head and each arm are considered 9% of total, and the chest and abdomen, the back and each lower extremity is considered to be 18% of total body surface. A more specific breakdown is shown in Figures 3-2 and 3-3. (Note the increased head size in the small child.)

The size or surface area of the body skin involved, the depth and location of injury, the patient's age, and the presence of associated injuries determine morbidity and mortality. Age and presence of associated injury now appear to be the most significant parameters of survival, since new aggressive approaches to the burn wound have decreased the role of the wound itself in morbidity and mortality.

Survival statistics are best for patients 10 to 30 years old whose burns are not complicated by smoke inhalation injury, since the latter markedly increases the mortality rate (Table 3-2).

Age becomes a major factor in the survival of burns with increased mortality seen in children less than 2 and adults more than 50 years old. An uncomplicated 50% total body surface burn in these populations has a mortality rate in excess of 50%. The higher death rate in small children results from a number of factors. First, the body surface area relative to body weight is much greater than that in adults, resulting in a comparably greater physiologic impact on the child. Second, an incompletely developed immune system decreases resistance to infection. Third, immature kidneys and liver diminish the ability to remove the high solute load from injured tissue, to produce new protein rapidly, and to utilize exogenous nutrients maximally. The inability of the elderly to tolerate stress due to preexisting cardiac, pulmonary, or other chronic disease, such as diabetes and general immune incompetence, increases mortality.

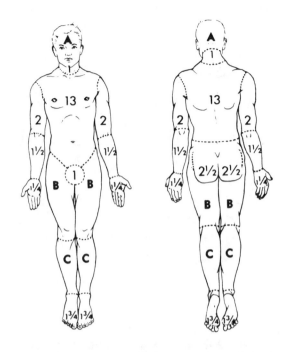

**Relative Percentages of Areas Affected by Growth**

| Area | Age | | |
|---|---|---|---|
| | 10 | 15 | Adult |
| A = half of head | 5½ | 4½ | 3½ |
| B = half of one thigh | 4¼ | 4½ | 4¾ |
| C = half of one leg | 3 | 3¼ | 3½ |

**Figure 3–2.** A normogram to determine percent of body surface area burn is shown for the adult.

## PRACTICAL APPROACH TO TREATMENT

The initial management of the burn wound is based on a knowledge of the skin anatomy and functional losses with injury. The major objectives are to decrease the potential of further local damage and decrease the systemic abnormalities that can be produced by the loss of the barrier function. The early treatment therefore focuses on:

1. Neutralizing the source of burn injury
2. Avoiding excess heat loss
3. Determining the extent of injury
4. Clean and debride the wound
5. Infection control
6. Maintain tissue perfusion

The early major cardiopulmonary disorders caused by the large burn and complicating injuries will be discussed in subsequent chapters.

**48** *Burn Trauma*

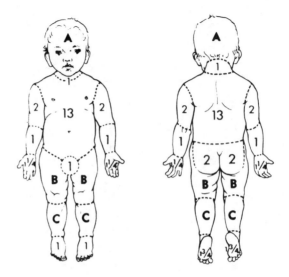

**Relative Percentages of Areas Affected by Growth**

| Area | Age | | |
|---|---|---|---|
| | 0 | 1 | 5 |
| A = half of head | 9½ | 8½ | 6½ |
| B = half of one thigh | 2¾ | 3¼ | 4 |
| C = half of one leg | 2½ | 2½ | 2¾ |

**Figure 3–3.** A normogram to determine percent of body surface area burn is shown for the infant and toddler.

**Table 3-2** Data Obtained From Specialized Burn Facilities for Mean Survival Rate (%) Comparing Age and Burn Size

| Burn Size (%) | Age (yr) | | | | | | |
|---|---|---|---|---|---|---|---|
| | 0–1 | 2–4 | 5–34 | 35–49 | 50–59 | 60–74 | >75 |
| 0–10 | >95 | >95 | >95 | >95 | >95 | 95 | 90 |
| 10–20 | 95 | >90 | >95 | >90 | >85 | 80 | 50 |
| 20–30 | 90 | 90 | 95 | 90 | 75 | 50 | 25 |
| 30–40 | 75 | 80 | 90 | 80 | 60 | 30 | <10 |
| 40–50 | 50 | 65 | 80 | 60 | 40 | 10 | <5 |
| 50–60 | 40 | 50 | 60 | 45 | 30 | <10 | <5 |
| 60–70 | 20 | 30 | 40 | 20 | 15 | <5 | 0 |
| 70–80 | 5 | 20 | 25 | 10 | 5 | 0 | 0 |
| 80–90 | 0 | <10 | 10 | <10 | <5 | 0 | 0 |
| 90–100 | 0 | <5 | <5 | <5 | 0 | 0 | 0 |

\* Total body surface burn, combined second and third degree.

## Neutralize the Source of Burn Injury

### Removal of Heat Containing Clothing

With a flame or scald burn, the clothing can retain heat for considerable periods of time. Rapid removal of burned clothing is therefore essential. If clothing is burned or melted into the tissues, just remove the loose surrounding fabric. The adherent clothing can be removed when further wound cleaning and debridement is performed after admission.

### Use of Cold Water

Cooling the burn wound has a number of advantages. First, immediate cooling will help neutralize retained heat, decreasing injury. Cooling also appears to stabilize skin mast cells, decreasing histamine release and resulting edema. These advantages are short-lived and cooling must be applied within seconds to minutes postburn to obtain these gains. Cooling also decreases pain from the irritated nerve endings of a partial thickness burn. This improvement can be seen anytime in the first several hours after injury. Deeper burns are relatively anesthetic and therefore do not need cooling.

Cooling has a number of major disadvantages as well. First, cooling will increase body heat loss through the burn wound. A decrease in body temperature is very deleterious in that the initial shivering that invariably occurs produces a marked increase in oxygen consumption and calorie demands at a time when oxygen delivery is compromised. Glycogen stores become depleted. Hypothermia will then develop and lead to a potentiation of the shock state. Rewarming is extremely difficult after a burn, not only because of the presence of hypovolemia, but also because of the inability of burned skin to vasoconstrict and minimize continued losses. Wet clothing or dressings markedly accentuate heat loss because the rate of loss of body heat in water is 25 times greater than in air. In addition, a wet burn dressing accentuates bacterial migration from the environment to the wound. The following guidelines should be used for *cool water treatment:*

    Indications:   Initial heat neutralization (minutes)
                         To control pain in superficial second degree burns (less than 15% total body surface)
    Contraindications:   For any third degree burn once heat neutralized
                                Any second degree burn with more than 15% total body surface

### Removal of the Burning Chemical

The burning process caused by chemical injury is the result of a chemical reaction in the tissue leading to protein denaturation and heat production. The tissue destruction will persist as long as the chemical is present even in minute amounts (Figs. 3-4, 3-5, 3-6). In addition, systemic toxicity as a result of the absorbed chemicals can occur, producing more morbidity than the surface burn. The injury produced by the more common caustic chemicals are described in Table 3-3. The chemical burn wound once identified is managed in most cases just like a thermal burn. However, since the burning process usually progresses, a several day delay before determination of the need for excision and grafting may be necessary.

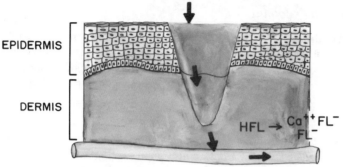

**PROTOPLASMIC POISONS**
**ALKALOIDAL ACIDS**

Tannic, Picric, Formic
Hydroflouric acid

EPIDERMIS

DERMIS

HFL → $Ca^{++}$ $FL^-$ / $FL^-$

**SYSTEMIC EFFECT**

Hepato-Renal
Bone Demineralization

**LOCAL EFFECT**

Protein Denaturation
Heat Production
Variable Depth

**TREATMENT**

Water Lavage
$Ca^{++}$ Gluconate (HFL)

Figure 3–4.

**CORROSIVES; DESICCANTS**

| Alkali | Phenol |
| --- | --- |
| NaOH | Phosphorus |
| CaOH | Sulfuric acid |
| KOH | |
| LiOH | |

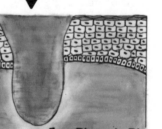

EPIDERMIS

DERMIS

Phenol, Phosphorus

**SYSTEMIC EFFECT**

Hepato-Renal
Neurological
Hematologic

**LOCAL EFFECT**

Liquifaction Necrosis
Heat Production
Tissue Saponification
Tissue Desiccation
Full Thickness Burn

**TREATMENT**

Remove Powder (phos, cement)
Particles (lithium)
Water Lavage (improvement beyond 1 hour)

Figure 3–5.

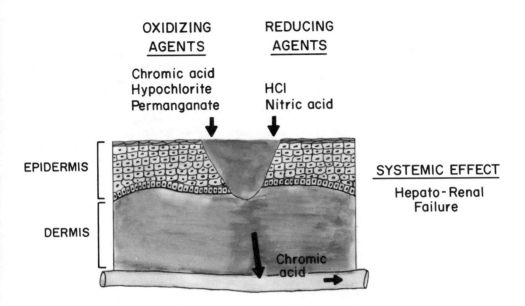

**Figure 3–6.**

**Table 3-3** Chemical Burns

| Agent | Pathophysiology | Treatment |
|---|---|---|
| General category of acids | Deep skin burn caused by tissue desiccation and protein denaturation. Injury may extend well below skin with concentrated acids. Acids, such as sulfuric, nitric, hydrochloric, cause local damage. Appearance tan to gray discoloration with extreme pain, a common finding | Vigorous water lavage up to 60 minutes after injury using warm water with extensive exposure to avoid hypothermia. Treatment should be based on the assumption that the burn will be much deeper than initial appearance indicates. Standard fluid resuscitation principles |
| Hydrofluoric acid | Deep skin burn, which can be extensive. Systemic effects due to hypocalcemia as a result of complex of $Ca^{++}$ to $Fl^-$ anion | Vigorous water lavage along with local injection of calcium gluconate as well as topical use of 2.5% calcium gluconate gel. Endpoint of local wound calcium is relief of pain. Monitor plasma calcium and replace, if necessary. |

**Table 3-3** Chemical Burns (*continued*)

| Agent | Pathophysiology | Treatment |
|---|---|---|
| General category of alkali | Deep skin burn caused again by tissue desiccation and protein denaturation from chemical reaction of alkali exposed to hydrated tissue. Alkali burns tend to be worse than acid burns, but systemic effects from absorption are not common. Appearance is tan to gray surface discoloration with characteristic extreme pain. | Vigorous water lavage for at least 60 minutes after injury and longer for lye burns, avoiding hypothermia during the lavage. Treatment should be based on the assumption that the burn will progress in depth. Standard fluid resuscitation principles |
| Gasoline immersion | Superficial skin injury: erythema<br>Systemic injury: from absorbed hydrocarbons<br>Renal: lipid degenerative changes to proximal tubules<br>Lung: surfactant denaturation, atelectasis, lipoid pneumonia<br>Central nervous system: edema producing seizures, coma<br>Liver: lipid degenerative changes, hepatitis | Water immersion<br><br>Aggressive maintenance of hydration and pulmonary support along with general critical care support |
| Phenol | Partial thickness burn: dull tan to gray color<br>Systemic injury from absorption, which is usually rapid with the rate and amount being directly proportional to surface area of exposure<br>Renal: Direct glomerular and tubular damage as well as indirect damage from precipitated hemoglobin<br>Hematologic: red cell hemolysis, decreased erythropoiesis<br>Central nervous system: seizures, comatose state<br>Liver: centrolobular necrosis | Spray or pour large volumes of water on surface. Do not swab or use small amounts of water, which will only increase surface area of exposure. After lavage, use a quick skin wipe with polyethylene or propylene glycol. Maintain urine alkaline with bicarbonate to decrease hemoglobin precipitation. Maintain excellent hydration and blood volume to support injured kidney and other organs |
| Tar | Superficial to deep skin burn, depending on the temperature of the tar when contacting the skin. No systemic absorption is usually present | Removal of tar to allow for burn wound management. Bacitracin or Neosporin ointment contain the emulsifier Tween-80, which is very useful in dissolving the tar. Apply and wash off several times a day until tar is removed. Avoid hydrocarbon solvents. Gentle mechanical debridement can also be used |

## Avoid Excess Heat Loss

With a deep burn, the barrier to the loss of water by evaporation is markedly impaired. The loss of the evaporation barrier also means loss of the barrier to *heat loss,* a fact extremely important to recognize in the resuscitation period. The normal protective mechanism of skin vasoconstriction is absent. Body heat is lost by the mechanisms of convection, conduction, and radiation, all of which are magnified after burns. Transfer of heat to a moving system such as air or water is known as *convection*. If body surface temperature is higher than air temperature, heat flows from the body to the air in the absence of a barrier until the gradient is gone. However, as the warmed air is soon replaced by cooler air, the gradient again increases, leading to further heat loss. Continuous air movement by a fan or by a laminar airflow unit, or an air fluidized bed can therefore play a major role in heat loss from the burn wound. Heat loss can be decreased by closing the wound with dry dressings, thereby limiting the air movement and decreasing the air-wound temperature gradient. The increased rate of loss of body heat in water occurs not only with wet dressings but also with hydrotherapy. Heat is also exchanged by direct contact with an object, e.g., bed or dressing table. This process is known as *conduction* and heat loss is again dependent on the temperature gradient. *Radiation* is emission of energy from the body surface as heat. The loss is dependent on body heat production, surface blood flow, and surface area. Radiation losses are increased postburn as a result of hypermetabolism and increased blood flow.

In summary, *increased heat loss postburn are:*

Convective losses: Increased in proportion to air-body temperature gradient accentuated by flowing air: breeze, fan

Conduction losses: Via surface in contact with skin accentuated by water or metal

Radiation losses: Relative to surface area and wound blood flow

The major burn patient must be placed in a warmed external environment to minimize heat loss. Wound debridement and washing should not be initiated on the large burn until the external temperature is controlled. The emergency room is often not the proper place for any substantial wound care. Once the heat source has been neutralized and the depth and extent of injury determined, the wounds should be covered with dry dressings until the problem of external heat loss can be controlled. Patients with burns of the magnitude that will lead to this problem should be transferred to the proper burn facility where more definitive wound care in a controlled environment can be provided. Controlled environment means a temperature greater than 80°F (depending on burn size) and humidity exceeding 30%.

## Determining the Extent of Injury

The history of the type of injury, i.e., scald, flame, explosion, and presence of smoke, will greatly assist in the determination of the magnitude of injury.

The depth and extent of injury can be determined using the characteristics previously described. However, exact determination will require cleaning of the wound and some debridement of nonviable epidermis. The wound can be categorized based on size, depth, age, and other complicating factors. The standard categorization used by the American Burn Association for critical, moderate, and minor burns is presented:

Major burns

1. Second degree burns involving >25% of total body surface
2. Third degree burns involving >10% of total body surface
3. Burns complicated by respiratory tract injury or fractures or involving critical areas, such as face, hands, feet, perineum
4. High voltage electrical burns
5. Lesser burns in patients with significant preexisting disease

Moderate burns

1. Second degree burns involving 15 to 25% of total body surface
2. Third degree burns involving 2 to 10% of total body surface
3. Areas above not involving face, hands, feet, perineum

Minor burns

1. Second degree burns <15% total body surface
2. Third degree burns <2% total body surface

## Cleaning and Debriding the Wound

The management of the burn wound itself is dependent on the status of initial cardiopulmonary function. Adequate control of the airway, gas exchange, and restoration of fluid loss must precede attempts at wound cleaning and debridement. The optimum environment for cleaning of the major burn is not the emergency room where temperature control and aseptic technique are difficult to maintain. In addition, the process can be time consuming, and using emergency rooms for this purpose is impractical. A relatively clean hospital area should be used where monitoring can be performed and resuscitation continued. A smaller burn can be managed in a clean treatment area. For all burns, the following components of care must be understood:

How to control pain
What to use for cleaning
What to debride
Where to clean: bed bath versus hydrotherapy

## Pain Control

As pointed out before, the deeper the burn, the less the pain, so that the full-thickness burn injury that is likely to have the greater hemodynamic instability will have the least discomfort. However, a burn is usually not totally uniform in depth and some partial thickness (second degree) burn is often present. The superficial second degree burn is the most painful and analgesics will be required before any cleaning can be performed. The increased burn-induced sympathetic discharge as well as the decreased blood volume with the larger injury will produce a relative decrease in skin and muscle blood flow. Except for the minor burn, *intramuscular narcotics are contraindicated* because of erratic absorption. *Intravenous narcotics are indicated* because of greater safety and better pain control. Start out with small intravenous doses, 1 to 2 mg morphine, 10 to 15 mg meperidine hydrochloride, and increase as required relative to the hemodynamic response. Fentanyl is also an excellent analgesic because of its rapid onset of action and short half-life.

## Cleaning Solutions

The solution used should be nontoxic yet effective for the organisms present. Chlorhexidine (Hibiclens), and povidone-iodone (Betadine), are the most commonly used agents diluted in sterile saline or water. The solution should be room temperature or greater, unless the burn is minor in size. Both agents come prepackaged for dilution in a basin of warm water or saline. *Chlorhexidine* is the *preferred* initial agent because it is very effective against the gram-positive organisms, which are the normal skin contaminant as well as somewhat effective against gram-negative organisms and fungus. Povidone-iodine solution is an effective bactericide against all three categories of microorganisms, but it frequently hurts on application and can be toxic to injured tissue if not diluted. Excessive absorption, if used on large burn surfaces, can lead to immunosuppression and other aspects of iodine toxicity.

## What to Debride

Loose tissue, broken blisters, and dirt should all be gently removed because they all add to subsequent infection risk. If the burn is partial thickness, removal of loose overlying epidermis results in exposure of underlying dermis. The injured dermis must be covered with a topical antibiotic, grease gauze, or temporary skin substitute to avoid desiccation, thus:

> Remove dirt, loose devitalized epidermis
> Leave large blisters intact on hands and feet
>    (Exception: if skin substitutes are to be used)

It is important to wash and gently mechanically debride the wound (gauze, cloth), not only to remove loose surface devitalized tissue, but also to determine better the true depth of the burn. Initial assessment before cleaning may be very inaccurate.

Large intact blisters (roughly greater than 4 to 5 cm in diameter) should be left intact initially if a skin substitute is not being used to protect the underlying dermis and decrease pain (Color plate 6, page 313). After 24 to 48 hours, breakdown of tissue and protein in the fluid will increase local osmotic pressure, leading to blister expansion. Debridement of larger blisters should take place at about 48 to 72 hours, or sooner if disrupted to avoid infection in the coagulated protein blister fluid.

### Role of Hydrotherapy Versus Sequential Cleaning (Bed Bath)

It is of the utmost importance that cardiopulmonary stability be maintained during the initial period after major burns. Wound cleaning must not impair the basics of resuscitation. Use of a hydrotherapy system for initial wound cleaning is only applicable to the moderate burn injury in which the wound itself is really the only major medical concern. It is well established that body immersion in a tank is contraindicated at this time if there is any cardiopulmonary instability. Also, there is an increased risk of bacterial cross-contamination from, e.g., perineum and other contaminated areas to clean burn areas. The patient should not be immersed during this period, but rather can be rinsed with water running from head to foot on a slanted board or shower. Sequential cleaning, meaning cleaning and wrapping of individual body parts separately, is ideal. This not only minimizes pain and hypothermia, but also ideal cardiopulmonary monitoring and support can be maintained during this period. The cleaning procedure can be done in a well-monitored treatment room or in the patient's bed. Advantages and disadvantages of both are presented in Table 3-4.

## Infection Control

Once the wound is initially debrided, control of potential infection in the injured tissue is the next priority:

    Tetanus Prophylaxis is required (American College of Surgeons Guidelines)

Table 3-4  Early Wound Cleaning

Sequential cleaning (bed bath)
  Indications: Major burn, especially with any cardiopulmonary dysfunction
  Advantages: Allows for adequate monitoring, minimizes stress, hypothermia, cross-contamination
  Disadvantages: Time consuming

Hydrotherapy (with top to bottom water runoff)
  Indications: Moderate heat burn or any severe chemical burn
  Advantages: Efficient removal of chemicals, expeditious removal of dirt, loose tissue
  Disadvantages: Impairs cardiopulmonary resuscitation, can lead to hypothermia, cross-contamination

Hydrotherapy (immersion)
  Not indicated for early wound cleaning, only later physical therapy

## Use of Prophylactic Systemic Antibiotics

Numerous studies have demonstrated that prophylactic systemic antibiotics in either the minor or major burn are of no benefit in decreasing the rate of wound infection. The relatively avascular deep burn will not receive a sufficient blood supply to provide adequate tissue antibiotic levels. In addition, any open wound will become colonized with bacteria. The only exception to the no prophylactic systemic antibiotics dictum would be low-dose penicillin for protection against β-hemolytic Streptococcus, especially if the patient is at particularly high risk for this organism, i.e., a carrier or having had recent exposure.

## Topical Antibiotics

Although the major problem with wound infection occurs over the next several weeks, the necessary information for appropriate decision-making on the use of these agents is required during the initial encounter with the patient. The indications for topical antibiotics are presented in Table 3-5. The rationale for their use is based on the fact that nonviable tissue is present that will act as a nidus for infection and the resulting decrease in blood flow markedly impairs the effectiveness of systemically administered antibiotics.

The deep wound must be protected from early bacterial invasion, which can rapidly convert the burn to a deeper injury. The use of topical antibiotics that are sufficiently water soluble to penetrate the burn eschar will temporarily control bacterial growth in the wound. The half-life of the currently available topical agents is only a few hours; therefore most agents should be applied twice daily to provide reasonable antibacterial protection. There are also considerable differences in the toxicity and the degree to which these agents penetrate the eschar. Because all topical agents retard wound healing to some degree and require frequent applications, small clean superficial burns are best managed by Xeroform gauze or a synthetic skin substitute, e.g., biobrane, if a closed dressing is feasible (an exception is the face). The least toxic and most broad-spectrum topical antibiotic is usually the first choice for initial management in the deep or large burn. The properties of the various available agents are more elaborately summarized in Chapter 22.

**Table 3-5** Topical Antibiotics

Absolute indications
  A deep second or third degree burn
  A superficial burn that is dirty and cannot be adequately cleaned
  A superficial burn in an area at high risk for infection or where skin substitutes are less useful, e.g., face, ears, perineum, feet
Relative indication
  A large superficial second degree burn >20%
  A superficial burn in a diabetic, elderly patient, or when there is increased infection risk (alternative: temporary skin substitute)
Not necessary
  Superficial burn <15%, which is in an area where treatment with grease gauze and an occlusive dressing or skin substitute can be achieved

A 1% silver sulfadiazine (Silvadene) cream is the first choice as an agent to be used on a relatively uninfected deep burn to be applied twice a day. Mafenide (Sulfamylon) is a more toxic agent but is the treatment of choice for the deep infected burn of small to moderate size. Bacitracin ointment, applied two to four times a day, is the agent of choice for superifical burns, especially to the face where a dressing is not applied. Xeroform gauze can be used for superficial burns where a dressing is applied.

## Closed Dressings or Open Exposure

The burn wound treated with topical agents can be managed open, i.e., without dressings, or closed, i.e., sealed by dressings. The decision to use either technique is based on the part of the body involved, on the depth of injury, on ease and comfort of care, and in part on personal preference.

Advantages of the open or exposure method are ease of application and less risk of surface bacterial proliferation compared with a wound closed with dressings. Disadvantages include increased discomfort with partial thickness burns, greater risk of wound desiccation, increased risk of bacterial cross-contamination, particularly if the wound dries and the crust crumbles with infected particles spreading to other areas (Table 3-6).

The closed (dressing) technique (Table 3-7) is the more common approach, particularly for outpatients. It requires more nursing time or patient self-care time, but comfort and appearance are usually improved. The usual approach is to apply the topical agent on fine or coarse mesh gauze followed by a soft, snug but not tightly wrapped gauze dressing. An elastic wrap on the surface helps to hold the dressing on and improve patient comfort.

Temporary skin substitutes also require the use of a dressing, at least initially, in order to allow for adequate adherence between skin substitute and underlying wound surface.

## Temporary Skin Substitutes

Drying of exudate on a superficial wound with resulting scab or eschar formation has been shown to retard reepithelialization. Wounds have been shown to reepithelialize more rapidly and with less pain and inflammation when occluded and a thin layer of wound fluid is maintained in contact with the surface. The sealed wound also creates a more favorable environment for wound defense mechanisms to clear surface bacteria. Heat and evaporative water losses can also be decreased. A number of temporary skin substitutes

**Table 3-6** Open (Exposure) Method

| | |
|---|---|
| Advantages: | Easier than use of dressing |
| | Less risk of closed space infection |
| | Applicable to areas difficult to apply dressings |
| Disadvantages: | Increased wound desiccation |
| | Increased discomfort and heat loss |
| | Increased risk of cross-contamination |
| Indications: | Burns on face, ears, perineum |
| | Superficial burns with less risk of desiccation |
| | Any deep burn (but consider disadvantages) |

Table 3-7  Closed (Dressing) Method

|  |  |
|---|---|
| Advantages: | Decreases risk of wound desiccation<br>Decreased heat loss<br>Decreased risk of cross-contamination<br>Debriding effect on wound<br>More comfortable |
| Disadvantages: | More time consuming and expensive<br>Increased risk of infection if not changed frequently |
| Indications: | Any deep burn as long as dressings are changed twice daily |

have been developed to improve healing of the partial thickness wound as well as to protect clean, excised wounds when not immediately autografted. The skin substitute allows for excision of an amount of burn tissue beyond that for which autograft is available, as the remainder can be occluded with the temporary skin while awaiting new donors. *Types of skin substitutes* include:

Biological:  Pigskin, amnion, cadaver skin

Synthetics:  Biobrane, Duoderm, Opsite

The ideal properties required of a temporary skin substitute have been well defined as follows:

Firm adherence to the wound surface

Safety (sterile, hypoallergenic, nontoxic)

Decreases evaporative water loss

Flexible and durable

Barrier to bacteria

Ease of application and removal

Availability—cost effective

Adherence to the wound is definitely the most important to maximize the reepithelialization rate as well as minimize inflammation and fibrosis. Also, the dressings must be permeable to water vapor and oxygen in order to avoid producing a totally anaerobic condition at the wound surface, yet be nonpermeable to bacteria. Elasticity and durability are also major advantages. The biochemical structure cannot be antigenic or toxic so as to cause a local rejection reaction or be at high risk for transmission of disease. There are two types of temporary skin. Biologic dressings, i.e., previously living tissue, including amniotic membranes, xenograft and homograft, or cadaver skin have been used for a number of years, although the latter because of limited availability is used primarily to cover excised wounds. A number of synthetic skin substitutes have recently been developed that have the advantage of ready availability, long shelf life, and minimal concern for disease transmission. Solid silicone polymers have been the most widely used because they are microporous and uniquely permeable to water vapor. Synthetic substitutes that depend on fibrin entrapment in the porous material for adherence appear to be less successful than those in which there is a direct chemical bond with the wound. The best available dressing is *biobrane,* which is made of a flexible silicone-nylon membrane bilayer on which is bonded collagen peptides. The collagen on the dressing is then chemically bonded to that on the wound by fibrin. The skin substitute should be applied to the wound after the initial cleaning. Adherence to the wound is usually excellent (Color plates 6,7 page 313). Although biologic substitutes are useful in the presence of modest infection, synthetic dressings adhere poorly to contaminated wound. After cleaning the wound by removal of any loose tissue and debris, the skin substitutes are applied to the wound surface under a little tension to provide a flat surface for better adhesion. Steri-strips or staples under anesthesia can be used to attach the dressing to the surrounding viable skin. The substitutes are held on the wound surface with gauze until firm adherence to the surface has occurred. The *wound surface must be clean* to avoid trapping a large bacterial load beneath the dressing. Temporary immobilization, of the area dressed with the skin substitute, will greatly assist in the adherence process.

Skin substitutes should be removed if poorly adherent after 24 hours, especially with any significant exudate buildup on the wound surface, to avoid a closed space infection. Initiation of topical antibiotics is usually indicated, if this occurs.

Table 3-8  Temporary Skin Substitute Versus Topical Antibiotics

Clinical advantages skin substitute
- Markedly reduces pain
- Decreased heat, water loss
- Decreases wound inflammation, drainage
- Prevents surface drying in superficial wounds
- Increases rate of epithelialization
- Decreases surface infection

Disadvantages
- Does not control deep infection
- Can seal bacteria in as well as out
- Pyrogen response with biologic dressing
- Biologicals can transmit infection

Indications
- Superficial second degree burn
- Clean, excised wound
- Skin donor sites

## Management of Specific Burn Areas

*Face*

Superficial burns of the face are best managed with a gentle wash or soak with mild soap two to three times daily. Wash is followed by application of a thin layer of bacitracin to keep the wound from drying as well as to maintain control of the predominantly gram-positive organisms on the face. Deeper burns will require a topical antibiotic cream with better eschar penetration. Silver sulfadiazine is the first choice, to be reapplied after a gentle wash two to three times daily. This agent can be applied without dressings or on a thin layer of fine mesh gauze. The latter is preferred because this prevents the cream from running into the eyes, nares, and mouth.

## Eyes

After initial vigorous (up to 12 hours) irrigation, superficial corneal burns should be managed like any corneal abrasion. Ophthalmic antibiotic ointment applied three to four times daily is indicated. An eye patch is then applied. Artificial tears every several hours will be required if the tear ducts are involved. Burns to the eyelids are managed in a similar fashion. As the lids retract with healing, a patch is often required at night along with the lubricant to avoid corneal drying. Tarsorrhaphy may be required with deep burns.

## Ears

Superficial burns to the ears can be managed like those to the face. However, external pressure should not be applied to the injured helix. The cartilage is already poorly vascularized and any compression will potentiate further injury. No pillows or any external pressure are allowed. In addition, the topical agent, silver sulfadiazine) or mafenide, must be applied multiple times a day, especially if any cartilage is exposed. Mafenide is the agent of choice for deep burns with a thick eschar. Chondritis is a major complication that requires an extensive (several weeks) course of systemic antibodies. Chondritis invariably leads to loss of cartilage and permanent deformity. Pseudomonas is the most common pathogen.

## Hands

Superficial burns of the hands can be effectively managed using Xeroform gauze with a thin layer of bacitracin followed by a soft gauze dressing. Temporary skin substitutes are also ideal and markedly decrease pain and improve motion. Topical antibiotics are necessary for deeper burns. Fingers should be wrapped separately to avoid any impairment of motion. Hands *must* be elevated for the first 24 to 48 hours to minimize edema. Escharotomies of hands and fingers must be adequate. Hand splints to maintain position of function are advantageous for superifical burns if pain is limiting motion. Motion, however, must be strongly encouraged. For deeper second and third degree burns, hand splints are *absolutely necessary* to avoid permanent loss of tendon function and development of flexion contractures. However, active and passive range of motion exercises should begin as soon as possible after injury, during which time splints are removed.

## Feet

Burned feet must also be elevated initially. An Ace wrap over a bulky dressing can be used when walking. Blood supply to the feet is not as good as that to face and hands, and therefore, better topical antibiotic coverage, e.g., silver sulfadiazine, is usually needed except in the very superficial burn. Twice a day cleaning and reapplication of the topical agent is needed. Because of the difficulty of function and of self-cleaning, foot burns of any significance should be admitted at least for the initial 24 to 48 hours until home care can be arranged.

*Perineum*

Superficial burns can be managed open with an antibiotic grease-based ointment that has a broad-spectrum coverage, such as Neosporin. Hospitalization is usually necessary, at least initially, for observation of urinary obstruction secondary to edema. Deeper burns by definition require admission with two to three times daily application of topical antibiotic cream, usually silver sulfadiazine. Open technique or closed dressing, with a loose diaper dressing, can be used.

## Impaired Distal Perfusion and Need for Escharotomy

As subeschar edema develops under the burn tissue, pressure increases. This is of particular concern in extremities with a circumferential burn where the increasing pressure cannot be dissipated by expansion of neighboring tissue. The pressure initially impedes venous return, which produces an increase in capillary hydrostatic pressure. Increased pressure markedly accentuates further edema production, raising pressure to a level that then impedes arterial blood flow. Injury to local lymphatics and veins impairs clearance of the edema fluid once formed.

Perfusion to the distal extremity must be closely monitored. Pain and color will be unreliable indicators of perfusion in the presence of a burn to the area. A warm extremity invariably indicates good flow during this period, but a cool skin does not always indicate that the problem is due to proximal burn constriction. Hypovolemia may well be the problem.

Steps for the *prevention and treatment of impaired distal perfusion* are as follows:

1. Remove constricting objects
2. Immediate elevation of burned extremities
3. Early escharotomies on circumferential third or fourth degree burn
4. Decreasing Doppler flow signal with adequate blood pressure or tissue pressure more than 25 mmHg means escharotomy is needed
5. Escharotomy must extend completely through the burn tissue
6. Hemostasis is obtained with pressure, cautery, or microcrystalline collagen

The monitoring of distal pulsatile flow initially by palpation and then by the use of a Doppler flowmeter is the most practical manner of assessment. Tissue pressure measurements using a small needle, similar to the method of measuring subfascial compartment pressure, can be done. This approach, however, carries a risk of infecting the subeschar space with surface bacteria and is not used routinely. A tissue pressure exceeding 25 to 30 mmHg indicates the need for escharotomy because this pressure exceeds capillary hydrostatic pressure. Superficial and, to a large extent, deep second degree burns have sufficient remaining dermal expansibility that severe vascular compression usually does not occur. However, once the underlying tissue edema has exceeded the expansibility of the burned skin, as can occur with excess fluid administration, an escharotomy will need to be performed. Immediate elevation of burned extremities before edema formation will usually control subsequent edema and decrease the need for escharotomies. In addition, rings, watches, or any circumferential nonelastic material must be removed on both burned and unburned extremities.

**Table 3-9** When to do an Escharotomy on Extremity Burn

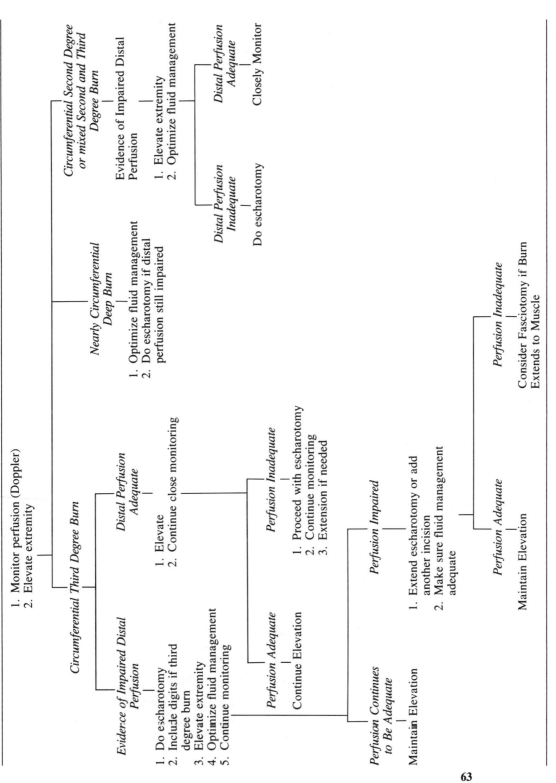

A decreasing distal flow with a proximal deep burn is an indication for an escharotomy (Table 3-9). The incision that is usually placed both medially and laterally on the involved extremity must extend completely through the nonviable tissue to subcutaneous tissue in order to allow release of the underlying tissue pressure (see Fig. 1-2). The best place for the incision is in the area of deepest burn because pain and bleeding will be minimal. Similar incisions on lateral and medial aspects of burned fingers, hands, and feet will be required with full-thickness burns to restore and maintain flow.

Cautery or microcrystalline collagen applied to the escharotomy site will usually control any minor bleeding. Suture ligatures will control any significant bleeding sites. Packing the wound, initially, with moist antibiotic soaked (bacitracin or neomycin) gauze will decrease bleeding. The dressing can be changed in 12 to 24 hours, after which a cream-based topical agent can be applied.

## Pitfalls in Early Wound Management

### *Prioritizing the Wound Ahead of Cardiopulmonary Function*

The excessive focus on early wound cleaning and debridement in the severe burn, especially inappropriate submersion in a tank of water, will inevitably lead to major complications. The basics of resuscitation cannot be violated.

### *Iatrogenic Hypothermia with Use of Wet Solutions*

The use of cold and wet on large total body surface burns and the attempted wound care in the absence of external heating devices will certainly produce hypothermia shivering and increased catechols. Once produced, it is very difficult to correct.

### *Failure to Elevate Burned Extremities Early*

With loss of veins and lymphatics, edema is rapidly produced by placing burned extremities in the dependent position. The edema cannot be readily corrected by elevation once developed. Escharotomies, which are not without morbidity, can often be avoided with early elevation.

### *Inadequate Lavage for Chemical Burns*

Lavage time is measured in hours, not minutes.

### *Failure to Perform Escharotomies When Indicated*

If there is a suggestion of impaired distal perfusion, do an escharotomy. Do not wait for the ischemia to get worse.

### *Underestimating the Amount of Full-Thickness Burn*

Often the epidermis, although devitalized, remains on the surface of a third degree burn, giving the impression of a very superficial burn. The magnitude of the dermal injury is not appreciated until the wound is cleaned and loose epidermis is removed.

# TREATMENT SUMMARY (0 TO 24 HOURS)

## Wound Management

1. Assure Adequate Ventilation and Perfusion
2. Remove Heat Source and Any Constricting items
3. Cool water for Small Second Degree Burns Only
4. Assess Size and Depth "Rule of Nines"
5. Tetanus Prophylaxis

### Patient Not Stable

1. Remove clothing
2. Cover with warm dry dressing
3. Wait until basics are controlled to initiate aggressive wound care
4. Do not put in hydrotherapy tank or move away from adequate monitoring

### Patient Reasonably Stable

1. Maintain warm external temperature during wound cleaning
2. Use adequate pain control (Small doses intravenous narcotics for major burn)
3. Chlorhexidine wash: Dilute contents of one packet in 1 to 2 quarts warm (85–90°F) water
4. Remove dirt, loose skin, may leave large blisters intact
5. Can use bed bath approach to hydrotherapy (do not immerse body in water to avoid cross-contamination)

#### Superficial Second Degree Burn

##### Wound Relatively Clean

1. Can use Xeroform gauze with dressing
2. Consider temporary skin substitutes: biobrane
3. Face: treat open with bacitracin
4. Perineum, feet use silver sulfadiazine
5. Elevate burned extremity

##### Wound Dirty

1. Use topical antibiotic silver sulfadiazine first choice
2. Elevate burned extremity

#### Deep Burn

1. Use topical antibiotic cream silver sulfadiazine first choice
2. Closed dressing technique, exception: face, perineum
3. Monitor perfusion to distal extremity

#### Third Degree Burn

1. Use topical antibiotic cream. Silver sulfadiazine: if wound not grossly infected. Mafenide for small to moderate-sized infected burn
2. Parenteral antibiotics if infected, not for prophylaxis
3. Closed dressing technique except face, perineum
4. Monitor perfusion, need escharotomy if circumferential third degree and any impairment in distal perfusion

65

# 4
# Transfer to Burn Facility

**DEFINITION OF A BURN CENTER**

The burn center must be capable of delivering all therapy required, including rehabilitation, and must perform training of personnel and burn research. Burn centers are generally found in association with hospitals of 500 beds or more, usually in university centers. No attempt has been made to differentiate between the expertise available and the severity of burns treated in burn units as opposed to burn centers. Burn centers do not provide treatment for only major burns. In fact, the center should also treat minor and moderate burns.

A burn center must contain a minimum of six beds and must have a designated director who is a board-certified general or plastic surgeon with one additional year of specialized training in burn therapy or equivalent experience in burn patient care. The head nurse of the facility may be a baccalaureate or registered nurse with 2 years of intensive care unit training, or its equivalent, plus a minimum of 6 months' experience in burn care. Fully trained and licensed or registered physical therapists and registered occupational therapists with a minimum of 3 months' training or 6 months' experience in burn treatment must be assigned regularly. A licensed dietician must also be assigned regularly.

**INDICATIONS FOR PATIENT TRANSFER**

Using these basic treatment settings, the American Burn Association has identified three treatment categories for burn patients: major, moderate, and minor burn injuries.

## Major Burn Injuries

This group includes second degree burns with a body surface area greater than 25% in adults (20% in children); all third degree burns with a body surface area of 10% or greater; all burns involving hands, face, eyes, ears, feet, and perineum; all inhalation injuries; electrical burns; complicated burn injuries involving fractures or other major trauma; and all poor-risk patients.

Major burn patients would normally enter the system at the site of injury and be transported to a hospital with a burn center. The choice of a hospital depends on distance and time, the patient's burn complications (respiratory condition, shock), and bed availability.

The American Burn Association emphasizes the importance of direct communication and transfer agreements among hospitals. If the seriousness of the patient's injury dictates transportation to the closest emergency department or special expertise hospital, then subsequent transfer to a hospital with a burn center should be arranged after establishing cardiopulmonary stabilization and intravenous fluid therapy for shock. Rehabilitation, including corrective surgery for cosmetic and functional deficiencies, completes the therapeutic circle.

## Moderate, Uncomplicated Burn Injuries

This second group includes second degree burns with a body surface area of 15 to 25% in adults (10 to 20% in children), third degree burns with a body surface of less than 10%, and burns that do not involve eyes, ears, face, hands, feet, or perineum. Excluded from the group are electrical injuries, complicated injuries (fractures), inhalation injuries, and all poor-risk patients (elderly patients and patients with an intercurrent disease).

Most of the patients in this group would receive emergency care at the site of the injury and be transported directly to either a special expertise hospital or to an in-depth expertise hospital with a burn center.

In certain situations involving transfer difficulties, a given hospital may have to assume the role of a special expertise hospital temporarily.

## Minor Burn Injuries

The third group includes second degree burns with a body surface area of less than 15% in adults (10% in children), third degree burns with a body surface area of less than 2%, and burns not involving eyes, ears, face, hands, feet, or perineum. It excludes electrical injuries, inhalation injuries (fractures), and all poor-risk patients.

The patients in this group may be treated at the scene of the accident by emergency medical technicians and transported to a hospital emergency department where definitive care begins. Definitive care includes follow-up care and discharge of the patient after complete recovery.

## HOW TO TRANSFER

The burn patient, as opposed to the multiple trauma patient with active blood loss, is unlikely to develop shock or airway obstruction in the first 30 minutes postburn. Therefore once oxygen is started at the scene to treat carboxyhemoglobin, two options are available:

> To transfer directly to burn facility if within 30 minutes

To transfer to local emergency room to initiate treatment, then to burn facility

The objectives of the interim emergency room admission are to: (1) secure an airway; (2) start fluid therapy and completely neutralize the heat source. These procedures should be performed before a long transportation. Safety during transfer is more important than speed. A warm environment with good monitoring equipment, ventilator, if necessary, and, of course, well-trained personnel. Within a 30-mile radius, ground transportation is usually adequate. Between 50 and 150 miles, the helicopter can save considerable time and should be used if a safe transportation can be provided.

# SECTION 2
# Postresuscitation Phase (2 to 6 Days)

The early postresuscitation phase is a period of transition from the ebb or shock phase to the flow or hypermetabolic phase. Major cardiopulmonary and wound changes occur that substantially alter the manner of patient care from that during resuscitation. In general, cardiopulmonary stability is optimal during this period because wound inflammation and infection have not yet developed. However, cardiovascular changes will only get worse with the upcoming hypermetabolism and sepsis unless the wound is aggressively managed. The early wound excision and grafting approach is initiated during this period because increased wound blood flow and infection have not yet peaked. Operative risks, especially blood loss and septicemia, are substantially less than that seen after inflammation and infection develop. The exceptions to this rule are the patient with severe smoke inhalation in whom major lung dysfunction is present or patients who are hemodynamically unstable.

Dramatic changes in the burn wound develop as neovascularization, colonization, and inflammation begin to evolve. Management begins with an understanding of these physiologic and metabolic changes.

# 5

# Pulmonary Abnormalities

There are five major abnormalities that can be seen during this period that will impair pulmonary function. Recognition of these potential problems will allow preventive measures to be initiated before severe dysfunction results. A major impediment to an aggressive surgical approach to the burn wound during this period is pulmonary dysfunction. The following topics are described in this chapter.

## GENERAL SECTIONS

>   Major Pulmonary Abnormalities
>> Continued Upper Airway Obstruction
>> Decreased Chest Wall Compliance
>> Tracheobronchitis from Inhalation Injury
>> Pulmonary Edema
>> Low Pressure Pulmonary Edema (Adult Respiratory Distress Syndrome)
>> Surgery- and Anesthesia-Induced Lung Dysfunction
>> Common Pitfalls
>> Summary of Pulmonary Abnormalities

A discussion of how to use and wean from ventilatory support is presented in Chapter 19.

## MAJOR PULMONARY ABNORMALITIES

### Continued Upper Airway Obstruction

*Pathophysiology*

Upper airway and facial edema caused by the heat-induced tissue and mucosal damage begins to resolve between 2 and 4 days, with superficial injuries. However, with full-thickness burns, edema, both external and in the oropharynx and larynx, will resolve more slowly. Occasionally, excision of deep neck eschar is necessary to allow expansion of the underlying soft tissue, which then restores venous drainage and allows edema resolution. The upper airway mucosal damage leads to increased production of oral secretions along with secondary bacterial colonization of the damaged tissue.

*Treatment*

Continued airway maintenance with an endotracheal tube may be required. Placement of the patient in the head-elevated position 30° to 45° will allow faster resolution of edema. Aggressive mouth care to avoid mucosal infection, particularly with anaerobes, is necessary because aspiration of the infected saliva will lead to airways infection.

The decision when to extubate is a difficult one because there is no good test for determining the adequacy of airway patency. Laryngoscopy to determine the presence of cord edema is helpful, as is deflation of the cuff after suctioning of the oropharynx, to determine if air moves around the tube. The latter test is useful if an air leak is present around the tube. However, the lack of an air leak may simply reflect a large tube in a small trachea. Edema of the false cords and oropharynx as well as external compression from a neck burn can also impair the airway even if minimal cord edema is present. Therefore one must be prepared to reintubate because no test of airway patency is foolproof (Table 5-1). Given this fact, extubation should not be performed unless reintubation is feasible. There is certainly a concern about maintaining a tube in place too long because laryngeal

**Table 5-1** Continued Management of Upper Airways Obstruction

*Increase Edema Resolution*

Maintain Head Elevation

*Minimize Nosocomial Infection*

Vigorous Oral Hygiene
(Add Nystatin Mouthwash if on Antibiotics)

*Minimize Airway Damage*

1. Avoid cuff overinflation
2. Monitor cuff pressure (<25 cm $H_2O$)
3. Avoid excessive tube movement

**When to Extubate**

*Evidence of Mucosal Edema Resolution*

1. Laryngoscopy

*Evidence of Adequate External Edema Resolution*

Patient Must Be Able to Be Reintubated if Necessary

*Evidence of Adequate Mechanics*

1. Can generate cough
2. No longer needs positive pressure

*Can Protect Airway*

1. Voluminous oral secretions not present
2. Sufficiently awake and alert

damage can result. However, loss of the airway can be fatal if residual edema substantially impedes reintubation.

## Decreased Chest Wall Compliance

*Pathophysiology*

The impaired expansibility of the chest wall caused by deep burns is improved but certainly not eliminated by escharotomy. A significant impairment in compliance will persist as a result of the loss of elasticity in burn tissue. In addition, tissue edema itself, which will remain for many days, impairs expansion and, in turn, decreases functional residual capacity and vital capacity. Work of breathing and energy requirements will remain increased. This process is particularly relevant for operative procedures requiring general anesthesia. The effect of impaired chest wall compliance on hemodynamic function will be accentuated with the use of an anesthetic that results in any element of myocardial depression, since the increased positive mean airway pressure is already impairing cardiac output. In addition, general anesthesia invariably impairs diaphragmatic activity, thereby further increasing the amount of positive pressure required to maintain a constant tidal volume. The process resolves as edema is reabsorbed in a partial thickness burn or as full-thickness burn is removed.

*Treatment*

Maintenance of a semierect position will assist in movement of edema away from the chest wall to more dependent tissues. Continued careful volume replacement will minimize further edema formation. Mechanical ventilator assistance with positive pressure may be needed to help maintain functional residual capacity and minimize atelectasis as well as diminish oxygen demands during this period of impaired energy stores. Early excision of the full-thickness wound will improve chest wall motion by removing both edema and noncompliant tissue (Table 5-2).

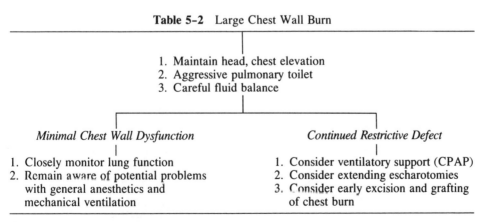

Table 5-2  Large Chest Wall Burn

1. Maintain head, chest elevation
2. Aggressive pulmonary toilet
3. Careful fluid balance

*Minimal Chest Wall Dysfunction*
1. Closely monitor lung function
2. Remain aware of potential problems with general anesthetics and mechanical ventilation

*Continued Restrictive Defect*
1. Consider ventilatory support (CPAP)
2. Consider extending escharotomies
3. Consider early excision and grafting of chest burn

CPAP: continuous positive airway pressure.

## Tracheobronchitis from Inhalation Injury

### Pathophysiology

The chemical burn to the airways results in a spectrum of clinical manifestations during this period. At the very least, a mucosal irritation will persist for several days causing a bronchorrhea, increased cough, and mucus production. The damaged ciliary function of the airways lining leads to a high risk for infection manifested first (in the next 3 to 4 days) by a bacterial tracheobronchitis followed by a bronchopneumonia. Bacterial colonization is inevitable. Characteristically with a severe injury, the damaged mucosa becomes necrotic at 3 to 4 days postinjury and begins to slough. Increased viscous secretions can lead to distal airway obstruction, atelectasis, and a high risk of a rapidly developing bronchopneumonia.

As airways inflammation and bronchial blood flow increases over the next several days, a diffuse interstitial edema can develop. Even modest volume overload will markedly potentiate the edema process. The magnitude of the pulmonary infection is in large part dependent on the status of host defenses and the aggressiveness of pulmonary support. The combination of the chemical lung burn and a body burn markedly potentiate the morbidity and mortality of either process (Tables 5-3, 5-4). If infection can be controlled and secretions cleared, the acute process will resolve over the next 7 to 10 days. However, the risk of infection persists for several weeks, extending well into the inflammation period.

### Symptoms

In the first several days after injury, remaining soot continues to be present in the airways secretions. Diffuse rhonchi are usually present, once inflammation develops. Wheezing also frequently persists as a result of continued bronchospasm and bronchial edema, the latter being the more prominent cause. Continued coughing and pulmonary toilet as well as the residual airways edema and some bronchospasm increase the work of breathing, which can lead to fatigue and hypoventilation. Secretions then become tenacious and

**Table 5-3** Pathophysiology of Chemical Tracheobronchitis (2 to 6 Days)

| *Large and Small Airways, Edema, Spasm* | *Increased Secretions* |
|---|---|
| 1. Decreased dynamic compliance | 1. Increased work |
| 2. Increased work | 2. Airways plugging by secretions |
| 3. Decreased functional residual capacity | 3. Increasing shunt (hypoxemia) |
| 4. Atelectasis and increased shunt (hypoxemia) | 4. Increased risk of infection (tracheobronchial colonization, pneumonia, sepsis) |
| 5. Parenchymal involvement | |
| 6. Increased risk of edema with any hypervolemia | |
| *Increased Minute Ventilation* | *Evidence of Sepsis Syndrome* |
| 1. Increasing dead space | 1. Lung inflammation |
| 2. Increasing carbon dioxide production | 2. Lung infection |

Table 5-4  Physiologic Definition of Acute Respiratory Failure

| Parameter | Normal Range | Respiratory Failure |
|---|---|---|
| Mechanics | | |
| Respiratory rate | 12–20 | >35 |
| Vital capacity (ml/kg body wt)* | 65–75 | <15 |
| $FEV_1$ (ml/kg/body wt)* | 50–60 | <10 |
| Inspiratory force (cm $H_2O$) | −(75–100) | <25 |
| Compliance (1/cm $H_2O$) | 0.1 | <0.02 |
| Respiratory rate | 12–18 | >30 |
| Oxygenation | | |
| $PaO_2$ (mmHg) | 100–75 (room air) | <70 |
| $P(A-a)O_2$ ($FiO_2 = 1.0$) (mmHg) | 25–65 | >450 |
| Shunt $Q_S/Q_T$ | 5% | >20% |
| Ventilation | | |
| $PaCO_2$ (mmHg) | 35–45 | >55† |
| $V_D/V_T$ | 0.25–0.40 | >0.60 |

\* Use ideal body weight.
† Exception is chronic lung disease.
$FEV_1$: forced expiratory volume in 1 second; $PaO_2$: arterial oxygen tension; $P(A-a)O_2$: alveolar-arterial oxygen tension; $FiO_2$: fractional inspired oxygen; $Q_S/Q_T$: shunt fraction; $PaCO_2$: arterial carbon dioxide tension; $V_D/V_T$: dead space to tidal volume ratio.

more difficult to clear. Rales compatible with an edema process will be noted in the most severe airways injuries, especially with concomitant volume overload. Evidence of bacterial tracheobronchitis is common, followed by bronchopneumonia in a substantial number of patients. The *characteristics of the symptom complex* are as follows:

Sputum changing from loose to mucopurulent

Evidence of necrotic tissue in sputum

Increased work of breathing

Altered gas exchange

Infiltrates on radiographs: Late finding

*Do not underestimate the magnitude of injury by initial presentation, since lung function may be deceptively good on day 2 only to deteriorate rapidly on day 3 to 4.*

## Diagnosis

Diagnosis of severity of injury is based more on the course of the disease process than on initial findings from laryngoscopy, fiberoptic bronchoscopy, or xenon scan, which basically only indicate that an injury is present. Chest radiographs during this period, in general, underestimate the severity of lung damage because the injury is usually initially confined to the airways.

Clinical evidence of continued respiratory compromise; namely, dyspnea, tachypnea, diffuse wheezing, and rhonchi precede radiographic changes. The first evidence on radiography of lung damage is usually that of either diffuse atelectasis, pulmonary edema, or bronchopneumonia. Altered gas exchange reflected in blood gas analysis and assessment of changes in sputum characteristics are useful parameters to monitor.

*Chest radiographic findings invariably underestimate the magnitude of the chemical inhalation-induced airways injury. Parenchymal changes are late findings.*

## Treatment

The clearance of soot, mucopurulent exudate, and sloughing mucosa is essential to avoid progression of the lung injury. An endotracheal tube may be necessary if clearance of secretions is inadequate. Ventilator assist may also be necessary if the patient is fatiguing and if gas exchange is worsening. (See Section 7 for assistance.) Continued readjustments in tidal volume, rate, and positive end-expiratory pressure (PEEP) are necessary to maintain gas exchange while minimizing barotrauma. Sedation (narcotic infusion) or paralysis may be necessary if the patient's spontaneous ventilatory attempts further impair lung function while on ventilator support. Bronchodilators, particularly those provided by aerosols, as described in Chapter 1, are also very helpful, along with frequent changes in position for postural drainage. Continuous rotating beds are ideal for the patient with an inhalation injury and a large body burn where side to side patient movement is difficult because of pain and stiffness from tissue edema (Figure 5-1). The constant postural drainage assists in removing airway plugs.

Infection surveillance is crucial during this early period in order to detect a bacterial bronchitis prior to development of a pneumonia. Sputum smears and monitoring of the character of the sputum are useful early guides. Systemic antibiotics are not given

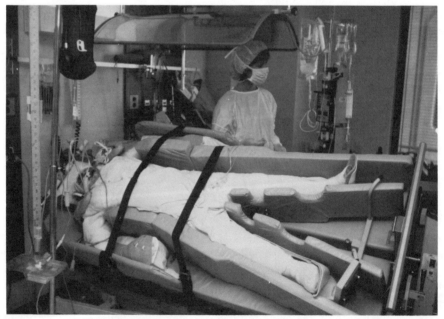

**Figure 5–1.** Rotating bed, which provides postural drainage after major burns, especially with smoke inhalation injury. Overhead heat shield maintains body temperature.

**Table 5-5** Treatment of Tracheobronchitis

| Increased Airways Resistance (Edema) | Increased Secretions; Bacterial Colonization |
|---|---|
| 1. Positive-pressure assist (CPAP) to increase functional residual capacity<br>2. Consider bronchodilators<br>3. Avoid congestive heart failure, volume overload<br><br>But Do *Not* Produce Hypovolemia in an Attempt to Correct Airways Edema | 1. Aggressive pulmonary toilet (postural changes extremely important)<br>2. Infection surveillance, daily sputum smear<br>3. Assess for antibiotic use, do not wait for radiographic findings of infiltrate before initiating empiric therapy if sputum indicative of infection |

CPAP: continuous positive airway pressure.

prophylactically but initiated when a bacterial process becomes evident. Do not wait until obvious radiographic evidence of bronchopneumonia is present because the process, once well established, will be difficult to reverse. Broad-spectrum antibiotics can be used until the specific sensitivities return and a more tailored antibiotic regimen can be instituted (Table 5-5).

## Pulmonary Edema

### Pathophysiology

The most common cause of pulmonary edema during this period is that from fluid shift-induced volume overload, especially in the presence of a smoke inhalation injury. An increase in pulmonary capillary hydrostatic pressure occurs leading to excess fluid crossing from plasma to interstitium (Table 5-6). Volume overload is frequently due to a combination of systemic resorption of tissue edema at a rate faster than that which can be cleared by the kidney and a continued excess infusion of salt-containing fluid at a rate faster than needed. The stress response and/or positive pressure ventilation will impair

**Table 5-6** Causes of Pulmonary Edema

Heart Failure, Hypovolemia (Especially After Inhalation)
Increased Capillary Pressure (Wedge >20 mmHg)
Accentuated by Severe Hypoproteinemia (<50% Normal)

*Physiologic Changes (Interstitial Edema)*
Increased Airway and Vascular Resistance
Increase Alveolar-Arterial Oxygen Gradient
Ventilation/Perfusion Mismatch
Mild Hypoxemia

(with Alveolar Flooding)
Increased Shunt, Hypoxemia, Work
Decreased Static Compliance, Functional Residual Capacity

renal clearance of the excess fluid by increasing antidiuretic hormone and aldosterone release and suppressing atrial naturietic factor.

Wedge pressure usually exceeds 20 mmHg in the early stages. Severe plasma hypoproteinemia (value less than 50%) will exaggerate the process, whereas a lesser degree of plasma hypoproteinemia is compensated for by a comparable decrease in interstitial protein content. The excess fluid crossing the plasma membrane will first migrate to the hilar area and accumulate in the loose interstitium around the larger airways and vessels. Dyspnea, diffuse rhonchi, and wheezing are the result of the interstitial edema process, whatever the cause. Only mild hypoxia is usually evident at this stage. The impaired oxygen exchange is in large part correctable by increasing the fractional inspired oxygen in air. The interstitial edema will also increase the lung stiffness (decreased static compliance) leading to a decrease in functional residual capacity.

If the edema process continues after the interstitium has filled with fluid, alveolar edema will occur. Edema in dependent lung occurs first. The alveolar flooding causes shunt fraction to increase, leading to significant hypoxemia as well as a decrease in lung volume and functional residual capacity. Compliance decreases and atelectasis increases, further increasing the shunt. Alveolar edema produces moist rales. However, these findings may be difficult to differentiate clinically from the bronchorrhea induced by an inhalation injury.

*Diagnosis*

The usual clinical findings seen with pulmonary edema are a reliable diagnostic clue (Table 5-7). If an inhalation injury has occurred, increased secretions, rhonchi, and wheezing are already present, making the determination of an added cardiogenic pulmonary edema difficult. Additional information utilizing a pulmonary artery catheter for determination of wedge pressure may be necessary.

*Treatment*

There are two main objectives of treatment:

>Maintain adequate oxygenation to systemic tissues
>Correct the process producing lung edema

**Table 5-7** Clinical Picture of Pulmonary Edema

Deteriorating Gas Exchange High Wedge Pressure, Low Proteins

*Radiographic Changes*

1. Bronchovascular cuffs
2. Blood flow redistribution
3. Septal lines (Kerley)
4. Cardiomegaly

(With Alveolar Flooding)

1. Alveolar consolidation
2. Decreased lung volumes
3. Pleural effusion

The optimum management for the pulmonary edema alone is "drying the patient out." However, this process may impair tissue oxygenation during this very vulnerable period for the wound and lead to problems greater than the lung edema. A relative hypovolemia will also increase operative risks. It is usually best to make appropriate adjustments in fluid infusion rate and protein replacement to minimize the progression of the process while utilizing positive pressure, if intubated (Table 5-8). Low-dose dopamine will assist in the diuresis by increasing blood flow and by its antialdosterone effects. The continued losses from the burn wound can result in a gradual decrease in blood volume. Therefore vigorous diuresis is normally not needed to correct the hypervolemia and actually is more likely to produce a hypovolemic state. If hypervolemia persists, furosemide can be used. If heart failure is present, as evident from a high filling pressure and low cardiac output, beta agonists can be added (see Section 7).

Those patients meeting the criteria for *acute respiratory failure* require endotracheal intubation and positive pressure ventilation. Positive pressure plus the addition of PEEP will redistribute the alveolar fluid so that some gas exchange can occur, leading to a decrease in shunt fraction.

The increased pressure will also impair preload and, in turn, decrease capillary pressure. Afterload reduction may be necessary to improve cardiac output. The edema process is usually readily reversible with control of capillary pressure or left-sided filling pressures. Mortality is dependent on the status of the underlying disease process.

## Low Pressure Pulmonary Edema (Adult Respiratory Distress Syndrome)

### Pathophysiology

Adult respiratory distress syndrome (ARDS) is a different disease process than that just described because an alteration in pulmonary microvascular permeability is present. Edema, which has a high protein content, occurs even in the presence of normal wedge

Table 5-8  Treatment of High-Pressure Edema

1. Increase monitoring
2. Maintain oxygen saturation >90%
3. Decrease fluid infusion rate
4. Avoid excess sodium administration

| Manage Heart | Manage Lung |
|---|---|
| 1. Preload reduction, decrease fluid infusion, low-dose dopamine, careful diuresis, if above not sufficient (avoid hypokalemia)<br>2. Add inotrope if necessary<br>3. Consider afterload reduction if heart failure persists | 1. If acute respiratory failure, add positive pressure with PEEP or CPAP |

CPAP: continuous positive airway pressure.

**Table 5-9** Comparison of High-Pressure (Cardiogenic) Versus Low-Pressure (ARDS) Edema

| High Pressure | Low Pressure |
|---|---|
| 1. Initiated by local process, namely, increased capillary pressure | Initiated by focus of inflammation-infection |
| 2. High wedge pressure capillary usually greater than 25 mmHg | Normal wedge pressure usually 10 to 15 mmHg |
| 3. Low protein edema | High protein edema |
| 4. Good correlation between increased water and increased shunt | Poor correlation; indication other factor involved in shunt |
| 5. Parenchymal involvement a later finding: interstitium first | Parenchymal involvement an early finding |
| 6. Rapid resolution (24 to 48 hours) | Slow resolution 4 to 7 days or longer |

pressure (10–15 mmHg). However, the radiographic appearance is somewhat different. A comparison is presented in Tables 5-9 and 5-10. Diffuse bronchopneumonia from an inhalation injury will also result in acute respiratory failure.

ARDS, which is highly lethal in the burn patient, is more prevalent in the inflammatory phase and will be described in more detail in that section.

*Treatment*

The same general treatment is provided as for acute respiratory failure (see Section 7). A more detailed treatment plan is described in the next section.

## Surgery- and Anesthesia-Induced Lung Dysfunction

Two processes, one due to wound manipulation and the second due to the anesthesia, can produce lung dysfunction with wound excision and grafting procedures:

    Mediator-induced lung dysfunction

    Volume overload

    Anesthesia-induced hypoventilation

**Table 5-10** Radiographic Characteristics of Pulmonary Edema

| High Pressure (Cardiogenic) | Low Pressure (Permeability) |
|---|---|
| 1. Redistribution of blood flow away from dependent lung | Normal vascular pattern |
| 2. Bronchovascular fluid cuffs without air bronchograms | Minimal to no fluid cuffs frequent air bronchograms |
| 3. Increased septal (Kerley) lines | Absence of septal lines |
| 4. Cardiomegaly | Normal size heart |
| 5. Pleural effusions | Infrequent effusions |

The manipulation of burn tissue during excision can produce at least a transient decrease in lung compliance from released tissue mediators such as thromboxane. A transient endotoxemia or bacteremia can also occur with its alteration in lung function. However, wound inflammation and infection are much less during this period than later, which is the reason why excisional therapy is safer during the 2 to 5-day period. Repeated excision and grafting procedures, especially on large body burns, usually results in a situation in which the patient is either recovering from an inhalation anesthetic or is preoperative. These patients often remain intubated between excision procedures if there is a concomitant inhalation injury and the burn is large. Most general anesthetics will cause a deterioration in an already marginal respiratory status, putting the patient at high risk for pneumonia and further lung failure during the subsequent phase of injury (Table 5-11). Muscle relaxants will further compound this problem. Ketamine anesthesia will help by decreasing some of the anesthesia-induced respiratory depression. Early recognition of the increased risks of a relative hypoventilation in the early postanesthesia period is essential. Ventilatory support systems should be added early to avoid the problem rather then attempting to treat the complications.

## Common Pitfalls

### Extubating Too Soon

Resolution of facial edema does not always correspond with resolution of airways edema. In addition, there are many pulmonary problems in the burn patient necessitating an artificial airway. Look at the whole picture!

### Underestimating the Lower Airways Injury

Once the initial airways edema is resolving, a quiet period (calm before the storm) is often present that predates the bacterial tracheobronchitis and resulting bronchopneumonia. An appreciation of impending problems will result in more aggressive preventive measures.

### Failure to Provide Adequate Postanesthetic Support

The major burn patient, especially one with a chest burn, requires a large work effort to maintain adequate ventilation. The work loading increases as hypermetabolism and increased carbon dioxide production results. A general anesthetic impairs diaphragmatic motion, decreases functional reserve capacity, decreases maximum inspiratory force, all

**Table 5-11** Pulmonary Effects of Anesthesia and Excision

| Excision | Anesthesia |
|---|---|
| 1. Release of mediators leading to bronchoconstriction and V/Q mismatch | 1. Decreased functional residual capacity and compliance |
| 2. Release of pyrogens leading to increased oxygen consumption and carbon dioxide production | 2. Decreased inspiratory force |
| | 3. Hypoventilation |
| | 4. Decreased clearance of secretions |

of which can result in significant postoperative pulmonary dysfunction. Muscle relaxants should be kept to a minimum. Ideal management is to maintain support, e.g., continuous positive airway pressure until full restoration of preoperative mechanics and gas exchange has occurred.

*Underestimation of the Effect of Chest Wall Stiffness on Lung Function*

Underestimation of the increased work of breathing created by a rigid chest wall even with normal lung parenchyma leads to fatigue, airway collapse, and secondary infection. This process is particularly prone to occur in the early postanesthesia period.

## SUMMARY OF PULMONARY ABNORMALITIES

1. Persistent Airways Obstruction
   Upper Airways Edema
   External Facial Edema
2. Persistent Restrictive Defect from Chest Burn
   Increased Work of Breathing
   Decreased Functional Residual Capacity, Atelectasis, Shunt
3. Tracheobronchitis from Inhalation Injury
   Decreased Compliance; Bronchiolar Edema
   Coarse Rhonchi, Increased Mucopurulent Sputum
   Airway Plugging, Atelectasis, Increased Shunt
   Secondary Airways Infection and Inflammation
   Impaired Gas Exchange
   Chest Radiographic Findings Underestimate Injury
   Parenchymal Infiltrates: A Late Finding
4. High-Pressure Pulmonary Edema
   High Capillary Pressure, Heart Failure
   Volume Overload Hypoproteinemia

   Leading to:
     Deteriorating Gas Exchange
     Radiographic Characteristics of: Cuffing Progressing to Alveolar
     Infiltrates Cardiomegaly, Pleural Effusions
5. Adult Respiratory Distress Syndrome
   Onset Usually with Sepsis
6. Surgery and Anesthesia Complications
   Mediator, Bacteria Release from Burn Wound During Excision
   Postanesthesia-Induced Hypoventilation

# TREATMENT SUMMARY (36 HOURS TO 6 DAYS)

### Airway Maintenance

1. Maintain artificial airway until face and neck edema and intraoral edema are adequately resolved
2. Perform Laryngoscopy or bronchoscopy before tube removal

### Maintain Pulmonary Toilet

1. Do not underestimate inhalation injury
2. Avoid airways plugging from inhalation injury; vigorous cough, suctioning, bronchodilators
3. Aggressive chest physical therapy
4. Avoid nosocomial pneumonia
   - Minimize airway obstruction
   - Minimize tracheobronchial aspiration
   - Maintain cough
   - Treat tracheobronchial infection early with specific antibiotics
   - Avoid excessive use of broad-spectrum antibiotics

### Maintain Adequate Gas Exchange

1. Avoid pulmonary edema from volume overload
2. Aggressively treat congestive heart failure (may need inotropes)
3. Avoid hypoventilation especially prevalent in perioperative period
4. Consider partial mechanical ventilatory assist, especially with frequent operative interventions

### Maintain Infection Control

1. Primary treatment is pulmonary toilet
2. Initiate antibiotics with early evidence of bacterial tracheobronchitis

# 6

# Maintaining Hemodynamic Stability

The following general areas will be discussed.

## GENERAL SECTIONS

Pathophysiology of the Postresuscitation Hemodynamic Response
- Fluid, Protein, and Red Blood Cell
- Fluid Gains
- Electrolyte, Acid-Base Abnormalities
- Systemic Metabolic and Hemodynamic Changes

Practical Approach to Management
- Type of Fluid
- Intravenous Access (Infection Control)
- What to Monitor
- Pharmacologic Support
- Common Pitfalls in Fluid Management
- Treatment Summary

## PATHOPHYSIOLOGY OF THE POSTRESUSCITATION HEMODYNAMIC RESPONSE

### Fluid, Protein, and Red Blood Cell Shifts

The postresuscitation period is again characterized by major fluid shifts, although of less magnitude than the first 36 hours. Red cell mass continues to decrease. Electrolyte and acid-base changes are more prominent, as are other biochemical changes with the transition from the ebb to the flow state (hypometabolism to hypermetabolism). The hemodynamic response will be quite different from that seen during the early phase and treatment is considerably different.

Edema in burned tissue is maximum between 24 and 30 hours after injury in the well-controlled fluid resuscitation. However, continued losses of fluid, protein and red cells are present in this period due to:

- Evaporative water loss
- Increased vascular permeability in burn tissue
- Hypoproteinemia-induced nonburn edema
- Loss from escharotomy and excision sites

## *Evaporative Water Loss*

The loss of skin integrity means loss of the barrier to water evaporation. Evaporation from the surface of the burn now becomes a major source of water loss that persists until the wound is closed. The loss is measured in terms of water vapor pressure measured at the surface. In normal skin, the vapor pressure is 2 to 3 mmHg, whereas on a full-thickness burn where the eschar is soft and hydrated, pressure is about 32 mmHg. The rate of loss is increased with increasing surface blood flow. A reasonable estimate of an average loss can be obtained from the following formula:

Evaporative water loss ml/hr $=(25+\%$ total body surface burn$) \times$ ($m^2$ body surface area)

When water passes from a liquid to a gas state, energy, known as the latent heat of vaporization, is required. This equals 580 kcal/L. Therefore not only is water lost, but so are calories.

## *Increased Permeability*

Although the edema process usually peaks during the resuscitation period, the increase in vascular permeability persists for days after injury until the basement membrane and endothelial cell layer integrity is restored. The continued increase in permeability is indicative of the fact that the initial edema process is due to more than an endothelial defect. Patent injured vessels will continue to lack plasma over the next several days, particularly from the wound surface, as in the partial thickness burn or the full-thickness scald in which vessels have not been heat coagulated. Continued protein losses appear less in the third degree flame burn in which surface vessels are coagulated. Increasing vascular hydrostatic pressure, will accentuate the edema process. Careful volume replacement, in particular during operative procedures, is necessary to avoid magnifying the edema.

## *Hypoproteinemia-Induced Nonburn Edema*

Most tissues, in particular the lung, can compensate for a decrease in plasma proteins of 30 to 40%, with a comparable decrease in interstitial protein content, thereby maintaining a constant oncotic gradient and no edema. The skin is less tolerance because of the normally very low interstitial protein content, which cannot decrease much further with hypoproteinemia. Systemic tissues will be more prone to edema with plasma protein levels less than 50% of normal, a value very commonly seen in the early postresuscitation period after a major burn, especially if no protein was given in the first 24 to 36 hours. The nonburn edema will persist, with resolution dependent on the status of plasma proteins and muscle activity level. Severe hypoalbuminemia will also diminish intestinal mobility and the binding of drugs and circulatory toxins.

## Blood Losses from Escharotomy: Excision

An incision through the burn eschar, especially an incision down to the fascial plane, will become a vent for the contained edema. Much of the fluid draining from these incised areas is sequestered edema. Surgical excision of burn tissue, especially to fascia, will essentially remove or allow drainage of all the contained edema as well as result in some new losses from the excision procedure.

## Loss of Red Cell Mass

Red cell mass can decrease markedly during this period due to the following factors:

>   Increased red blood cell breakdown
>   Decreased red blood cell production

A large portion of the red blood cell mass is exposed to heat with a large flame burn, a long exposure to scald, or an electrical burn. In addition, many absorbed chemicals will increased red cell fragility. Increased lipid peroxidation of the red cell membrane is well described after burn injury. Hematocrit characteristically decreases to levels of 30 to 35 or lower at several days postburn. If there are additional external losses or hemolysis is evident during the early period, hematocrit will decrease more rapidly and to a greater degree. Part of the reason for decreased red blood cell mass is the shortened red blood cell half-life and clearance of injured cells. Also, as plasma volume is restored over the next several days, the red blood cell distribution space will increase and hemoglobin decrease. Besides increased breakdown, there is also a decreased production by the bone marrow, characteristic of any chronic injury state. The exact nature of this impaired production is not known. Red cell production does not return to normal until after the wound is closed. Therefore the decreased red blood cell mass will not correct by itself, as is the case with a transient whole blood loss in an otherwise healthy host. In addition, losses from escharotomies and blood drawing become more evident during this period when blood volume is restored.

## Fluid Gains

Intravascular fluid and protein are also gained during this period as edema fluid is resorbed and interstitial protein in nonburned tissue returned via lymphatics. The *factors determining rate of edema resorption* are:

>   Adequacy of lymphatic vessels and veins
>   Restoration of burn tissue blood flow
>   Muscle activity improving venous return
>   Water clearance from kidneys

Intravascular fluid is gained, during the postresuscitation period, from the absorption of edema fluid. The rate of absorption is variable and depends on many factors, including burn depth and subsequent lymphatic damage. Interstitial protein needs to be cleared by functioning lymphatics, whereas water can cross the endothelial barrier from interstitium to plasma. Edema resorption is much more rapid in superifical burns when lymphatics are intact. The process begins at about day 2 or 3. Edema resorption is much slower after full-thickness injury due to the lack of local lymphatics and venules. In addition, fibrin deposition in the burn edema produces a gellike state that requires some fibrinolysis before resorption. Restoration of blood and lymphatic flow to the wound is required. The rate of edema resorption can be impaired by an increase in capillary pressure with high central venous pressures retarding venous and lymphatic return. However, a hypovolemic state is not going to accentuate fluid resorption from sequestered burn edema fluid. Increased muscle activity will improve venous return and lymphatic function. The magnitude of the tissue edema is not a valid reflection of the circulating volume and should never be used to judge the rate of fluid replacement.

The adequacy of clearance by the kidneys of the fluid gains is dependent on a number of factors.

Salt solution is essential in the resuscitation period to maintain adequate plasma volume. Isotonic or hypertonic solutions used during this period, however, produce a large increase in total body sodium, which is difficult to eliminate. Subsequent evaporative water or urine losses will be hypotonic. A relative salt overload and hypernatremia will then develop, leading to further water retention.

Any impairment in renal perfusion will, of course, impair glomerular filtration rate. Heart failure often occurs during this period in the elderly patient population. In addition, stress-induced antidiuretic hormone and aldosterone release will accentuate water and $Na^+$ resorption and $K^+$ loss.

## CHANGING PATTERN OF FLUID GAINS VERSUS LOSSES DURING POSTRESUSCITATION PERIOD

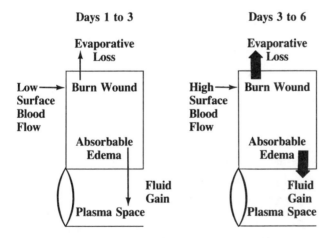

### Electrolyte, Acid-Base Abnormalities

*Hyponatremia* in the range of 130 mEq/L is commonly seen in the early postresuscitation period, especially if lactated Ringer's solution ($Na^+$ = 130 mEq/L) is the predominant fluid used. The process usually corrects itself as evaporation losses increase water relative to sodium losses.

*Hypernatremia* in the range of 145 to 150 mEq/L is also commonly seen if water losses through evaporation and urine, exceed sodium losses. The process will correct itself slowly if $Na^+$ intake is decreased and free water is increased.

*Hypokalemia* in the range of 3 to 3.5 mEq/L is also quite common, especially with the reinstitution of glucose infusion during this period because of the shift of $K^+$ back into the cells.

*Hyperkalemia* is not very common despite hemolysis and tissue breakdown as long as renal function is adequate.

*Respiratory acidosis* is a common occurrence with the combination of a pulmonary injury and increased carbon dioxide production.

*Respiratory alkalosis* can occur with overventilation, usually seen in attempts to decrease shunt fraction by increasing tidal volume and rate rather than PEEP.

*Metabolic acidosis* reflects impaired perfusion if lactic acidosis is present (increased anion gap) or hyperchloremic acidosis due to excessive $Cl^-$ intact.

*Metabolic alkalosis* is commonly seen with the use of large volumes of lactated Ringer's solution or if bicarbonate is given during the resuscitation period.

## Systemic Metabolic and Hemodynamic Changes

### Metabolic Changes

The *ebb phase,* or hypometabolic phase, characteristic of the initial burn shock period begins to be transformed to the *flow phase,* or hypermetabolic state, over the next 3 to 5 days. The specific properties of burn-induced hypermetabolism will be discussed in depth in the next section. It is important, however, to recognize this transition during the postresuscitation period. The *flow phase* is characterized by

> Increased oxygen consumption ($>$100 to 140 ml/min/m$^2$)
> Increased body temperature
> Increased gluconeogenesis
> Increased anti-insulin hormones (decreased glucose tolerance)
> Increased catabolism (increased ureagenesis)

The increase in oxygen consumption usually peaks 5 to 10 days postburn. The transition to the flow state also initiates an increase in body temperature that increases further with burn wound pyrogen release. The characteristic 1° to 2°F increase in body temperature makes it more difficult to diagnose the presence of infection. Glucose utilization increases, carbohydrate being the principal fuel of the hypermetabolic state. High levels of catechols, cortisol, and glucagon are present as well as increased levels of insulin, with the anti-insulin effect predominating. In most patients, a gradually increasing carbohydrate infusion is well tolerated as long as supply does not exceed demand. However, hyperglycemia is commonly seen in the prediabetic patient with a large burn. This patient population is characteristically obese or elderly, or both. The increased catabolism will also lead to increased urea production, especially if inadequate glucose calories are being provided. Increased urea nitrogen production needs to be distinguished from decreased urea clearance.

Water deficit = ideal total body weight (0.6 × ideal body weight) − ideal total body weight × 140 mEq/L / serum $Na^+$

## Urine Output

The restoration of blood flow to the burn tissue after resuscitation will result in the resorption of a large load of osmotically active particles, comprised of solutes from disrupted cells and fragments of denatured proteins. Normal daily solute load is about 600 mOsm, and the kidney can usually concentrate urine to a level of about 600 mOsm/L (isotonic, i.e., 300 mOsm/L = 1.010). The solute load with reperfusion and with onset of hypermetabolism will be significantly increased. This process results in an obligate solute diuresis manifested by the increased output of high specific gravity urine. This increased osmotic load is very evident in second degree burn blisters, which increase in size and pressure over a period of days. An increase in urine output can be mistaken for fluid resorption and hypervolemia unless the specific gravity is also followed carefully (Table 6-1).

# PRACTICAL APPROACH TO MANAGEMENT

Understanding of the physiologic and metabolic changes during this period is the key to successful management because errors in judgment will be minimized. The major decisions are what type of fluid and how much to give and what to monitor.

## Type of Fluid

A common management error is to continue to infuse isotonic crystalloid during this period when major losses of sodium do not occur. A 5% glucose containing solutions with a low sodium content is the primary initial replacement fluid for evaporative and urinary losses during this period (Table 6-2). The glycogen stores have been depleted by this time and exogenous glucose will be required, especially for obligate users, such as the brain and red blood cells. The addition of 20 to 30 mEq/L of potassium will usually be necessary once glucose and other nutrients are initiated to keep up with urinary $K^+$ losses as well as $K^+$ shift into cells with protein synthesis and carbohydrate infusion. The high fluid requirements in large burns needed to replace evaporative losses of a large burn make it easier to give the needed increased calories and nitrogen.

Nutrient infusion should begin as soon as the patient becomes glucose tolerant, i.e., in the first 48 to 72 hours, while waiting for gastrointestinal motility to return and to begin enteral feeding. The administration can be initiated through a peripheral vein. The osmolarity of the solution limits peripheral vein alimentation. Solutions with an osmolarity up to 600 mOsm/L can safely be given through most veins. Solutions up to 900 mOsm/L can be given in larger veins, such as the antecubital. The osmolarities of basic nutrient solutions are listed in Table 6-3. Thus, a 3% amino acid solution (30 g/L of protein) and a glucose solution of 5 to 10% can be infused along with a 10% fat solution.

**Table 6-1** Changes in Urine Output During Post Resuscitation Period

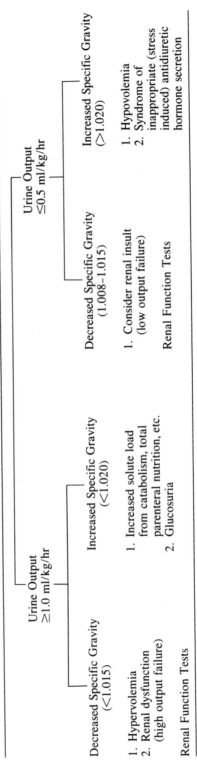

- Urine Output ≥1.0 ml/kg/hr
  - Decreased Specific Gravity (<1.015)
    1. Hypervolemia
    2. Renal dysfunction (high output failure)
    
    Renal Function Tests
  - Increased Specific Gravity (<1.020)
    1. Increased solute load from catabolism, total parenteral nutrition, etc.
    2. Glucosuria

- Urine Output ≤0.5 ml/kg/hr
  - Decreased Specific Gravity (1.008–1.015)
    1. Consider renal insult (low output failure)
    
    Renal Function Tests
  - Increased Specific Gravity (>1.020)
    1. Hypovolemia
    2. Syndrome of inappropriate (stress induced) antidiuretic hormone secretion

**Table 6-2** Fluid Replacement

Type of Fluid to Use
|
Replace

| Evaporative Urine Losses | Red Blood Cell Losses | Surgery Losses |
|---|---|---|
| Hypotonic Salt Solution Add $K^+$, Calories and Protein | Packed Cells Maintaining Hematocrit $\geq 30$ | Red Blood Cells Plus Plasma (Not More Crystalloid) |

*Protein Losses*

Nutrition Plus Albumin

*Fluids of Choice*
1. Use low salt-glucose containing
2. Add increased amounts potassium
3. Add nutrients: glucose, amino acids, lipid
4. Maintain albumin above 2.5 g/dl
5. Maintain adequate red blood cell mass (hematocrit $\geq 30$)

---

The fat solution decreases the total osmolarity. A sufficient volume can usually be given during this period to provide up to 75% of the calculated caloric and protein requirements by a peripheral vein. The specifics of nutritional demands and management are discussed in detail in Section 3.

Sufficient volume to maintain adequate tissue oxygen transport to tissues is necessary. This determination will be assessed by the *monitors* that are used. A constant fluid infusion is preferrable to bolus volume loading because transient increases in pressure will continue to accentuate losses through burn tissue. The rate of infusion will require frequent readjustments throughout this period to compensate for both fluid losses and fluid gains. Even though evaporative losses are fairly constant, the rate of edema mobilization varies considerably based on a variety of cardiopulmonary parameters, as previously described. In addition, frequent surgical procedures with creation of new wounds in the form of donor sites as well as losses of whole blood will require frequent readjustments in volume replacement. Since multiple access sites are often a problem, it is often most practical to administer the anticipated free water, potassium, and nutrients together at a constant infusion predicated on the mornings assessment of the status of fluid shifts. Additions, such as protein and red blood cells, can then be supplemented.

The protein deficit caused by the losses into burn tissue and blood loss from wound excisions, should be carefully restored to levels that allow maintenance of adequate oncotic pressure and protein binding. Do not infuse proteins, however, if hypervolemia is already present. A value for albumin of greater than 2.5 g/dl is reasonable. It is

**Table 6-3** Comparative Osmolarity of Nutrition Solutions

| Solution | Osmolarity* (mOsm/L) | Nonprotein Energy (kcal/L) | Nitrogen (g/L) | Protein (g/L) |
|---|---|---|---|---|
| Dextrose 5% | 250 | 180 | | |
| Dextrose 10% | 500 | 360 | | |
| Dextrose 25% | 1250 | 860 | | |
| Amino acid 2.8% | 280 | | 4.5 | 28 |
| Amino acid 4.3% | 430 | | 7.0 | 43 |
| Fat emulsion 10% | 140 | 1000 | | |
| Fat emulsion 20% | 290 | 2000 | | |

* A solution of 600 mOsm is safe; 900 mOsm results in increased phlebitis.

unreasonable to assume that albumin will be made by the liver in adequate quantities once nutrient is initiated, because albumin synthesis is markedly diminished in favor of acute-phase protein synthesis. It is also unrealistic to ignore extremely low levels of albumin, especially when restoration of blood volume and gastrointestinal motility is expected. Even though albumin solutions do not restore the globulin losses, the risks of fresh frozen plasma use outweight benefits except for clotting abnormalities. The role of gamma globulin replacement remains unclear.

*Do not infuse plasma proteins if hypervolemia is present, unless additional pharmacologic support such as a diuretic is to be added.*

It is also frequently necessary to replace red cells during this period, both the cells lost initially through hemolysis and those lost directly through, for example, escharotomy sites and wound excision procedures. In addition, heat-injured red cells have a shortened half-life and the production of new red cells is significantly impaired with burn injury. The hematocrit should be kept at least in the low 30s to optimize the carrying capacity and delivery of oxygen to tissues. Also, maintenance of a reasonable red blood cell mass, preoperatively, is essential to minimize operative morbidity, and red blood cell loss can occur very rapidly very early in the procedure.

## Intravenous Access (Infection Control)

A peripheral line remains the first choice of access. This site should be changed from the original intravenous puncture if started in an emergency room setting. Conservation of peripheral sites is necessary; therefore additional intravenous lines not absolutely needed should be removed, as should any invasive monitoring catheters once they are no longer essential.

*Rules to Follow to Avoid Cathether Sepsis*

1. The intravenous catheter is inserted using sterile technique. The date and time of insertion is written on the dressing and charted in the patient's record. All central catheters should be removed when *no longer medically indicated* due to the severity of the complications of sepsis and thrombosis.

2. All catheters peripheral or central through *burn tissue* must be rotated every 48 hours until they can be permanently removed and placed through clean tissue.
3. All peripheral lines through *nonburned tissue* should be rotated to a new site every 3 days.
4. Insertion by percutaneous puncture rather than surgical cutdown is always the preferred method of insertion.
5. It is preferred that all arterial catheters be changed every *4 days* to minimize infection.
6. Central venous catheters inserted through a peripheral vein (arm or leg) should be treated as peripheral lines, i.e., should be changed *every 3 days*.
7. Triple lumen catheters should be used only when the patient has the need for a multiple use central venous access, e.g., infusion of multiple incompatible medications, with or without hyperalimentation, or central venous pressure monitoring. These catheters are not indicated if a single central venous access for simple hyperalimentation or intravenous drug administration is all that is required.
8. The optimal duration of catheter placement for central venous catheter is not yet clear, but based on available date, pulmonary artery (Swan-Ganz) catheters and any central catheters inserted through an introducer in nonburn skin should be replaced in a new site *every 4 to 5 days*, if feasible. Central catheters placed through burn tissue must be removed as soon as possible.
9. The practice of changing central catheters in the same site using a guide wire should be discouraged if done as an infection control measure. If there is a need to replace a central catheter because of suspected catheter-related sepsis, but there are extenuating circumstances that make insertion of the catheter in a new site very difficult or hazardous, it is possible (but not preferred) to change the catheter in the same site using a wire. The catheter tips is then cultured. If these cultures indicate that the older catheter was infected, the new catheter must be removed from the infected site and access reestablished at a new, clean site.

*It is clear that following these rules may not be feasible in massive burns. However, in the vast majority of burn patients, most of these rules are feasible with proper planning beginning at the time of admission. Early grafting of potential access sites will help solve the same problem once the next phase is entered.*

## What to Monitor

The assessment of the adequacy of perfusion (oxygenation) and fluid and electrolyte balance can be difficult unless one has a good understanding of what is happening to the patient. Oxygen consumption will gradually increase, i.e., oxygen demands increase with transition from *ebb to flow*. The same parameters are monitored as before. However, interpretation of some of the specific physiologic values is different from comparable changes during initial resuscitation.

## All Patients

*Intake-output:* Intake will continue to exceed measured output (urine) at least for the first several days. Consider, however, that the major output, namely, wound surface and evaporative losses, cannot be accurately quantitated.

*Body weight:* Anticipate a gradual decrease toward but not to preburn levels as edema is very gradually mobilized. Therefore the absolute value of body weight cannot be used during this transition period to reflect blood volume. However, if weight is increasing during this period, excess fluid and, especially, salt are being given.

*Arterial pressure:* Maintain at a level (usually more than 90 mean) for adequate perfusion. In general, the absolute value in this period is affected by many more variables than during the (0 to 36 hour) period. The effects of pain, elevated temperature, narcotics, and increasing metabolic rate on the measured value must be considered. *An arterial line* is usually not necessary unless large surgical procedures are done with no access to noninvasive assessment. A line may be needed for blood gases, although a pulse oximeter can be used quite easily to measure oxygen saturation of hemoglobin.

*Pulse rate:* Rate usually decreases in the first 1 to 2 days compared with that seen with the initial resuscitation phase. Pulse then begins to increase again as the *flow* phase evolves. One must consider the effects of increase in temperature, pain, etc., which again alter the value unrelated to blood volume.

*Temperature:* Anticipate gradual increase of 1° to 2°F over normal due to hypermetabolism. Further temperature increases are common with wound manipulation.

*Urine output:* The value will usually exceed 0.5 ml/kg/hr as edema fluid and solute load are mobilized. Urine output may not reflect adequacy of perfusion because an increased solute load diuresis will increase output even if fluid intake is inadequate. However, changes in output do reflect changes in the physiologic and metabolic status; the key is to make the correct interpretation.

*Electrocardiogram:* Continuous monitoring of the heart is indicated in high-risk patients.

*Arterial blood gases:* Monitor as needed to maintain arterial oxygen tension greater than 80 mmHg and arterial carbon dioxide tension less than 50 mmHg. Arterial carbon dioxide tension will often vary, depending on acid-base balance.

*Electrolytes:* Electrolyte studies should be obtained daily during the initial large fluid shifts.

*pH, acid-base balance:* The pH and acid-base balance should be monitored to assess perfusion and to avoid excessive alterations in pH, particularly alkalosis, which will affect oxygen unloading from hemoglobin.

*Creatinine, blood urea nitrogen:* Changes in blood urea nitrogen relative to creatinine are very useful in sorting out the status of the exchangeable total body water space, i.e., the rate of evaporative loss. Consider, however, the effect of catabolism, and nutrient infusion on the blood urea nitrogen. A transient increase in blood urea nitrogen and creatinine is commonly seen in massive burns due to an initial renal hypoperfusion injury.

*Plasma proteins:* Severe hypoproteinemia is common. Maintain albumin more than 2.5 g/dl to assist in maintenance of plasma volume.

*Prothrombin time, partial thromboplastin time, platelets:* Monitor these parameters, especially if early excision is planned. Use fresh frozen plasma and platelets as needed (see Section 7).

## Additional Measurements in Selected Patients

*Central venous pressure,* if elevated more than 15 mmHg, indicates either hypervolemia or impaired venous return, e.g., from PEEP. A low to normal value is not particularly helpful in the assessment.

*Pulmonary artery wedge* pressure, as above if elevated more than 15 mmHg, indicates heart failure, hypervolemia, or simply positive-pressure ventilation. Wedge measurement is usually only required in the elderly or the patient with significant continued cardiopulmonary dysfunction where one cannot assess volume status. Most patients do not require this measurement. In addition, infection risks increase as even unburned skin becomes colonized due to neighboring burn wound colonization.

*Cardiac output:* Since oxygen demands begin to increase in the major burn, a value of cardiac output adequate to 0 to 36 hours now becomes inadequate. Cardiac output is usually double normal by the end of this period in patients with burns in excess of 30% of total body surface. One must be cautious about interpreting the adequacy of a value of cardiac output if not compared with other parameters.

*Oxygen consumption:* An increase in oxygen consumption of between 50 and 100% of normal is expected by the end of this period. The predicted value is comparable to the predicted percent increase in metabolic rate relative to burn size and age. A value too low indicates inability of the patient to maintain sufficient oxygen delivery.

*Hematocrit, hemoglobin:* An increasing value in hematocrit or hemoglobin indicates hypovolemia, whereas a decreasing value is expected. Hematocrit should be maintained greater than 30, especially if surgical excisions are being performed or if impaired oxygen delivery is evident.

*White blood cells:* An increase may be stress related if in the range of 15,000 to 18,000. Value of 20,000 or more usually indicates infection. A low value of less than 5000/mm$^3$ may be silver sulfadiazine-induced or a sign of severe sepsis. No treatment is necessary for silver sulfadiazine-leukopenia.

## Pharmacologic Support

Congestive heart failure is commonly seen in the fluid resorption period in the elderly. Salt load, excessive antidiuretic hormone, and aldosterone release can impair water clearance from edema resorption. Digitalis is not recommended during the initial resuscitation period but can be used now as long as adequate K$^+$ is being given. This agent is not the optimum inotrope. A very effective agent to maintain glomerular filtration rate and increase both Na$^+$ and water loss is low-dose dopamine (1 to 3 μg/kg/min). The agent is very safe with few complications at this dose range. In the case of increased filling pressures and a catechol-induced tachycardia (flow phase), the inotrope of choice is often dobutamine. In the case of a severe sepsis syndrome with a marked decrease in systemic vascular resistance and hypotension, volume loading and mid- to high-range dopamine would be the agent of choice. The alpha agonists, such as norepinephrine, should be reserved only for severe systemic hypotension (mean pressure less than 80 mmHg) not controlled by fluid and inotropes (see Section 7).

**Table 6-4** Pharmacologic Support of Burn Patient

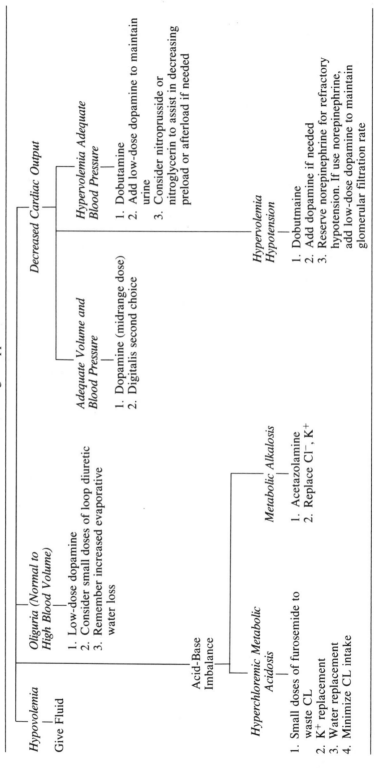

```
                                    Pharmacologic Support of Burn Patient
                                                    |
         ┌──────────────────────────────────────────┼──────────────────────────────────────────┐
    Hypovolemia                          Oliguria (Normal to                        Decreased Cardiac Output
         |                                High Blood Volume)                                   |
    Give Fluid                                                                  ┌──────────────┴──────────────┐
                                  1. Low-dose dopamine                   Adequate Volume and          Hypervolemia Adequate
                                  2. Consider small doses of loop diuretic    Blood Pressure                Blood Pressure
                                  3. Remember increased evaporative
                                     water loss                         1. Dopamine (midrange dose)   1. Dobutamine
                                                                        2. Digitalis second choice    2. Add low-dose dopamine to maintain
                                                                                                         urine
                                                                                                      3. Consider nitroprusside or
                                                                                                         nitroglycerin to assist in decreasing
                                                                                                         preload or afterload if needed

                                                                                                        Hypervolemia
                                                                                                        Hypotension

                                                                                                      1. Dobutmaine
                                                                                                      2. Add dopamine if needed
                                                                                                      3. Reserve norepinephrine for refractory
                                                                                                         hypotension. If use norepinephrine,
                                                                                                         add low-dose dopamine to maintain
                                                                                                         glomerular filtration rate

                    Acid-Base
                    Imbalance
         ┌──────────┴──────────┐
  Hyperchloremic Metabolic   Metabolic Alkalosis
       Acidosis
                              1. Acetazolamine
  1. Small doses of furosemide to    2. Replace Cl⁻, K⁺
     waste CL
  2. K⁺ replacement
  3. Water replacement
  4. Minimize CL intake
```

\* Also see Section 7 on Pharmacologic Support.

Diuretics may be helpful during this period if fluid retention and hypervolemia are problems. Remember that the amount of tissue edema does not accurately reflect blood volume. Small quantities of a loop diuretic, e.g., 10 to 20 mg furosemide, will often initiate a controlled diuresis. In addition, $Cl^-$ excess can be excreted in cases of hypercholeremic metabolic acidosis as long as $K^+$ is replaced. Acetazolamide is a useful agent to correct the metabolic alkalosis (Table 6-4).

## Common Pitfalls in Fluid Management

### Assessing Plasma Volume Using Extent of Edema

A common error is overestimating plasma volume because of the magnitude of edema present. Continued plasma loss into the burn eschar and from the burn surface will persist for several days.

### Continued Isotonic Salt Infusion for Replacement

Although plasma losses persist, the major loss (outside of debridement) is evaporation. Salt loading, at this time, is disadvantageous. Excess fluid clearance will be impaired with continued infusion of $Na^+$ excess.

### Underestimation of Evaporative Losses

Initially during this phase, evaporative losses are often compensated for by the resorption of edema fluid, lulling the novice into underestimating actual losses. When the edema well runs dry, so does the patient.

### Using urine Output to Assess Perfusion

A number of processes occur during this period that make urine output difficult to interpret. Increased urine output may be due to hypervolemia or an increased solute load (especially with onset of nutrition). Urine osmolality must be assessed to determine which is happening. A urine output of 1 cc/kg/hr with a specific gravity of 1.030 is not adequate. Oliguria may well be due to congestive heart failure or syndrome of inappropriate secretion of antidiuretic hormone.

### Using Hemoglobin to Assess Blood Volume

A decreasing hemoglobin level does not necessarily mean plasma expansion from edema resorption nor does it necessarily mean a source of hemorrhage. Heat-injured red blood cells will be rapidly cleared from the circulation, decreasing red blood cell mass.

### Keeping Monitoring Lines in Place Too Long

Now is the time to remove invasive monitoring lines, i.e., while the patient is stable and before septic thrombophlebitis.

## TREATMENT SUMMARY

### Monitoring Guidelines

1. Blood pressure: Anticipate considerable variability during fluid shifts with hypertension evident in approximately 10%
2. Pulse: Initially decreases toward normal values only to increase again during flow phase. Glucosuria common with onset carbohydrate infusion
3. Urine output: Anticipate considerable variability. Low specific gravity usually seen initially with hypervolemia-induced diuresis. High specific gravity with clearance of increased osmotic load. Maintain more than 0.5 cc/kg/hr
4. Electrocardiogram: Anticipate sinus tachycardia
5. Temperature: Anticipate gradual increase in temperature to one to two degrees above normal, with spikes after wound manipulation
6. Blood gases: Continued risk of hypoxemia, hypercapnia, especially with smoke inhalation
   pH, acid-base: anticipate variety of acid-base abnormalities resulting primarily from electrolyte disorders
7. Wedge: Measurement not usually required during this period unless congestive heart failure present or with severe pulmonary dysfunction
8. Hemoglobin: Anticipate gradual decrease due to decreased half-life, decreased production, increased losses
9. White blood cells: Variable response, leukocytosis second degree burn.
   Leukopenia seen with silver sulfadiazine
10. Electrolytes: Hyponatremia, hypokalemia most common
11. Blood urea nitrogen, creatinine: Anticipate increasing blood urea nitrogen with combination of dehydration, catabolism, protein infusion
12. Plasma proteins: Remain decreased, especially albumin
13. Coagulation: Initial thrombocytopenia common, which corrects over several days. Prothrombin time, partial thromboplastin time usually become normal

# SUMMARY (PATHOPHYSIOLOGY)

## Fluid, Protein, Red Blood Cell Shifts

### Fluid and Protein Losses

1. Increased permeability burn tissue persists; plasma loss from surface second degree burn
2. Nonburn edema from low protein content
3. Evaporative water loss increases with surface blood flow estimate milliliters per hour = [(25+ % total body surface burn) × m² surface area]
4. Losses from surgical incisions, excisions

### Changes Red Blood Cell Mass

1. Increased red blood cell breakdown
2. Increasing plasma volume
3. Decreased red blood cell production
4. Added losses; blood tests, surgery

### Fluid Gains

1. Edema resorption dependent on: Status of lymphatics, veins, plasma protein status of burn tissue blood flow, Muscle activity increasing reabsorption
2. Further fluid gains due to: Initial salt loading; impaired urinary diuresis (increased antidiuretic hormone, aldosterone)

Use of isotonic crystalloid to replace evaporative water losses

### Electrolyte Changes

Hyponatremia: 36 to 48 hours Due to Hypotonic Fluids Usually Above 130 mEq/L
Hypernatremia: 3 to 7 Days Due to Water Loss Exceeding Na$^+$ Loss
Hypokalemia: With Onset Glucose Infusion Due to Increased Renal K$^+$ Loss
Hyperkalemia: Due to Renal Impairment

### Acid-Base Changes

Respiratory Acidosis: Related to Status of Ventilation
Hyperchloremic Metabolic Acidosis: Excess Sodium Chloride
Lactic Acidosis: Not Common if Adequate Fluid Intake
Respiratory Alkalosis: Common with Mechanical Ventilation
Metabolic Alkalosis: Common (36 to 48 hours) After Large Load of Lactated Ringers Solution or Bicarbonate

### Systemic Metabolic Changes

1. Increasing oxygen consumption (>140 ml/min/m²)
2. Increasing body temperature
3. Increasing levels, catechols, cortisol, glucagon may be continued glucose intolerance
4. Catabolism with increased urea production, increasing blood urea nitrogen common

### Systemic Physiologic Changes

1. Increasing cardiac output
2. Persistent tachycardia
3. Decreasing systemic vascular resistance
4. Urine output usually increasing due to both increased volume and increased solute load
5. Marked increase in body weight

# MAINTENANCE OF HEMODYNAMIC STABILITY (36 HOURS TO 6 DAYS)

## All Major Burns

1. Infuse glucose (5 to 10%) in low salt crystalloid to replace evaporative loss minus gain from edema resorption
2. Replace plasma protein losses, albumin >2.5 g/dl. Be careful if patient already hypervolemic
3. Assure adequate oxygen delivery, maintain oxygen saturation 95% or greater, hematocrit greater than 30 cardiac output more than 1.5 times normal
4. Begin nutritional support: Calories and protein can use peripheral vein and enteral route instead of central line
5. Monitor pulse, blood pressure, temperature, urine, body weight, input and output, electrocardiogram, acid-base electrolytes, complete blood count, blood urea nitrogen, creatinine, albumin
6. Maintain urine output greater than 0.5 ml/kg/hr.
7. Maintain temperature greater than 37.5.

If Hemodynamic Stability Not Achieved

*Hypervolemia*

Consider

1. Gentle diuresis, low-dose loop diuretics
2. Inotropes; best choice, dopamine, dobutamine

*Low Flow State: Volume Status? Hypervolemia, Congestive Heart Failure, Hypovolemia*

Consider

1. Increasing monitors. Add: wedge pressure, cardiac output, oxygen consumption
2. Use beta inotrope, dopamine, dobutamine

*Increased Systemic Vascular Resistance, Hypertension Impaired Perfusion*

Consider

Low-Dose Dopamine Vasodilator

# 7

# Daily Care of the Burn Wound

The wound undergoes dramatic changes during these next several days as inflammation develops. In addition, the onset of wound colonization and the potential for wound infection increases during this period. Of particular importance is the potential for change in the *zone of ischemia,* that area of tissue that is injured but still viable on admission. Changes in local wound microcirculatory blood flow, as a result of vasoactive inflammatory agents or local infection, can convert the zone of ischemia to a *zone of necrosis*. This process, termed "wound conversion," is most commonly seen in the deep second degree burn and can occur even with optimum management. Processes such as wound desiccation, hypovolemia, increased tissue pressure, hypothermia can all accentuate the potential for conversion and must be controlled. The most common cause, however, is local infection. For deep second and third degree burns, the optimum timing for removal of the devitalized tissue and wound closure is during this period, i.e., before onset of inflammation and infection. The term "early excision" really means within the first postburn week.

These specific burn wound changes will be discussed, as will the approaches to wound management both for superficial and deep burns.

> Pathophysiologic Changes
> > Changes in the Burn Wound
> > Epidemiology of Burn Wound Infection
> > Diagnosis of Wound Infection
> 
> Practical Approach to Treatment
> > Infection Control Policy
> > Daily Care of the Burn Wound

## PATHOPHYSIOLOGIC CHANGES

### Changes in the Burn Wound

The burn wound changes dramatically during this 6 to 7 day period as neutrophil infiltration occurs, followed by macrophage infiltration. The relatively inert burn wound 24 hours postburn changes to a focus of intense inflammation at about 7 to 10 days in the full-thickness burn and several days sooner in the partial thickness burn. The rate of onset of inflammation is dependent on the blood flow to the wound, with inflammation occurring more rapidly in the more superficial burn.

> A marked increase in wound vascularity is seen beginning at about day 3 to 5 in the partial thickness and day 7 to 10 in the full-thickness burn. The neovascularization is initiated and essentially parallels the degree of acute inflammation.
>
> Bacterial colonization and infection become much more prominent beginning about 7 days postburn than during the early postresuscitation period of 2 to 6 days. Increased vascularity, leads to an increasing release of inflammatory mediators. Bacteria and bacterial by-products can more readily enter the circulation during wound manipulation. In addition, blood loss with wound debridement will be in direct proportion to the vascularity of the wound.

### *Superficial—Midthickness Second Degree Burn*

Wound erythema and pain are produced almost immediately after injury by vasoactive inflammatory mediators, especially the prostaglandins. As blood flow increases, so does the degree of inflammation and the delivery of inflammatory cells to the wound surface. A thin superficial eschar usually develops, which is made up of coagulated extravasated protein and wound exudate. Plasma leakage can persist for days from the wound surface. Initial application of an adherent temporary skin substitute will eliminate much of the plasma leak and surface coagulum as well as the collection of surface white cells whose release of proteases can damage remaining viable and new tissue formation. Topical antibiotics will usually increase the amount of surface exudate and coagulum. The adherent exudate is removed with dressing changes, leaving an erythematous, pink, and very painful wound base that then begins to epithelialize and close over the next 7 to 14 days. Pyrogen release with elevated temperature is typically seen even in the absence of infection. Infection risks are relatively low with this depth of burn due to preservation of dermal blood flow along with the added neovascularization. Adequate blood flow allows for improved local immune defenses. The delivery of adequate oxygen to the wound is crucial because oxygen is needed both for healing and neutrophil killing of surface bacteria. The patient who is also severely immunosuppressed due to the magnitude of injury, extremes of age, or the presence of other systemic illnesses, such as diabetes, is at further risk of infection. Burns in poorly vascularized areas, such as over the joints, feet, ears, are also at increased risk of infection even with a relatively superficial burn.

### *Deep Second Degree Burn*

The deep burn develops a more prominent eschar during this period. (Color plates 8A, 8B page 314). The eschar is made up of: (1) the nonviable upper dermis, which initially remains adherent to the lower dermis; (2) surface coagulated protein; and (3) residue from topical antibiotics. The yellow- to white-appearing adherent eschar can give the wound an appearance indistinguishable from that initially seen with a full-thickness injury. The thickened eschar also decreases the wound sensation, making it extremely difficult to distinguish the deep second degree from a conversion to a third degree burn. Often the determination can only be made during early tangential excision if this approach is selected or when the eschar begins to seperate at about 10 to 14 days.

The subeschar tissue changes dramatically as neutrophil infiltration at 2 to 3 days is followed by an intense macrophage infiltration turning the relatively inert tissues into an inflammatory focus with peak inflammation, usually occurring at about 7 to 10 days postburn. Both vasodilation and neovascularization are responsible. The marked increase in vascularity essentially parallels the increase in wound inflammation. White cell proteases begin to liquify and macerate the eschar. Some bacterial colonization is usually evident in 2 to 3 days but invasive wound infection is not common during the first week unless the initial wound was grossly contaminated and initial wound debridement and topical antibiotics were delayed. *Conversion* characteristically occurs during this period as injured ischemic dermis becomes nonviable with local vasoconstriction or occlusion of dermal vessels.

## Third Degree (Full-Thickness) Burn

The wound surface appears to be much dryer with less surface exudation because of the initial coagulation of surface vessels. Frequently, thrombosed vessels can be seen on the wound surface. The exception is the third degree scald burn where surface vessels remain patent and leak plasma for days, even with the full-thickness necrosis of surrounding soft tissue. The thick, firm eschar, initially dehydrated from the thermal injury by flames or intense heat, begins to soften as the topical antibiotic cream restores tissue moisture. Eschar softening is also the result of beginning inflammation with white cell protease release. In general, the inflammatory response is delayed, in onset, over that seen in the less deep burn as the impaired blood flow limits inflammatory cell migration and hyperemia. Impaired oxygen delivery to the eschar impairs local immune defense as bacterial killing by neutrophils is impaired. Increased vascularity begins in the subeschar space toward the end of the first week.

## Onset of Wound Healing

The burn wound, unless immediately excised and grafted, begins the secondary healing process, i.e., healing of an open wound during this period. The response of the underlying viable tissue to the burn can be divided into four components.

1. Inflammation; neutrophils and platelets followed by macrophages
2. Infiltration and replication of fibroblasts and endothelial cells leading to neovascularization
3. Increased collagen synthesis
4. Epithelial cell replication and migration leading to wound closure in second degree burns

The first cells to arrive are the neutrophils from the remaining intact blood vessels. The initial attraction of neutrophils to the wound is caused in part by the local release of chemoattractants. The latter come from activation of the complement, clotting, and kinin cascade. In addition, platelets release a number of mediators that attract inflammatory cells and mesenchymal cells, which will be used for new vessel growth and fibroblast stimulation. Platelet-derived growth factor is one such agent. Neutrophils begin to lyse necrotic tissue, softening the eschar. Neutrophils can also control surface bacterial growth. This process requires oxygen and a lack of available oxygen retards local defenses as well as subsequent new tissue formation. These cells, however, do not appear to activate the healing process itself. This process appears to be initiated by platelets through release of growth factors and by the macrophages. These cells arrive hours to several days after the neutrophil. Macrophages at the surface respond to the hypoxic environment by releasing angiogenesis factors that are chemoattractants for mesenchymal cells for new blood vessel formation. Clusters of endothelial cells grow out toward the wound edge, forming new capillary buds. Macrophages deeper in the wound release fibroblast-stimulating factors referred to as macrophage-derived growth factors. The rate of fibroblast proliferation and in turn new collagen and ground substance deposition is directly dependent on the adequacy of local oxygen supply as well as the supply of amino acids, nutrients, and the vitamins and trace minerals necessary for healing, among them zinc and ascorbic acid (Table 7-1).

Epithelialization also begins during this period. Epithelial cells at the wound edge begin to divide and proliferate, as do epithelial cells in skin appendages in the wound base. The new cells in response to signals from the macrophages migrate across the wound. Once the surface is closed in the second degree burn by the thin layer, continued cell division results in further thickening, although a deeper second degree burn has no rete pegs to anchor the epidermal-dermal attachment.

Retardants of healing during this phase include the presence of eschar, the lack of wound blood and nutrient supply, and an excess of phagocytizing neutrophils on the surface, e.g., in response to infection or dead tissue, which results in local release of enzymes and oxygen radicals. To summarize, the *retardants of healing* are:

1. Eschar
2. Low blood flow, decreased oxygen, decreased nutrients
3. Surface build-up of exudates, including phagocytizing cells and cell by-products

**Table 7-1** Wound Healing

Inflammatory Response
Neutrophils, Platelets, Macrophages
↓
Release of Growth Factors

Angiogenesis Factor
1. Release stimulated by low tissue oxygen tension at surface
2. Initiates new vessel growth

Fibroblast Stimulating Factor
Macrophage-Derived Growth Factor
1. Increases collagen and ground substance deposition
2. Rate of deposition directly proportional to amount of available tissue oxygen

Epidermal Growth Factors
1. Increase epithelial cell division
2. Increase rate of migration

The wound healing process is, however, most sensitive to a decrease in perfusion. All the other factors are important but adequate blood flow is essential. The excised and grafted wound during this period essentially bypasses much of the exaggerated inflammatory response, characteristic of any necrotic tissue. The graft adheres to underlying dermis, fat, or fascia, which has only modest changes. Primary healing then results with sheet grafts or a modified secondary healing with meshed grafts.

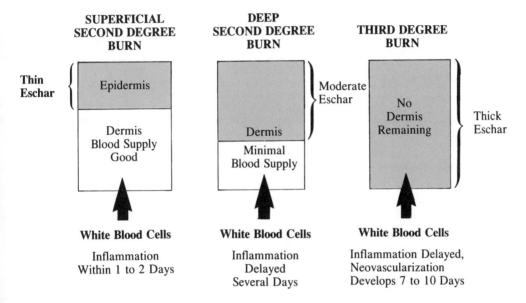

Bacterial colonization also begins in this period. Adequate levels of topically applied antibiotics in the subeschar space are more difficult to attain with the thicker eschar because of impaired penetration. Spontaneous surface sloughing due to loss of integrity of the thick eschar begins toward the end of this period. The rate of eschar sloughing is accentuated by wound bacteria, which create an additional stimulus to inflammation and local protease release. As with second degree burns, invasive infection is not common in the first several days unless initial gross contamination was present.

## Evaporative Water and Heat Loss

As wound blood flow increases, so does water and heat losses. This process is particularly true for the deep second degree burn. The superficial second degree burn still has some remaining skin barrier and the third degree burn, until eschar separation, has a limited perfusion. The heat and water losses are further accentuated by the increase in core temperature, which develops with the onset of hypermetabolism. The specific estimation and replacement of water is described in Chapter 6.

## Epidemiology of Burn Wound Infection

The burn wound is a major site of infection for three reasons: (1) loss of the skin barrier; (2) presence of dead tissue; and (3) systemic immunosuppression (Table 7-2). The stratum

**Table 7-2** Causes of Burn Infection

| Impaired local defenses | Impaired systemic immune defenses |
|---|---|
| 1. Loss of outer skin barrier | 1. Decrease in phagocyte and lymphocyte function |
| 2. Impaired local blood flow | 2. Decrease in humoral immunity |
| | 3. High-risk environment for nosocomial infection |

cornium is a relatively impermeable barrier to bacterial invasion through the skin. When this barrier is removed, microorganisms can more readily invade the underlying tissues.

## Impaired Local Defenses

With the loss of the outer skin barrier, bacteria can populate the burn wound. Most of these early colonizing bacteria are endogenous. They are either present in the heat-injured skin, especially in hair follicles, glands, etc., or they reside in the nares and oropharynx. Perineal and stool organisms are, of course, also present in large numbers and are a source of infection. The bacteria find their way to the wound by migration in wet dressings, water immersion, by way of hand contact, and to a lesser extent via aerosolized particles. The impaired blood flow to the surface of the burn results in decreased local immune defenses because oxygen is required for white blood cell bacterial killing. In addition, the decreased blood flow decreases the ability of phagocytes and opsonins to reach the wound. The wound also releases a number of immunosuppressive substances that lead to impaired systemic immunity as described next.

## Impaired Systemic Immune Defenses

Systemic host defenses are significantly impaired after a major burn. A number of specific white cell abnormalities have been defined. The function of the T lymphocyte, the cell responsible for cell-mediated immunity, is clearly impaired. Lymphokines responsible for T-cell function include interleukin-2 and macrophage-activating factor. The T cell participates in a direct cytotoxicity reaction destroying microorganisms (and foreign tissue) and also via initiating antibody production through activation of the B lymphocyte. The lack of a normal antibody response because of impaired B cell activation will then affect the killing of bacteria by way of the humoral system. In addition, suppressor factors are released, such as prostaglandin $E_2$, which further alter lymphocyte function.

Monocyte or macrophage defects that occur include a decrease in interleukin-2 production and an impaired antigen presentation to the lymphocyte on the macrophage surface.

Phagocyte cell function is also impaired. The phagocyte, i.e., neutrophil and macrophages, in order to be effective, must be able to migrate to the site of infection, a process known as chemotaxis, to phagocytize and then to kill the bacteria. Chemotaxis and phagocytosis require complement activation and release of complement fragments C3a and C5a to be effective. An increase in complement consumption is seen postburn, again, probably due to the large burn wound and the large surface of evolving inflammation. The complement consumption can lead to depletion of complement components. Intracellular killing of the bacteria requires the release of oxygen radicals via myeloperoxidase activity. This process is also impaired in the burn phagocyte.

**Table 7-3** Impaired Cell-Mediated Immunity

1. Altered skin test reactivity (anergy)
2. Increased allograft survival
3. Decreased T-cell response to mitogen
4. Decreased T-cell number and response to antigen
5. Increase in suppressor relative to helper T-cell

*Released lymphocyte suppressor substances*
Prostaglandins (in particular, $PGE_2$)
Cutaneous burn toxin (collagen fragment)
Endotoxin
Corticosteroids

*Alterations in humoral defenses*
1. Decreased immunoglobins
2. Decreased fibronectin
3. Decreased first degree antibody response

Early changes also occur in the humoral system (Table 7-3). The immunoglobulin G (IgG) class, which is responsible for opsonization of particles and bacteria, is decreased initially, in part due to loss into the burn wound. Proteins of the IgA and IgM series decrease to a lesser degree. The response is transient, normal levels being restored within several days. A similar early decrease occurs in plasma fibronectin, the factor necessary for the clearance of particulate debris by the reticuloendothelial system. As with the other components just described, this decrease is transient as levels return to or above baseline within several days, only to decrease again when sepsis occurs, typically in the inflammatory phase (Table 7-4).

*Environmental Factors*

Movement via hand contact by patient and personnel of organisms from area to area on the patient or between patients is the major factor leading to bacterial contamination of the wound. This process is particularly prevalent with non-nursing personnel, who, in

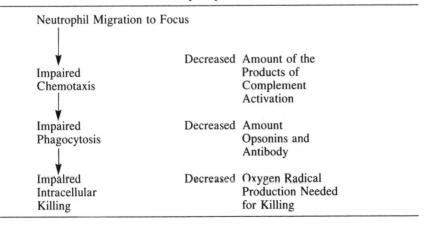

Table 7-4 Decreased Polymorphonuclear Function

general, are less compulsive about standard infection control techniques. The problem can be markedly attenuated by enforcement of hand washing between patients and avoidance of breaks in standard aseptic techniques. Aerosolized bacteria from drying wound crusts, airborne by turbulent airflow, is another known method of cross-contamination. Common sources are vents and airflow systems not regularly dusted and disinfected. Hydrotherapy equipment is a known source of contamination. A warm, moist environment and the repeated use of the same equipment for multiple patients with little time for decontamination are known factors. The addition of hypochlorite to the wash water does *not* sterilize the water. Thus, the *environmental factors leading to bacterial contamination* are:

1. Hand to wound cross-contamination
2. Wound to wound contamination by water
3. Airborne to wound contamination
4. Invasive catheters: Intravenous lines, arterial lines, urinary catheter
5. Endotracheal tubes, respiratory therapy equipment

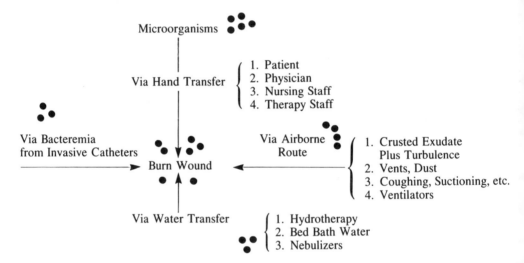

The intensive care needs of the burn patient and the burn unit environment will also increase infection risks. All objects in the patients environment become potential reservoirs for wound contamination. The most dangerous on the list are invasive catheters and tubes. Septic thrombophlebitis remains a major, but preventable, cause of burn sepsis. The decreased number of available intravenous sites due to burn increases the potential for maintaining peripheral and central lines for periods in excess of 3 to 5 days. After 3 days, virtually all peripheral catheters have bacteria in their skin tract or on the tip. In addition, monitoring catheters, arterial lines, Swan-Ganz cathers, etc., run the same risk. Endotracheal tubes, although necessary for pulmonary support, will increase the risk of oropharyngeal colonization, the bacteria that, in turn, will find their way to the lung and the wound. Urinary catheters are also high risk for infection. There are, in addition, resistant strains of microorganisms found in hospitals, especially critical care or burn units, that reside within equipment, drains, and the personnel. The combination of these environmental risk factors and the immune compromised host leads to a never-ending challenge to care providers.

## Diagnosis of Wound Infection

In order to assess the wound for infection, a definition of infection must be well understood. Burn wounds are never sterile even in the presence of topical agents or systemic antibiotics. The presence of the bacteria only on the wound surface or in the nonviable tissue, itself, is termed *colonization*. Colonization may be with a single type of organism or with multiple organisms types. Although endotoxin may be released locally and some absorbed, the bacteria, themselves, are not invading underlying viable tissue. "Infection" of the wound, or local wound sepsis, is the term used to indicate beginning invasion of the underlying viable tissue. With progression, the viable tissue and its blood vessels are invaded and *septicemia* develops. Endotoxemia can also produce a picture of sepsis, and endotoxin absorption can occur without the need for bacterial invasion of blood vessels. The risk of infection overcoming local defenses is high when the blood flow in the subeschar space is marginal, as occurs before neovascularization and granulation tissue formation. After several weeks, when the highly vascularized granulation tissue develops at the interface, local resistance to invasive infection will increase. Inflammation of the wound will be present as a result of the response to the nonviable and injured tissue.

The most common organism involved in wound infection particularly in the first week, is *Staphylococcus aureus*. β-hemolytic Streptococcus infection can also be seen early but the organism is recovered in less than 5% of burn patients. Infection with gram-negative organisms is more evident after the first week. *Pseudomonas aeruginosa* is present on the wound of approximately 20 to 30% of burn patients. *Escherichia coli*, Proteus, or Klebsiella are also noted in about 25% of burn wounds. Enterococcus and *Candida albicans* are microorganisms that are now seen with increasing frequency. Each is now seen in the wound of about 50% of burn patients (Table 7-5).

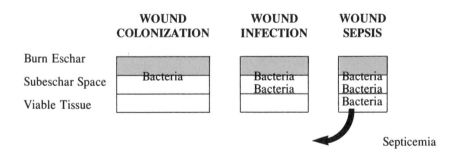

Table 7-5  Percent Recovery From Burn Wounds

| Organism | % of Patients |
|---|---|
| *Staphylococcus aureus* | 85 |
| β-hemolytic Streptococcus | 5 |
| *Pseudomonas aeruginosa* | 25 |
| *Escherichia coli* | 40 |
| Enterococcus | 55 |
| *Candida albicans* | 40 |

The clinical diagnosis of a wound infection can be quite difficult. Fever leukocytosis, tachycardia, and intermittent temperature spikes are characteristically seen in the burn patient with or without infection. A sudden accentuation of these abnormalities can be taken as an indication of an infection some place. Common characteristics of invasive burn infection (burn wound sepsis) relative to the most common organisms involved are presented in Table 7-6.

A conversion of the burn wound in the first several days is usually not bacterial in origin and may actually not be deepening at all but simply a build-up of surface exudate. After this time, however, conversion is usually due to increased bacterial content, particularly *S. aureus*, during the first week. Wound purulence is a reliable indicator of infection only if the purulence is in the subeschar space. What looks like purulence on the surface when the dressing is initially removed is often simply surface exudate mixed with residue of the topical antibiotic. Exudate is especially prominent with silver sulfadiazine. Wound inspection is more valid after the previously applied topical agent and surface exudate have been wiped off.

Surface cultures of the wound will invariably grow some bacteria. It is impossible to distinguish a surface bacterial colonization from that of a wound infection by the results of surface cultures. However, identification of the type of bacteria colonized on the surface is useful information in allowing assessment of the effectiveness of the topical agents being used. Cultures are taken after the wound exudate has been removed. The wound is colonized and subsequently infected most commonly by *S. aureus* in the first week, with gram-negative organisms being more prevalent beginning in the second week.

The most reliable method of diagnosing a burn wound infection is the bacterial analysis of the burn wound biopsy. A small full-thickness portion of eschar is removed using a punch biopsy instrument or scalpel. The biopsy must include some underlying viable subcutaneous tissue. Two techniques can then be applied. The quantitative bacterial count of the biopsy material is one method. It has been established that $10^5$ organisms per gram of tissue is the bacterial load that is preinvasive. The same quantitation is considered to indicate infection in the urinary tract, i.e., greater than 100,000 organisms per ml. Less than $10^5$ is indicative of colonization, whereas $10^5$ or greater indicates infection with a high potential of progressing to wound sepsis. The

Table 7-6 Diagnosis of Burn Wound Infection

| Systemic Changes | Colonized or Clean | Wound Infection |
|---|---|---|
| Body Temperature | Increased | Variable |
| White blood cell count | Increased<br>Mild left shift | High or low<br>Severe left shift |
| Wound appearance | Variable: may appear purulent or benign | Purulence may be present or wound surface may appear dry and pale |
| Bacterial content | | |
|   Surface | Scant to large amount | Variable |
|   Quantitative | Usually $<10^5/g$ | Usually $>10^5/g$ |
|   Biopsy | No invasion of normal tissue | Invasion of normal tissue by organisms |

Table 7-7  Most Common Organisms in Burn Infection

| Organism | S. aureus | P. aeruganosa | C. albicans |
|---|---|---|---|
| Wound appearance | Loss of wound granulation | Surface necrosis Patchy black | Minimal exudate |
| Course | Slow onset 2 to 5 days | Rapid onset 12 to 36 hours | Slow–days |
| Central nervous system | Disorientation | Modest changes | Often no change |
| Temperature | Marked increase | High or low | Modest changes |
| White blood cells | Marked increase | High or low | Modest changes |
| Hypotension | Modest | Often severe | Minimal change |
| Mortality | 5% | 20 to 30% | 30 to 50% |

diagnosis of wound infection indicates the need for systemic antibiotics. The pitfalls of this method are an overestimation of infection when only superficial eschar is obtained for analysis. A reproducible technique of obtaining an accurate sample of eschar is essential for the validity of this method. The second and more reliable technique is that of histologic inspection of the biopsy, sectioning the sample so that the interface between viable and nonviable tissue is seen. Bacterial invasion of viable tissue indicates true infection rather than colonization and the need for systemic antibiotics. Routine monitoring of the wound with biopsies every 3 to 4 days will provide continuing information on microbiologic changes in the wound.

## PRACTICAL APPROACH TO TREATMENT

The primary objective of treatment is prevention. Prevention focuses on two areas: controlling the environment in which the organisms are apt to be transmitted, and controlling or removing the burn wound that will become the focus of infection.

### Infection Control Policy

Infection control is a major component of burn management (Table 7-8). Virulent antibiotic-resistant organisms on the healing or freshly grafted wound can lead to a marked delay in healing and loss of graft. Movement of organisms from dirty to clean areas or to other noninfected patients will lead to a significant increase in morbidity and mortality. An infection control policy is necessary for any burn unit or intensive care unit managing burn patients. A standard policy is presented.

### Daily Care of the Burn Wound

The nonsurgical wound care during this period is a continuation of the care initiated in the immediate postburn period.

**Table 7-8** Full Burn Precautions

Purpose
1. To control transfer of microorganisms that can lead to infection or colonization by personnel and patients by direct contact with wound and heavily contaminated articles, such as dressings or sputum
2. To prevent contact between potentially pathogenic microorganisms and burn patients with seriously impaired resistance

Criteria
1. All patients with burns greater than 15% total body surface area unhealed or ungrafted or complicating illness, e.g., pulmonary dysfunction, which makes the patient prone to infection
2. All patients with grossly infected burns
3. All patients with deep partial thickness or full-thickness facial burns or other burns being treated open, until healed or grafted

Specifications
1. The patient is to be housed in a private room
2. The nurse assigned to give direct care to the patient is to:
   Wear scrub clothing at all times

   Wash arms and hands thoroughly with an antibacterial soap solution (e.g., chlorhexidine) at the start of each shift

   Wash hands thoroughly on entering and leaving the room; arms to be washed once they have come in contact with contaminated objects

   Wear cap, mask fully covering the hair, gloves, and plastic burn apron to enter the room.

   Wear long sleeve isolation gown tied in the back for burn care; a plastic burn apron is to be worn in addition if there is much wound exudate or if wet dressings are used.

   Discard cap, gloves, apron, gown, and mask in plastic lined waste container before leaving the room; discard isolation gown in covered linen receptacle before leaving the room.

   Double bag all linen using red outer bag

   Double bag all trash
3. All other health care personnel (i.e., physicians, physical therapists, charge nurse, or those entering more than one burn patient's room during the day) are to:
   Wash hands thoroughly on entering and leaving the room

   Wear long sleeve isolation gown tied in the back, cap fully covering the hair, mask, and clean gloves to enter the room; a plastic burn apron is to be worn in addition if there are wet dressings or much wound exudate during burn care.

   Gloves, cap, mask, and apron are to be disposed of in a plastic lined waste container before leaving the room; the isolation gown to be discarded in a covered linen receptacle before leaving the room.
4. All visitors are to follow the steps outlined in 3 and are to be so instructed
5. Special instruments are to be washed with an appropriate disinfecting agent, placed in Visi-peel packages labeled and placed in the dirty utility room for reprocessing
6. Medical equipment (i.e., scales, monitors, ventilators, chairs, etc.) are to be disinfected with an appropriate disinfecting agent before being removed from the patients room.

## General Principles

There are a number of general rules regarding burn care that must be followed (Table 7-9).

*First,* cardiopulmonary monitoring, considered to be indicated before burn care, should continue during burn care. The addition of medications for care itself can only lead to a potential for further instability.

*Second,* invasive catheters, such as vascular, urethral, must not become wet at the skin site or be submerged in water. These catheters are at high risk for being a source of *systemic* infection.

*Third,* the patient must not be allowed to lose large amounts of heat. Overhead heaters, warm water, and the unwrapping and wrapping of individual body parts, rather than total patient exposure, are methods to avoid heat loss.

*Fourth,* the risks of cross-contamination must be controlled. Risks of transmission from environmental sources, such as equipment, are minimized by prior decontamination, wrapping, etc. Risks related to transmission from personnel are minimized by wearing of caps, mask, gloves, and a gown. Transmission from a dirty wound to a clean wound can be minimized by exposing and cleaning these areas separately with a different setup, i.e., change of water, gowns, and gloves. Preferably, the less infected areas should be done first and rewrapped before approaching dirtier areas.

The *fifth* principle is that adequate stress management, analgesia and sedation, should be initiated before initiation of burn care. It is much easier to control pain and anxiety by pretreatment than it is to treat once it develops. In large burns, intravenous narcotics are the treatment of choice. Short-acting sedatives, such as midazolam (Versed) can give antianxiety relief without a long "hangover." Antipyretics given before burn care can attenuate the fever seen after wound manipulation. Pretreatment of the dressing change with an antipyretic is indicated in patients who demonstrate a marked temperature spike, i.e., >103°F, after wound care. Acetaminophen, 600 mg orally or 1200 mg through the rectum, is useful. Ibuprofen, 600 mg orally, is a far superior drug for controlling temperature.

The *sixth* principle is that the dressing should be comfortable but should not totally impair motion and muscle activity (exception: a new graft). Sufficient dry gauze should be applied to allow for absorption of drainage. Then an elastic bandage wrapped distal to proximal should be applied over the gauze, especially on extremities, to decrease venous stasis and also minimize continued dependent edema formation. The patient also needs to maintain joint motion and muscle activity to avoid stiffness and atrophy. Early ambulation, i.e., as soon as cardiopulmonary function allows, is indicated.

## Superficial Second Degree Burn

The superficial second degree burn can be managed with a temporary skin substitute, such as biobrane, once wound adherence has occurred, only the outer layer of gauze needs to be changed, usually once a day when it becomes saturated with plasma from the wound surface. Areas not covered with skin substitutes are usually managed in several ways. Loose epidermis and remaining blisters are debrided. Areas such as the face and ears are then treated open, usually with an ointment such as bacitracin to maintain wound moisture as well as control the predominantly gram-positive bacteria. The open areas are usually gently washed two to three times a day with a dilute chlorhexidine solution to remove crust and surface exudate. Areas such as the hands, upper and lower extremities, and

Table 7-9  General Principles of Daily Burn Care

| *Do Not Discontinue Monitoring Considered Indicated Before Burn Care!* | *Avoid Hypothermia* | *Avoid Cross-Contamination* | *Assure Adequate Control of Pain and Anxiety and Hyperthermia* |
|---|---|---|---|
| Do Not Allow the Catheter Sites to Become Wet and Therefore Potentially Contaminated | 1. Warm room<br>2. Heat lamps<br>3. Warm wash water<br>4. Do not expose entire body at one time if burn is massive | 1. Wear caps, masks, gown, gloves; wash hands before and after<br>2. Expose, clean, and rewrap less infected areas first<br>3. Look for sources of bacteria in equipment used | 1. Premication with narcotics and short-acting sedative<br>2. Use intravenous route<br>3. Consider antipyretic pretreatment |
|  |  | *Wound Dressing*<br>Use Comfortable but not Immobilizing Dressing as Muscle Activity Is Important!<br>(Exception: New Grafts) | *Wound Infection*<br>1. Monitor wound flora<br>2. Wound biopsy, if eschar is thick enough<br>3. Adjust topical agents and isolation technique accordingly |

trunk can be treated with a grease gauze impregnated with antibiotic ointment, usually bacitracin. The grease gauze is covered with several layers of dry absorbant gauze. If the grease gauze appears well adhered to the superficial wound with no underlying exudate, the gauze does not need to be changed, as is the case with a donor site dressing. If some exudate is present, the dressing should be removed, the wound gently washed with dilute chlorhexidine, and the dressing reapplied. Exceptions would be the dirty wound that has not been totally cleaned of initial dirt and debris or the perineal or buttock wound. These wounds are best managed with a broad-spectrum topical antibiotic, such as silver sulfadiazine, changed twice daily. Again, the wound should be gently washed to remove any nonviable tissue and exudate (Table 7-10).

## Deep Second to Third Degree Burn

Initial nonsurgical management is primarily that of daily debridement along with twice daily application of a water-soluble topical antibiotic. Silver sulfadiazine is the agent of first choice unless there is evidence of a wound infection, in which case mafenide would be a consideration. As with the superficial wound, gentle washing with a dilute chlorhexidine solution is indicated with at least one of the two dressing changes. Simple reapplication of the topical agent is usually done with the evening change. After washing, any devitalized tissue should be removed. A more vigorous attempt at eschar removed, with scissors and forceps removal of loose eschar, is required compared with the more superficial burn. Sharp dissection at this stage is reserved more for the full-thickness injury because exposure of any underlying viable dermis can lead to desiccation and conversion to a deeper injury.

The full-thickness burn requires a more aggressive paring down of the eschar to allow better penetration of the topical agent if early excision and wound closure are not going to be initiated. The wound is less vascular during this period, and therefore significant blood loss is less likely than during a later period. This process of eschar shaving is known as "sequential tangential excision." A Goulian dermatome and Weck blade is ideal for shaving down the eschar. Thin layers of eschar are removed using the guards on the dermatome, which allow depths of .008 to 0.020 thousandths of an inch. Excision should not be carried down into viable bleeding tissue, but rather a thin layer of eschar should be left to protect underlying viable tissue. Viable tissue should not be exposed unless it is to be occluded by a graft or a skin substitute because desiccation of the tissue with reformation of eschar is likely to occur. The thin eschar can be penetrated by the topical agents. This procedure can be performed at the bedside or on a slant board in a hydrotherapy tank, avoiding total body immersion. A simple bed bath setup using a sterile field and clean basins of wash and rinse wash and rinse solution is ideal. This bedside approach is particularly useful for the patient with invasive catheters in place where contact with water, as in a hydrotherapy tank, would increase the risk of contamination. Low-dose ketamine, 4 to 5 mg/kg intramuscularly, can be used if the patient is not intubated and there is a concern about respiratory depression. Narcotics in moderately high doses can be used for this procedure if the patient is intubated. Impregnation of the topical antibiotics on fine mesh gauze improves the surface eschar debridement because some adherence to the underlying eschar occurs that debrides loose tissue when the gauze is removed.

Although infection is not particularly common in the first several days postburn (unless the burn was heavily contaminated or inadequately cleaned), the wound bacterial

**Table 7-10** Specific Principles of Daily Burn Care For a Superficial Second Degree Burn

Aggressively Remove Loose Epidermis, Blisters, etc. in First Days

| *Areas Covered with Temporary Skin Substitutes* | *Areas Covered with Grease Gauze* | *Areas Treated Open with Bacitracin* | *Areas Treated with Topical Antibiotics (Silver Sulfadiazine)* |
|---|---|---|---|
| 1. Change outer dry gauze covering daily to remove collected exudate<br>2. Roll out small pockets of exudate from beneath substitute<br>3. Can leave open without dressing once drainage has ceased<br>4. Remove skin substitute if exudate extensive or if nonadherent and switch to grease gauze method or topical antibiotic if infection considered | 1. Inspect daily<br>2. If gauze adherent and no exudate, simply change outer dry gauze<br>3. Change dressing, wash surface and reapply if exudate present<br>4. Use topical antibiotic if infection considered | 1. Reapply two to three times daily<br>2. Gently wash off crusts, exudate, especially on face and neck | 1. Usually perineum, buttock area or wound with dirt, tar debris still present<br>2. Change twice daily, wash and debridge once daily and simply reapply the topical agent at the second change |

**Table 7-11** Specific Principles of Daily Burn Care for Deep Second and Third Degree Burns

Daily Washing and Debridement Along with Twice Daily Application of Topical Antibiotics

*Deep Second Degree Burn*

1. Debride loose eschar after washing wound surface (Exception: Plans for early excision and graft)
2. Avoid exposing viable dermis with sharp dissection as desiccation can then occur
3. Closely observe for evidence of conversion or subeschar pockets of exudate
4. If present: Unroof pockets and biopsy wound for assessment of invasive infection
5. If present: Consider changing topical agent to mafenide in involved areas and begin systemic antibiotics

*Third Degree Burn*

1. Daily wash and debride loose eschar
2. Shave down thick eschar with sharp dissection (sequential tangential excision), avoiding excision to viable tissue
3. Closely observe for evidence of subeschar pockets of exudate
4. Unroof pockets and biopsy wound to determine presence of infection necessitating systemic antibiotics
5. If present, consider changing topical agent to mafenide along with removal of overlying eschar

flora should be monitored with surface cultures. The information on the organisms present will assist in the assessment of the adequacy of the topical agent being used as well as provide epidemiologic information, especially important in controlling resistant hospital-based organisms (Table 7-11).

# 8
# Early Wound Excision and Grafting

Early excision and grafting should be considered as a treatment option for all burns that will not heal by primary intention within 3 weeks. Full-thickness burns will by definition require grafting unless smaller than 3 to 4 cm in diameter. The more rapidly the wound is closed, the better. Burns less than 30% of total body surface can be, at least theoretically, rapidly closed because adequate donor sites are available. Larger burns will be more difficult, if not impossible, to completely graft early. Deep partial thickness burns are also difficult to assess clearly as to time of healing. Considerable judgment and assessment skills are therefore essential for this approach to yield optimal results.

The topics to be discussed in this chapter include both the indications and the general and specific techniques used.

> General Principles of Early Excision
> Types of Surgical Excision
> > Tangential (Sequential) Excision
> > Excision to Fascia
> 
> Obtaining Skin Grafts (Donor Sites)
> Grafting and Dressing the Wound
> Surgical Approach Based on Burn Size
> Management of Specific Burn Areas

## GENERAL PRINCIPLES OF EARLY EXCISION

There are two key judgments that are required. The first is determination of cardiopulmonary stability and operative risk. The second is the judgment as to the potential morbidity of the wound itself if not rapidly closed. This judgment takes into consideration wound depth, functional loss, and the risk of the inflammatory wound on the host. Thus, the *key judgments as to role of excision* are:

1. Cardiopulmonary stability and operative risk
2. Magnitude of burn injury considering depth, area involved, potential morbidity of allowing wound inflammation to occur

The first judgment, weighing risk versus benefit, requires considerable experience and an in-depth knowledge of the resources to be used. The resources consist not only of the operative team, but also the anesthesiologist who must be experienced in the anesthetic management of the burn patient. Of extreme importance is an experienced team to manage the patient and the wound in the postoperative period. Any significant complications in an already severely compromised patient is apt to lead to severe morbidity or mortality. The second judgment also requires considerable experience in defining what the risk is of not excising the wound. One must project ahead 7 to 10 days as to the ability of the patient to tolerate intense wound inflammation, infection, and hypermetabolism. A key component of this assessment is defining wound depth, i.e., what will heal and what will not heal. The following *facts which can aid in decision-making:*

1. Infants and the elderly tolerate burn inflammation and infection poorly.
2. Burns in infants and the elderly are usually deep.
3. Pulmonary dysfunction from smoke inhalation will be accentuated by burn-induced hypermetabolism, inflammation, and infection.
4. Burns tend to get deeper over the first several days as a result of necrosis of ischemic areas.
5. Burns caused by direct contact with flames, hot grease, chemicals, or electricity are invariably deeper than first appearances would suggest.
6. Burns on the low back, scalp, palms, and soles usually have sufficient remaining dermis to allow primary healing in 3 to 5 weeks.
7. Small burns that are deep dermal or even full thickness are not life-threatening, and therefore, there is much more flexibility as to timing of surgery based on the risks to the patient.
8. Large full-thickness burns are life-threatening until closed.
9. Large burns, which are mostly superficial with small scattered components of deeper injury (2 to 3 cm in diameter), usually heal satisfactorily by primary intention and excisional therapy for the deep areas.

There are a number of general principles that apply to all methods of excision and grafting. The *first* is that the patient must be hemodynamically stable before considering excision. Pulmonary function can be impaired, but the patient must be able to be safely moved to the operating room and back, preferably using a portable ventilator. An alternative solution is to perform the procedure in a special procedure room in or near the burn unit. *Second,* the potential for significant blood loss must be recognized and adequate amounts of red cells, plasma, and platelets, if indicated, be available before starting treatment. Preoperative planning should also include systemic perioperative antibiotics considering the burn at this stage to be a clean but contaminated wound. The initial organisms of concern are gram positive; therefore a first generation cephalosporin is usually the drug of choice. The *third* principle is that patient transport and movement can be very dangerous and must be carefully performed. One of the major risks of anesthesia and surgery during this period relates to patient movement:

*Major risks*

1. Transport to and from the operating room
2. Movement to and from bed to the operating table
3. Positioning on the operating table

Movement to and from the controlled intensive care unit environment results in potential risks to cardiopulmonary stability. The ideal system is the use of a portable ventilator if the patient requires mechanical ventilator support. If not available, the pulmonary function of the patient on the mechanical ventilator should be matched as closely as possible using an Ambu bag. Hypo- or hyperventilation may result which can lead to major blood gas abnormalities during the 10- to 15-minute transport time. Obviously, performing the procedure in a burn unit operating room, assuming that a complete operating room is present, is ideal, but is not practical except for very large units. Pulse oximetry has improved the safety of transfer by allowing a continuous measure of oxygen saturation. Hypercapnia is a potential problem in that the increasing ventilatory requirements are frequently underestimated by transporting personnel. The ideal system is the use of a portable ventilator matching the settings used in the patient's room. Movement to and from the patient's bed runs a major risk of displacing tubes and lines. It is difficult to secure tubes and lines with tape or sutures because of the burn itself, the burn exudate, and the use of topical agents. Accidental endotracheal extubation could be fatal in the patient with deep burns to the face and neck. Although less risky but still a problem is positioning for the surgical procedure. Movement after the procedure runs the risk of dislodging skin grafts and dressings.

A solution to the movement problem is to perform the operative procedure in the patient's own bed. This can be done very easily in the standard bed, kinetic bed, air bed, etc. Two plastic sheets placed from top to bottom, each covering half of the bed, are placed beneath the patient before movement to the operating room. Beneath the sheets can be placed an elastic dressing pinned to the corners of the bed as well as clean gauze dressings. These can be used for a circumferential dressing to hold on flank, chest, abdominal, and buttock grafts, etc. When the procedure is completed, the plastic sheets can be removed from side to side along with debris, blood clots, etc. The clean dressings beneath are now available for wrapping around the patient. The intensive care unit or general floor patient bed is also wider than the operating room table and therefore easier for positioning. In addition, a traction frame can be fixed to the bed for elevation of extremities, etc., rather than having to suspend traction from the operating room ceiling.

The *fourth* principle is that major pulmonary abnormalities in the burn patient can be readily accentuated with general anesthesia if preplanned safeguards are not initiated. Adjustments in management of anesthesia must be made based on a clear understanding of these changes. Pulmonary support is a major problem as patient's oxygen consumption and carbon dioxide production began to increase. Stiff lungs and increased dead space often require special mechanical ventilatory needs, which must be prepared for and met in the operating room. These include the needs for providing positive end-expiratory pressure (PEEP) and increased minute ventilation. The anesthesiologist must also recognize the restrictive component to ventilation caused by a chest wall burn and the burn edema. Chest wall compliance will be significantly decreased.

The *fifth* principle is that hypothermia must be avoided during surgery. The operating room and fluids used must be warmed to avoid severe hypothermia, a major hazard, particularly if coagulation is as crucial as it is with excisional techniques. The operating room temperature should be maintained between 75 and 85°F. The *sixth* principle is that the stress induced by anesthesia and surgery must be limited to that which the patient can safely tolerate. The time in the operating room should be carefully controlled, again to minimize hypothermia and to minimize postoperative risks because the major burn patient is a potentially very unstable patient. It is better to do several moderate operative procedures 1 or 2 days apart than one massive procedure. The exception is children, i.e., older than 5 years old, who tolerate large excision procedures much better than adults. A reasonable operating time limit, including anesthesia, is 2 hours. A shorter period is indicated for elderly or compromised patients. Total blood loss per procedure should be restricted to avoid development of a coagulopathy. Blood loss should not exceed 60% of estimated total blood volume at any one operation. One can stay within this limit if appropriate timing is used and attention is paid to hemostasis during the procedure. Two operating teams, working simultaneously, are required with large excisions. One team is responsible for obtaining the skin grafts and maintaining hemostasis from the donor site. The other team is responsible for excising the wound, maintaining hemostasis, and closing the wound. Donor blood is dwindling in quantity and therefore attempts at minimizing blood loss are mandatory.

The *seventh* principle is that blood loss should be replaced with blood products rather than crystalloid in the major burn patient. The patient already has massive edema and red cell production will be markedly depressed until the wound is healed, especially in a massive burn. It is therefore unrealistic to assume that red blood cell mass will quickly return to baseline by increased production. In fact, a significant anemia will occur postburn without added external losses due to decreased red blood cell lifespan and decreased production. Large fluid shifts and a potential for hypervolemia are occurring at this time and therefore replacement of blood loss with an equal amount of blood products minimizes the risk of under- or overshooting replacement. Adequate monitoring of cardiopulmonary function is essential. Frequently, there is decreased availability of monitoring sites and therefore urine output, acid-base balance, body temperature, and electrocardiogram may be the only available monitors. Filling pressures at this stage will usually remain low to normal even with adequate perfusion, because a leak is still present. An increase in filling pressures indicates excessive volume or heart failure. The patient may well be mobilizing edema fluid. An assessment of blood loss must be done by the surgeon with experience in this determination, for much of the loss can be hidden from the anesthesiologist. Continued communication is necessary. A short anesthesia period is another safety valve in cases in which monitoring is marginal.

The choice of anesthetic agents is dependent on a number of variables. An inhalation agent can be used if an element of cardiac depression can be tolerated. Nitrous oxide and a narcotic is another very useful technique. The required dose of the narcotic is usually quite high, given the tolerance that develops with continued use for dressing changes. Narcotic anesthesia is usually used in patients who will remain on the ventilator at least for 12 to 24 hours postoperation. New donor sites will result in a significant increase in pain. Ketamine is another useful and very commonly used agent, especially in patients in whom maintenance of spontaneous ventilation is preferred. An increase in oxygen consumption will occur with ketamine due to increased sympathetic activity. Bad dreams and excitation are common problems seen in the postoperative period. Addition of diazepam attenuates the hyperexcitability caused by the ketamine.

It is also important to recognize that the tissue oxygen demands return to and often transiently exceed the demand before anesthesia. The wound inflammation can magnify any blood flow redistribution caused by general anesthesia, leading to an oxygen debt.

Carbon dioxide production also increases dramatically in the early postoperative period as opposed to the nonburn patient. Any hypothermia will initiate an extreme catechol release as well as increased caloric expenditure to generate the heat required by the hypothalamic temperature regulatory center. It is therefore best for the major burn patient to return to the burn unit rather than be placed in the recovery room because of the temperature-controlled environment in the unit.

Timing of excision relative to changes in the wound itself is crucial to minimize risks. Blood flow to the burn wound is markedly increased beginning several days after injury and peaking between 5 and 14 days. The increasing blood flow, which parallels the development of wound inflammation, is present in the viable tissue beneath the eschar. A significant increase in blood loss should be expected with wound excisions after 5 to 6 days. Clotting abnormalities at this stage will be a major problem.

In addition, colonization of the wound develops during the first week and manipulation of the colonized or infected wound runs an increasing risk of bacteremia. Because of these facts, the size of the planned excision must be determined based on a clear understanding of increasing risks of blood loss and bacteremias (Table 8-1).

## TYPES OF SURGICAL EXCISION

There are two types of surgical procedures to remove the eschar: tangential excision and excision to fascia. There are also several types of grafts and dressing techniques, which will be described.

### Tangential (Sequential) Excision

The principle is to excise the wound in thin layers using a blade held at a very acute angle with the skin surface. The objective is to remove only the nonviable tissue, sparing, in particular, as much viable dermis as possible in the case of the deep dermal burn. The dermis contains the elasticity in skin. In addition, the viable dermal surface is an excellent base for grafting. Fat is a less attractive bed for skin grafting because of decreased vascularity as well as the difficulty of determining viable fat on inspection Table 8-2).

The excision is performed with a hand-held dermatome using guards of variable thickness (0.008 to 0.020 inch) to help control depth of excision (Figs. 8-1, 8-2, 8-3; color plates 9, 10, page 315). A back and forth motion is utilized for cutting with very little forward force (Fig. 8-4). Control of depth is based not only on the gauge of the guard, but also on the angle of the blade in relation to the surface. A sharp blade is needed for this approach, and frequent blade changes are required. A Goulian or a Watson knife is used, depending on the area being excised. The Watson, being larger, is used for larger flatter surfaces, whereas the Goulian is used over curvilinear areas, e.g., over bony prominences or on fingers, toes, neck, and, occasionally, face. Excision over bony surfaces can be aided by injecting saline beneath the eschar to flatten and push the wound surface away from the bone. The endpoint of excision is brisk punctate bleeding and a completely viable wound base. Viable dermis is white and shiny in color. One or two large bleeders can make the wound look red, so careful inspection and considerable experience is needed to assess the adequacy of the wound bed. Injured fat is particularly difficult to diagnose. Any fat that is dark yellowish-brown in color should be removed. Healthy fat is light yellowish in color and shiny (Color plate 11, page 316). It is easy to underexcise, leaving a poor bed for graft take. In addition, it is easy to excise too much tissue, thereby removing potentially viable dermis. Overexcision would be particularly detrimental if done on hands, neck, or face, or over joint surfaces. It is very difficult to detect accurately the proper endpoint of this technique using tourniquets to control bleeding and therefore tourniquets are usually not used. Blood loss can then be a major problem and rapid control of bleeding is of critical importance. The procedure must be approached with this fact in mind. Timing of the procedure is therefore very important. The burn wound becomes very hypervascular beginning 3 to 5 days postinjury, with blood flow peaking at 7 to 14 days. Tangential excision of large burns should be attempted either *before* 5 days, i.e., onset of hypervascularity, or after a layer of granulation tissue has formed, when the grafts are applied on the granulation tissue itself. Between this time, only small body surface areas can be excised using this approach due to the risk of massive blood loss.

The procedure itself should be performed by excising small burn areas at a time (150 to 300 $cm^2$), controlling hemostasis in each excised area before continuing on to other areas. Usually, a maximum of 18 to 25% of total body surface can be excised at one time. Normally, this much is only feasibly excised on the first operation if done 1 to 3 days postburn. Later excisions are usually limited to 9% total body surface or less because of blood loss. The punctate bleeding from dermal vessels is best stopped by application of the skin graft, especially if meshed 1.5 to 1. The exposed collagen on the dermal surface of the graft stimulates hemostasis. Granulation tissue is composed of masses of small capillaries that will bleed when abraded but the bleeding is punctate and usually stops with pressure. The vessels just beneath the surface, feeding the granulating bed, have dramatically increased in size, compared with normal subdermal vessels. The addition of pressure for 2 to 3 minutes substantially diminishes the bleeding. Other approaches include application of topical thrombin or a solution of 1/10,000 epinephrine. If epinephrine or thrombin is used, one must be assured of the adequacy of the wound bed before their application, since bleeding ceases, making a subsequent assessment very difficult. Microcrystalline collagen can also be applied, but a coagulum is left on the wound surface, which should be removed before graft placement. Larger vessels, particularly those encountered with excision to fat, need to be individually cauterized or suture ligated. Bleeding is much more difficult to control within the fatty tissue layer because severed vessels retract into the tissue. Because skin graft application is an effective hemostatic agent, grafts should be taken before beginning the excision. This sequence also allows for control of bleeding from the donor sites before beginning the excision.

Once the wound is excised, the wound bed must be closed. Usually, immediate application of skin grafts is performed. The mesh, used with tangential excision, is usually no greater than 1.5 to 1 to avoid any excessive exposure of viable tissue, especially fat, which can then desiccate and form new eschar. A temporary skin substitute is required if a wider mesh is used or if an area is excised and not grafted. Any neighboring burn must continue to be treated with an antibacterial agent.

The advantages and disadvantages of tangential excision are listed in Table 8-3.

**Table 8-1** General Principles of Excision

### Anesthesia Considerations

#### Preexcision
1. Patient must be hemodynamically stable
2. Adequate blood products must be available, the amount determined by the procedure planned
3. Perioperative antibiotics are indicated; first choice is first generation cephalosporin

#### Airway
1. Depolarizing muscle relaxants contraindicated
2. Consider awake intubation with local anesthesia
3. Carefully secure tube

#### Maintain Ventilatory Needs
1. Peep to maintain functional residual capacity and decreased shunt, especially after inhalation injury
2. Maintain necessary minute ventilation (may exceed 25 L)
3. Modify equipment as needed preoperatively
4. Increased oxygen and carbon dioxide consumption must also be provided during transport

#### Choice of Agent
1. Inhalation agent although usually satisfactory is usually not the agent of choice for repeated procedures
2. Nitrous narcotic very useful, but consider increased narcotic tolerance when dosing patient and consider that postoperative ventilatory assist may be needed
3. Ketamine plus mild sedation useful for patients who cannot tolerate further cardiovascular instability

## Adequate Monitoring

May need to use more noninvasive methods: Oximeter and end-tidal carbon dioxide, if catheter sites not available

## Hemodynamic Stability

1. Have blood in the room before starting
2. Give blood products for blood loss
3. Give crystalloid only for evaporative losses

## Maintain Temperature

1. Warm room >80°F
2. Warm fluids

## Surgery Considerations

1. Timing is crucial relative to safety of the procedure (early excision means less blood loss)
2. Limit operative and anesthesia time to 2 hours
3. Limit blood loss to less than 60% of total blood volume
4. Consider performing procedure with patient in unit bed rather than moving to operating room table

**Table 8-2** Tangential (Sequential) Surgical Excision

*Indications and Timing*
1. Deep dermal or full thickness (small to moderate in size)
2. Very early (1 to 5 days) or very late (granulation tissue)

*Technique*

| Excision | Hemostasis | Coverage |
|---|---|---|
| 1. Thin slices (0.008 to 0.012 inch) Goulian or Watson dermatome | 1. Pressure followed by cautery or ligature of major bleeders followed by immediate application of mesh graft | 1. Meshed graft 1.5 to 1 is the best |
| 2. Back and forth motion with depth controlled by guard and angle of blade to skin surface | | 2. Sheet grafts: face, neck |
| 3. Endpoint: white shiny dermis or light yellow shiny fat along with brisk bleeding | 2. Additional treatment includes use of epinephrine 1:10,000 or topical thrombin or wound surface | 3. Wide mesh (3:1) is used only in case of limited donors |
| 4. Excise 150 to 300 $cm^2$, stop and control bleeding before continuing | | 4. Skin substitute on nongrafted excised wound or when wide mesh is used |
| 5. Be careful about under- or overexcision | | |
| 6. Maximum excision 18% total body surface, days 1 to 3 and 9 to 10% total body surface beyond day 3 | | |

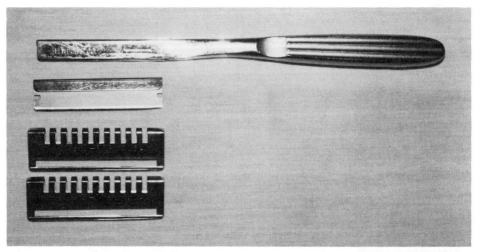

**Figure 8–1.** Goulian dermatome with different guards and Weck blade, used for excisions on small areas.

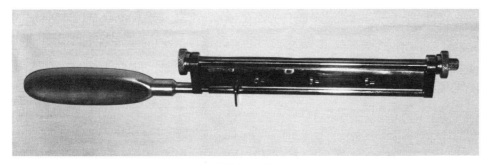

**Figure 8–2.** A Watson dermatome is shown, which is used for larger excisions.

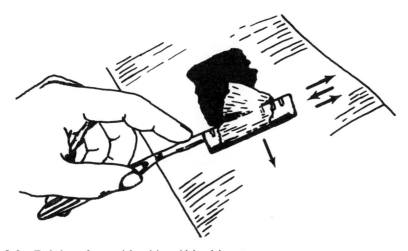

**Figure 8–3.** Technique of tangential excision with hand dermatome.

## Excision to Fascia

Excision of the burn wound to fascia is used in cases of very large full-thickness burns or with small deep burns that extend well into the fat or underlying tissues (Table 8-4). This approach is used in the large burn with limited donors for the following reasons. *First*, the endpoint of excision is well defined and graft take is always excellent. Therefore less

**Table 8-3** Tangential Excision

| |
|---|
| Advantages |
|     Optimal functional and cosmetic result |
|     Can be performed rapidly |
| Disadvantages |
|     Large blood loss |
|     Difficult endpoint to define |
|     Easy to excise too much or too little |
|     Need more donor skin for coverage |

**Table 8-4** Excision to Fascia

*Technique*

*Indications and Timing*
1. Large full-thickness burns
2. Smaller burns if extending well below dermis
3. Very early (1 to 7 days) postburn

*Excision*
1. Extends to fascial layer using sharp dissection, tension, and cautery
2. Be careful to avoid injury to major nerves
3. Do not expose fascia over joints or expose tendons, leave some soft tissue behind
4. Taper edges and suture approximate to fascia at edges
5. Limit excision to ≤20% total body surface on first excision, with much less area on subsequent excisions

*Hemostasis*
1. Pressure, cautery, and ligatures of larger vessels
2. Punctate bleeding not encountered unless excision is done late

*Coverage*
1. Meshed grafts 1.5 or 3:1
2. Cover wide mesh or ungrafted areas with skin substitute: Biobrane, cadaver, pigskin
3. Suture skin substitute to skin edge

experience is required to define an adequately excised wound surface. *Second,* wide meshed skin grafts can be used because the fascia appears to be less vulnerable to desiccation than fat or dermis when covered with a skin substitute. *Third,* a large excision, when performed early, can be done in most body areas (exception being the face and perineum) with only modest blood loss. In the case of the very deep small wound, excision to this depth or deeper is required because of the extent of the injury itself. It can take weeks for a third degree burn to slough the eschar spontaneously and develop a granulation tissue bed.

Excision is performed using a combination of sharp dissection, constant tension, and electric cautery. The vessels encountered at the fascial plane are fewer in number and larger in size and are much easier to control with cautery and ligatures. If performed in the first several days, the edema fluid separates fascia from overlying subcutaneous tissue, making excision very easy. The major bleeding occurs from the wound edge. This bleeding can often be better controlled and the exposure of fat on the wound edge minimized if the skin edge is sutured to the fascia. This form of marsupialization can also decrease the total size of the wound as the edges are pulled toward the middle. Excision of up to 18% of body surface can be performed with 1 to 2 U of blood loss. Total excision per operation should be limited to 18 to 20% of total body surface. Tourniquets are also applicable in cases of extremity excision, especially if delayed for several days, because the endpoint is an anatomic one rather than punctate bleeding.

Fascial excision becomes less feasible with time after injury. The reabsorption of edema over 5 to 7 days and the increase in wound blood flow increases the difficulty and risks. Beyond 7 days when the eschar is heavily colonized and the subeschar space is infected, fascial excision can be very dangerous. Complications of bleeding and septicemia will be much higher with time postburn. It is important to remember that this procedure is usually performed on large burns, and therefore patients tend to be at greater risk for perioperative problems.

There are number of disadvantages to this approach that must be outweighed by the advantages (Table 8-5). The major disadvantage is a potential impairment in long-term function to the excised and grafted areas, especially extremities. Distal edema becomes a problem because of removal of superficial veins and lymphatics. However, in many cases they have already been heat destroyed. In addition, removal of cutaneous nerves will lead to impaired sensation, although sensation on any skin graft is decreased compared with normal skin. There is, however, a significant risk of injury to other superficial nerves that

**Table 8-5** Excision to Fascia

Advantages
    Can be done rapidly with much less blood loss
    Well-defined endpoint of excision
    Can be done using tourniquets
    Can use wide mesh grafts
    Can readily excise areas and cover with skin substitute

Disadvantages
    Risk of injury to nerves
    Risk of increasing distal edema
    Risk of exposing joints, tendons
    Cosmetic defect

have motor function. In addition, exposure of the relatively avascular fascia near joints along with potential exposure of tendons will result in a nongraftable surface that is now prone to desiccation. Coverage of this area becomes a major problem. Because of this problem, some soft tissues are left behind over joints to cover tendons and protect the joint itself. Mesh grafts or skin substitutes are applied in these areas. The second problem of fascial excision is cosmetic, since a rim of tissue remains at the edge of the excised and nonexcised tissue producing a balloonlike effect, especially on the extremities. Tapering of the excision at its endpoints can help decrease this problem. Fat normally does not regenerate between fascia and skin grafts; therefore the cosmetic defect is persistent, particularly in the obese patient. Frequently, a combination of fascial and tangential excision is used in the patient to maximize benefits of early wound closure and minimize complications. Excellent graft take and reliability of excision endpoint outweighs these disadvantages in the massive burn.

Once excised, the fascial surface must be covered. Since donor sites are usually limited unless the wound is small, 3 to 1 meshed grafts are used (Color plate 12, page 316). Skin substitutes, either biobrane or cadaver skin, are very effective in occluding the fascial wound until the mesh fills in (7 to 10 days) or until new donor sites become available with rehealing (10 to 14 days). The biobrane, pigskin, or cadaver skin can be sutured to the remaining skin edge using a continuous running suture. The skin substitute should also be tacked down to the fascia with through and through sutures spaced every several inches, at least until adherence has occurred.

Two operating teams are required for large excisions in order to diminish blood loss with careful control while expediting the procedure.

## OBTAINING SKIN GRAFTS (DONOR SITES)

Donor sites are obtained wherever unburned skin is available (exception: face, hands). Preferred areas are thighs, buttocks, and abdomen. However, large burns have limited donors and other areas need to be used, e.g., arms, lower legs, back, and soles of feet. Split-thickness skin can also be removed from the chest. One has, however, to recognize that impaired chest expansion will result secondary to pain and the tight healing wound. The scalp is an excellent donor site when needed. As opposed to most other areas that require 14 days or more to heal sufficiently before reuse, scalp heals in 7 days and can be reharvested 3 to 4 times. The only area in which color match between donor and recipient site is of significant concern is the face and neck. Upper chest, upper back, and scalp are a good color match for face and neck. Split-thickness skin can be removed using a variety of dermatomes. Air pressure driven or electric powered dermatomes are the most common. Free hand skin grafts can also be obtained using the Goulian or Watson, a dermatome used for tangential excision.

The best instrument for obtaining the skin graft is an electric Pagett. A Brown dermatome is also commonly used, but is not as good. The length and width of the graft obtained will be dictated by the width of the dermatome guard, the dimensions of the donor area, and whether meshing is to be used. The plastic board used for the standard Tanner mesh unit is a standard length and width (8 by 3 inches). Injection of saline beneath the dermis will greatly assist the removal of split-thickness skin from areas around changes in contour or from the scalp.

Graft thickness is dependent on the size of the burn and the potential need for reharvesting the same donor site, the area to be grafted, and the donor site to be used. The ideal thickness for most areas to be grafted is 0.012 inch for the adult. Slightly thicker grafts (0.012 to 0.014 inch) would be ideal for face, neck, hands, and over joints because less scarring and more pliability would be anticipated for a thicker graft that contains more dermis. A donor site 0.012 inch will require approximately 10 to 14 days to reepithelialize and about 21 days or longer before it can be used again. A second use of this area will be limited because of concern over producing a full-thickness injury. A donor site where a thick graft is obtained usually cannot be used again. A thinner donor site, 0.010 inch, will often be ready for reuse in 14 days where another graft of 0.01 inch thickness can be obtained. Since fewer epidermal cells are present with a reuse donor, a less wide mesh is usually used. Skin graft thickness is also dependent on the thickness of the donor skin. Children and elderly patients have a thinner dermis and therefore a thinner graft, i.e., 0.008 to 0.010 inch, is usually obtained to avoid major morbidity at the donor site. In addition, areas such as inner arms and legs have thinner skin, and adjustments need to be made in the dermatome when obtaining skin grafts from these areas.

Bleeding from a donor site is similar in amount to that of tangential excision of a fresh, deep dermal burn, i.e., diffuse, punctate, and profuse. Bleeding from a reuse donor is even more profuse and again an analogy can be made with tangential excision of a hyperemic wound. Because blood loss will be substantial, hemostasis at the donor site should be controlled before pursuing wound excision. The ideal situation is the use of two teams, one whose role is to obtain skin grafts and maintain hemostasis. Pressure followed by application of fine mesh gauze or Xeroform gauze, again followed by pressure (1 to 2 minutes), is usually adequate to control bleeding. As with the excised wound, topical thrombin or dilute epinephrine solution can also be used.

A number of dressings can be used on donor sites. Fine mesh or grease gauze is porous and allows the initial bleeding to exit from the wound surface as well as the exit of blood and plasma that leak during the postoperative period. Gauze, however, is not flexible and is not sufficiently occlusive to control pain. In fact, ambulation or motion is very difficult with donor sites covered with these dressings. In addition, there are minimal to no antibacterial properties, increasing the potential for infection if nearly open burn wounds are present. Application of moist antibiotic-moistened gauze over the Xeroform for 24 to 48 hours assists in removal of blood beneath the dressing as well as provides antibacterial protection. Dilute bacitracin, neomycin, or mafenide solutions have been used with success. After 2 to 3 days, the donor site should be left exposed and the dressing allowed to dry. The exception would be if an open wound is adjacent, in which case the antibacterial solution should continue or the wound should be occluded from nearby burn. Gauze dressings are applied over the donor site covered by an outer moderate compression dressing to maintain hemostasis. The outer dressings are changed daily until the wound can be exposed to air. Grease gauze impregnated with antibacterial ointment, e.g., scarlet red, provides some protection against infection, but it also impairs removal of clot or exudate because of the multiple layers of gauze used. An effective alternative dressing is a skin substitute, such as biobrane or polyurethane dressing such as Opsito. The skin substitute will provide a seal, thereby eliminating the risk of external infection as well as diminishing pain. In addition, biobrane is flexible, thereby improving efforts at motion and ambulation. Disadvantages, however, are that excellent hemostasis must be obtained before application. In addition, these dressings have no antibacterial properties. This is less of a problem with biobrane if adherence to the wound is good. Dry dressings and moderate compression maintain hemostasis while allowing optimum wound adherence over the first 24 to 48 hours. The inner donor site dressing is gradually removed at 10 to 14 days with reepithelialization.

A number of complications can occur in the donor site. Infection can occur, which can result in deepening and possibly conversion of the wound to full thickness. Infection is usually evident from surrounding cellulitis. Systemic antibiotics as well as topical antibiotics are required for treatment. Blistering and continued breakdown are also seen, especially with deep donors or donors in small children or the elderly. Healing usually occurs in time. Hyper- or hypopigmentation may persist for long periods of time and may be permanent. Hypertrophic scarring is seen, especially in dark-skinned persons and with deep donor sites (Table 8-6).

## GRAFTING AND DRESSING THE WOUND

### Skin Graft Placement

It is best to place grafts on the wound at the time of excision. Since the graft itself controls hemostasis and protects the wound, it makes little sense to wait 24 to 48 hours until bleeding has stopped. This approach requires an additional procedure and there is a significant risk of the wound bed becoming desiccated or reinfected.

The skin grafts are best handled by placing the dermis side up on a mesh board. Even if skin meshing is not going to be performed, a number of small slits should be placed along the skin lines to allow efflux of any blood or plasma that collects. Leave meshed skin on the mesh board until ready to use to keep the interstices flat. Grafts are best placed longitudinally in most areas and transversely across the joints to match the normal skin lines and forces during movement. Lay the mesh board on the excised surface skin dermis side down and then peel it off the board directly onto the wound surface. It is better to have a slight overlap of skin on the wound rather than to leave excised wound uncovered. Hypertrophic scarring will result and most evident at the edges of the graft, especially if a ridge of open wound is left to heal primarily. The plastic mesh board is also a good surface for cutting the skin to conform to difficult wound shapes. A heavy scissors can easily cut the plastic board and graft. It is important to avoid the edges of the graft from rolling up, thereby preventing skin adherence in this area. Adjacent grafts should be carefully approximated. Sutures can be used but are very time consuming. Staples or Steri-strips usually work very well.

### Dressing the Excised Wound

The dressing applied over the grafted area must accomplish two goals. First, it must protect the graft from environmental insults, in particular desiccation and avulsion as well as infection. Infection is most likely to develop from nearby areas of open wound. Secondly, the dressing must immobilize the area and allow graft vascularization to occur, i.e., graft take. To summarize, the *role of dressing* is as follows:

1. Must control environmental hazards especially desiccation and avulsion, and
2. Must immobilize the grafted area

**Table 8-6** Donor Sites

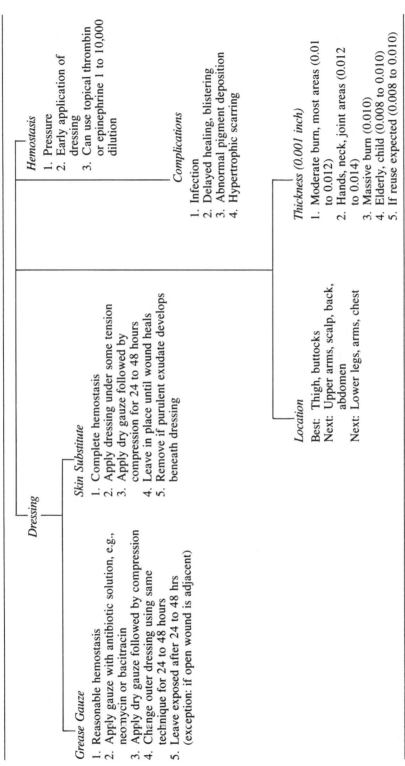

*Dressing*

*Grease Gauze*
1. Reasonable hemostasis
2. Apply gauze with antibiotic solution, e.g., neomycin or bacitracin
3. Apply dry gauze followed by compression
4. Change outer dressing using same technique for 24 to 48 hours
5. Leave exposed after 24 to 48 hrs (exception: if open wound is adjacent)

*Skin Substitute*
1. Complete hemostasis
2. Apply dressing under some tension
3. Apply dry gauze followed by compression for 24 to 48 hours
4. Leave in place until wound heals
5. Remove if purulent exudate develops beneath dressing

*Hemostasis*
1. Pressure
2. Early application of dressing
3. Can use topical thrombin or epinephrine 1 to 10,000 dilution

*Complications*
1. Infection
2. Delayed healing, blistering
3. Abnormal pigment deposition
4. Hypertrophic scarring

*Location*
Best: Thigh, buttocks
Next: Upper arms, scalp, back, abdomen
Next: Lower legs, arms, chest

*Thickness (0.001 inch)*
1. Moderate burn, most areas (0.01 to 0.012)
2. Hands, neck, joint areas (0.012 to 0.014)
3. Massive burn (0.010)
4. Elderly, child (0.008 to 0.010)
5. If reuse expected (0.008 to 0.010)

Sheet grafts can be managed in two ways. The most common is the application of grease gauze (Xeroform) or fine meshed gauze followed by dry gauze and moderate compression. Grafts can also be left open if there is no exposed wound not grafted. This approach is best used on face and neck. The exposure method has limited use in other areas, since the grafted area needs to be immobilized in some fashion. The usual method of immobolization is the use of a firmly placed gauze dressing followed by a compression dressing and splint. Skeletal traction can also be used, although this method is usually not necessary and further hampers patient mobility, which should be initiated in 3 to 4 days.

There are a number of techniques used for dressing mesh grafts, depending on the size of the mesh and the area grafted. A 1.5 to 1 mesh is best managed by application of a single layer of grease gauze or fine mesh gauze followed by gauze moistened in an antibiotic solution. The most common solutions used are bacitracin, 25,000 U, or neomycin (0.1 to 1 g/L of saline). Any combination of antibiotics in solution can be used. However, it must be remembered that some absorption will occur, so there needs to be concern for potential toxicity. Povidone-iodine solution is a drying agent and should not be used initially to cover new skin grafts. The advantages of the antibiotic solution are to: (1) help remove blood and wound exudate from beneath the graft by acting as a wick; (2) protect the area between the mesh from desiccation; and (3) protect the skin graft from bacteria in any adjacent ungrafted wound. A cream base antibacterial will lead to further wound inflammation and graft maceration and is not indicated for initial protection. The inner gauze dressing can be kept moist by placing several soft rubber catheters above the gauze through which the solution can be injected every 8 to 12 hours. An outer dry gauze dressing is then applied, followed by a compression dressing. The grafted area needs to be immobilized. A nearby joint can be immobilized using a fabricated splint or a soft splint, such as a pillow wrapped around the extremity with an elastic bandage. The outer gauze dressings should be changed daily to remove blood and exudate. The burn wound is contaminated and should be managed like a contaminated wound rather than completely occluded for any prolonged period. The innermost grease gauze dressing is usually left in place for 3 to 5 days before changing.

Wide meshed grafts, i.e., 3 to 1, can be managed in a similar fashion. However, there is an increased risk of desiccation of tissue between the mesh, especially if the wound surface has any exposed fat. Placement of a skin substitute, i.e., biobrane, pigskin, or cadaver skin, over the wide mesh protects the interstices. Porous biobrane or meshed, but not opened, pigskin, or cadaver skin allows for the drainage of blood and exudate. Wet dressings are needed, as is some compression until the dressing has adhered to the tissues.

Excised but not grafted wounds need to be covered with a skin substitute because the surface will invariably desiccate with an attempt at wet dressings alone (Table 8-7). In addition, the skin substitute restores the barrier to heat and evaporative loss as well as invasive infection.

## Skin Substitutes

Cadaver skin is an excellent temporary skin because it not only protects the wound from desiccation but also has antibacterial properties, probably from the exposed collagen. It is in short supply and has the risk of disease transmission. Cadaver skin can revascularize and essentially "take" to the excised wound bed in the immunocompromised host. It can undergo a rejection if left on too long. Usually, allograft should be changed every 7 to 10 days because it can adhere and be difficult to remove if left on longer. The major difficulty with allograft is its extremely short supply and great expense. Because of these two facts, cadaver skin should be reserved for the young, salvageable patient with a massive burn. Pigskin is also useful but is not nearly as good as allograft. Pigskin does not revascularize but dermal elements can be incorporated into the wound, leading to increased inflammation. Pigskin should be changed more frequently than allograft. Biobrane has the advantage of not being degraded or rejected. However, if left on an excised wound for more than 14 days, biobrane can also become very adherent and difficult to remove.

## SURGICAL APPROACH BASED ON BURN SIZE

### Massive Full-Thickness Third Degree Burn

For the massive (more than 60% total body surface) full-thickness burn, early excision to fascia is indicated when the patient is hemodynamically stable (best time is usually 48 hours postburn). The first excision procedure is usually the easiest to perform. Excision of chest and abdomen (18%) is a first priority because it is fast and removal of the thick noncompliant eschar can improve pulmonary function. The wound is grafted with 3 to 1 mesh followed by biobrane (or grease gauze). Donors are approximately 0.01 inch in thickness. On day 4 to 5, the lower or upper extremities are excised (total not to exceed 18%), followed in 1 to 2 days by the remainder of extremity burn. Areas excised but not grafted because of lack of donors can be covered with skin substitutes awaiting new donors. The back can also be excised early, but the back having thicker skin often has viable dermal elements. Tangential excision is therefore more appropriate for this area. Hands, neck, and face, which need tangential excision and more skin, are left for later, i.e., 2 to 3 weeks, when donor sites become available and the patient is in less of a life-threatening situation. Paring down of the eschar in these areas is indicated to improve control of bacterial growth.

### Massive Burn, Mixed Second and Third Degree

The full-thickness burn is excised to fascia and covered with mesh (usually 3 to 1) graft. Donors are 0.01 inch in thickness. Management of partial thickness burn depends on availability of donors. Tangential excision with coverage of 1.5 to 1 grafts is ideal but may not be feasible. Partial thickness burns not excised in the first 6 to 7 days should be treated with daily debridement and dressings until the area heals or granulation tissue forms. Grafts can then be placed with less risk of bleeding or dissemination of bacteria. The exception would be small areas that are cosmetically or functionally important.

### Small to Moderate Deep Dermal or Full-Thickness Burns

Early tangential excision is indicated, covering important functional and cosmetic parts first. Fascial excision is indicated if burn extends well into fat. Grafts are 0.012 inches in thickness or greater for areas such as the face and neck.

Table 8-7  Dressing the Excised Wound

| Sheet Grafts | Mesh Grafts 1.5 to 1 | Mesh Grafts 3 to 1 |
|---|---|---|
| 1. Grease gauze plus dry gauze dressing plus compression<br>or<br>open without dressings<br>2. Area needs to be immobilized<br>3. Change dressings daily | 1. Grease gauze or fine mesh<br>2. Add inner gauze layer moistened with antibiotic solution keeping moist for 2 to 3 days<br>3. Add dry gauze layer<br>4. Area needs to be immobilized<br>5. Change gauze dressing daily<br>6. Remove grease gauze at 3 to 5 days (earlier if hematoma or exudate present) | 1. Same technique as described for 1.5 to 1<br>or<br>skin substitute: biobrane, pigskin, cadaver skin<br>2. Remove grease gauze or skin substitute at 5 to 7 days, when mesh filling in or before if evidence of infection |

*Excised Not Grafted Wound*

Use Skin Substitute Followed by Gauze and Compression Until Skin Substitute Is Well Adherent to Wound Surface

## Burn Plus Inhalation Injury

If the burn is life-threatening, then early excision is indicated, even though some pulmonary dysfunction is present. Severe lung dysfunction or hemodynamic instability is a contraindication to excision. The lung dysfunction is usually most severe initially, i.e., in the first 24 to 36 hours, with bronchospasm and then at about 6 to 7 days with onset of severe inflammation and infection. The best time for surgical intervention is usually between days 2 and 3 and days 6 and 7.

## MANAGEMENT OF SPECIFIC BURN AREAS

### Chest and Abdominal Wall

*Massive Deep Burns (More Than 60% Total Body Surface)*

This area is a high priority for early fascial excision of full-thickness burn if a large component of full-thickness burn is also present in other areas. The wound is grafted with 3 to 1 mesh and covered with Xeroform gauze and antibiotic moistened dressing or a temporary skin substitute. It is advantageous to suture the remaining skin edges to the fascia to cover any exposed fat as well as diminish the cosmetic defect. The umbilicus should be spared if possible. The areas of greatest concern are usually the axilla and the posterior skin edge. It is easy to find oneself deep in the axilla when making the transition from a fascial plane to the axillary fat. It is much safer to skirt around the axilla with the fascial excision and tangentially excise the axillary burn. Placement of sheet grafts or 1.5 to 1 mesh grafts over the infraclavicular areas is also advantageous in preparation for subsequent use of these sites for central lines. Central access is a major problem with neck and chest burns. A moderate compression dressing is applied, usually placed on the bed before excision to avoid disturbing the grafts by having to roll the patient. Deep partial thickness burns are not excised to fascia. Tangential excision and grafting are also not feasible because of the large amount of donor skin required. Removal of the outer layer of eschar can improve infection control. However, viable dermis should not be exposed unless it is to be covered with graft or skin substitute.

*Moderate Burns (30 to 50% Total Body Surface)*

A similar approach as described with massive burns is often needed if most of the burn is full thickness. It is also helpful to save skin donor sites for functional areas, such as over joints, arms, and legs.

*Small Burns (Less Than 30% Total Body Surface)*

Excision to fascia is indicated for deep third degree burns that extend into fat using 1.5 to 1 mesh coverage. Tangential excision and grafting are preferred if char is not present and adequate donor sites are available. Tangential excision to debulk the eschar can be done to improve infection control. However, viable dermis should not be exposed unless the wound is going to be closed by grafts or skin substitutes.

## Neck

### Massive Burns

This area is not high priority for early excision unless the need for a tracheostomy is anticipated. Often patients with deep neck and chest burns have severe smoke inhalation as well. In this case, excision and coverage with 1.5 to 1 mesh or preferably a sheet graft is done. A tracheostomy can then be performed through the graft. The grafts can usually be treated open so it is easier to inspect and remove any clot. The grafted neck needs to be maintained in some extension to avoid contracture formation. This can be done with a blanket roll behind the shoulders.

### Small to Moderate Burn

This area now becomes a higher priority for early excision, usually by tangential excision. If char is present, a sharp excision to or below the platysma is the optimal approach. Again, the neck should be placed beyond neutral in extension.

## Breast

The management of the breast burn is determined by the size of the total burn and the patient's age and medical condition. The small deep dermal burn involving the breast is managed by tangential excision, cautiously sparing areolar tissue. The areola is thick and is usually not burned full thickness unless char is present. Primary healing of the deep dermal burn (i.e., greater than 3 weeks) will usually result in considerable hypertrophic scarring. Moderate body surface burns in the young patient are treated by tangential excision and grafting unless the burns extend well into breast tissue. In the deep massive burn or in the elderly with full-thickness burns to breasts, a mastectomy is often required. The elderly patient has considerable fibrous tissue with diminished blood supply to the breast. An adequate endpoint using the tangential excision approach often cannot be found and graft take will be poor. The elderly patient, in general, tolerates the burn wound and any infection very poorly. Expediting complete wound closure with mastectomy and skin grafts may well be life-saving in this patient population.

## Axilla and Posterior Shoulder

### Massive Burn

Usually significant burns of the axilla also involve the posterior shoulder and lateral chest wall. Excision and grafting of this area are best performed after the chest has been excised and grafted and the patient is more stable. It is better to skirt around the axilla if a chest wall excision to fascia is being performed because it is very easy to remove too much axillary tissue and end up with a large axillary defect. The axilla, fortunately, is often spared. The eschar can be debulked awaiting granulation tissue for later grafting or a delayed excision and grafting can be performed using 1.5 to 1 mesh or sheet. It is easier to hold the graft in place if the surrounding tissue has been previously grafted or covered with a skin substitute. The arm needs to be maintained in abduction. Soft splints such as pillows are usually the most feasible approach.

### Small to Moderate Burn

Axillary coverage usually follows higher priority areas, such as hands and feet. The uneven fatty tissue of the axilla makes it difficult to graft before neovascularization. Also, the axilla and the posterior shoulder are difficult to immobilize. An airplane splint attached around the opposite shoulder, chest, and abdomen is ideal for the burn localized to the one arm, axilla, and shoulder. Motion should resume in about 4 to 5 days after surgery.

## Lower Extremities

### Massive Burns

The lower extremities with third degree burns are the second priority area for excision to fascia because they are large in surface area. However, they are a little more difficult to excise than chest and abdomen. As opposed to chest, back, and abdominal wall, the legs are more prone to functional impairment as a result of fascial excision. There is an increased risk of distal edema and of potential nerve injury compared with tangential excision. In addition, there are several areas that are very difficult to graft with fascial excision. These include the anterior tibial area, the popliteal fossa and the ankle, especially over the achilles tendon. The upper lateral thigh at the fascia lata can also be difficult to cover. In addition, a cosmetic defect at the upper extent of the excision will also occur. Certain modifications are necessary to minimize complications. The saphenous system should be preserved, if possible, to minimize edema. Care should be taken to avoid injury to nerves. Some fatty tissue should be left over the tibia (if possible), around the knee and over the achilles. Often, a deep burn extends in to the fascia over the tibia and into the achilles because no subcutaneous tissue is present in these areas. Be aware of the saphenous vein as it exits the fossa ovales. It should be spared if some tributaries are still open. However, if it is to be ligated, the distal vessel should be removed. Do not leave a clotted saphenous vein in place because it is a potential source of infection. One leg should be excised at one procedure. This will often require two teams if the procedure is to be performed in a reasonable period. It is only possible to excise both legs if one is to be covered with skin substitute rather than autograft since this can be done quite rapidly. However, excising both legs is usually in excess of that which can be done safely unless this procedure is the first procedure and it is done in the first 2 to 3 days, using two teams. A note of caution is that a circumferential third degree burn acts like an entire leg tourniquet compressing the vasculature beneath. When the eschar is removed, the available vascular space increases and more blood needs to be replaced than is actually lost. Leg excision to fascia can be performed under tourniquet. Be prepared to replace both blood loss from surface bleeding as well as from the blood volume expansion of the underlying soft tissues with tourniquet release. The dorsum of the foot should not be excised to fascia because tendons will be exposed. It is better to excise this area tangentially at a later date or simply pare down the eschar and wait for neovascularization.

The leg grafts need to be protected using skin substitutes or wet dressings, as previously described. The leg also needs to be elevated and immobilized. Skeletal pins and traction is one approach. However, an alternative approach is equally effective. The legs can be suspended using broad soft padded slings behind posterior thigh and posterior calf using the same standard weights and pulley system attached to a bed traction frame. The feet should be positioned in neutral with foot splints well padded over the achilles. The patient's legs can be easily taken down from the traction for exercising and when the patient is rolled. External compression is required for months because of the impaired venous drainage so as to avoid dependent edema. Deep dermal burns to the legs are treated with topical agents. Paring down of the eschar can be done in deeper areas. Grafting may be necessary later, i.e., in several weeks, when donor sites used in excision and grafting of higher priority areas become available again.

*Moderate Burns*

Excision to fascia is still indicated if higher priority areas, such as hands, face, and feet, will be utilizing the majority of donors in this early period. Fascial excision is also indicated if the burn extends well into fat or if the burn patient is elderly. The elderly patient usually has thin donor skin that can only be used once, as well as poor peripheral blood flow. Concerns over leg cosmesis are outweighed by the life-threatening nature of a burn of this size. Tangential excision is used in the young patient with third degree leg burns if other higher priority areas have sufficient available donor skin. Deep dermal burns are excised early if they can be grafted using 1.5 to 1 mesh. Grafting at a later date with reused donor sites may be the better alternative.

*Small Burns*

Excision to fascia for extremely deep burns may be needed. In general, the preferred approach is tangential excision with coverage using 1.5 to 1 mesh on flat surface and sheet grafts over joints.

## Foot

Burns of the feet are very difficult to manage. Poor blood supply makes the foot a difficult area to allow to heal primarily and also a tricky area to graft. Tangential excision with use of 1.5 to 1 mesh grafts is usually required because the thin layer of viable tissue beneath deep burn desiccates easily with a wider mesh graft. Exposure of tendons is a major problem in this area. Fortunately, loss of flexor tendons on the foot from an extensive burn leads to less morbidity than a similar tendon loss on the hand. Tangential excision is more difficult on the foot.

The endpoint of excision is more difficult to define than in other areas with greater blood flow. The endpoint is usually defined by a white shiny tissue base. Bleeding may be minimal, especially on the sides of the feet. Considerable experience is necessary to avoid going too deep compared with not going deep enough. Deep burns to the toes (exception the large toe) are difficult to excise and graft and therefore the wounds are left to either granulate or demarcate.

Burns to the soles are rarely full thickness. The outer eschar can be removed and the wound base allowed to reepithelialize.

## Upper Extremity

### Massive Deep Burns

Surgical management of the upper extremity is much more complicated than the lower extremity because of the major functional concerns for hand, wrist, elbow, and axilla. The arms are a lower priority to excise to fascia than chest, abdomen, or legs because of the smaller surface area (each arm is 9% total body surface). If excised to fascia, a 3 to 1 mesh not completely opened is preferred for upper and lower arms and a 1.5 to 1 mesh over elbow, wrist, and hands. A skin substitute can be placed over excised areas until donor sites are available if available donors have been used for coverage of large surface areas.

As with the lower extremity, there are several areas, namely, wrist and elbow, that should not be excised to fascia unless the burn clearly extends to this depth. Extreme caution is required with excision around the elbow to avoid injury to the ulnar nerve. Exposing tendons in these areas will also present a major problem for coverage. Some soft tissue should be left in these areas, especially over the olecranon. These areas should also be covered with 1.5 to 1 mesh or a sheet graft. In addition, the cephalic and basilic vein should be preserved if they are patent. Clotted veins should be removed. A tourniquet can be used for fascial excision. The upper arm and shoulder can then be excised when the tourniquet is removed.

After excision and coverage, the arms should be elevated. The elbow needs to be splinted in extension. The splint can be applied over the antecubital space or posteriorly over the olecranon. The former is preferred in most cases because pressure is then not applied over the olecranon, an area particularly prone to breakdown. The wrist also needs to be maintained in 30° to 40° of extension. Skeletal traction using pins can also be used for this purpose. The grafted arm should be immobilized for 3 to 4 days, after which some elbow and wrist motion should begin, with a more aggressive approach to physical therapy beginning about 5 to 7 days. Compression should be applied to the arm to minimize distal edema. Edema will increase the risk of skin breakdown.

### Moderate to Small Burn

Tangential excision with preservation of viable tissue is preferred if donor sites are available. This approach clearly requires more skin than fascial excision because a narrower mesh is needed to avoid desiccation of fat between the mesh. If there is a problem with the amount of donor skin, it is better to save the skin for the hands, neck, and over the joints, and use a fascial excision with a wider mesh on the upper arm and forearm. Tangential excision with 1.5 to 1 mesh is preferred for deep dermal burns. Coverage in this fascia with reuse donor sites usually leads to a better cosmetic result than allowing the deep dermal burn to heal. Positioning and splinting is the same as just described.

## Hand

### Massive Deep Burns

The hand burn becomes a lower priority, even though hand function is of major concern in a burn of this size. However, the initial concentration should be on excision of large burn surfaces. Unfortunately, it is difficult to excise and graft a third degree burn between 7 and 21 days when new donor sites now become available. The hand becomes very vascular beginning at about 7 days and is difficult to excise to any defined endpoint because copious bleeding makes it difficult to inspect the tissue. Although blood loss is significant, it is considerably less if one can remain above the now very large dorsal vein. Excision under tourniquet requires considerable expertise because an inadequate removal of nonviable tissue or removal of excessive amounts of viable tissue is apt to occur when the bleeding endpoint is not directly visualized. The other alternative is waiting 14 to 21 days until a granulation tissue bed has developed upon which the grafting can be performed. If a significant delay in closure is anticipated, paring down the eschar will help control infection. Deep dermal burns should be treated with topical antibiotics until adequate skin is available for grafting.

## Moderate to Small Burn

The hand is now a high priority for excisional therapy. Early excision and grafting is indicated for dorsal hand burns not expected to heal by 3 weeks. This decision is easier with full-thickness burns but is less obvious with the deep dermal burn. Factors such as increasing age and chronic disease will substantially slow the rate of healing. Early excision is not indicated for fourth degree burns. Aggressive removal of eschar to viable tissue can lead to exposed tendons and bone that will not accept a graft. A flap or pedicle graft will be required and complete excision should not be performed unless one is prepared to perform the more complex procedure at this time or have ample cadaver skin available to hold the wound until the definitive procedure can be performed. Pins can be placed in the proximal interphalangeal and metacarpophalangeal joints to hold proper position in these cases of extensive burn. The dorsum of the hand and the fingers are the areas most commonly excised and grafted. Palmar burns are usually not full thickness, and paring down of the eschar and awaiting primary healing is usually successful. Dense scar may develop on the palm as a result. Skin grafts on the palm will lead to decreased sensation in an area where sensation has a critical function. The hypothenar and thenar eminence, as opposed to the palm, often have a full-thickness burn because skin over these areas is not nearly as thick as the center of the palm.

The hand excision, as opposed to areas such as chest or proximal extremity, requires considerable experience and surgical expertise. It is extremely important that nonviable tissue be removed but viable tissue be preserved, since there is very little soft tissue present between skin and tendons. Early excision in the presence of edema but before inflammation gives one the best opportunity to excise only dead tissue. Visibility is a major problem after 4 to 5 days because significant bleeding makes the determination of endpoint more difficult. It is, however, more difficult to determine an endpoint if a proximal tourniquet is used, since all the clues used to determine viability, such as tissue color and punctate bleeding, are missing.

Excision is performed using the Goulian dermatome for fingers and hand. The web spaces may need to be excised using a scalpel to shave the eschar, since this area is difficult to reach with the Goulian. It is essential that the tangential excision not be carried too deeply into the finger because tendon will be exposed or distal blood flow impaired. One should avoid the large venous plexus on the dorsum of the hand if at all possible. Not only will bleeding be profuse but venous return will be impaired. Burns extending through this system are usually fourth degree and long-term function will be markedly impaired due to the damage to underlying structures. It is best to excise one finger at a time, control bleeding, and place a graft rather than attempt to complete excision of the whole hand before coverage because blood loss will be excessive. Grafts can be applied longitudinally from the dorsum of the hand to the endpoint of the finger excision. The graft can then be cut to fit the web space, avoiding excess skin in this space or webbing will result. Another alternative is to place the grafts transversely covering the entire dorsum. Then individual grafts can be placed on each finger meeting the hand graft at the metacarpophalangeal joint. This latter approach is useful if there is also thenar or hypothenar involvement, since this area can be covered in one piece with a transversely placed graft. Each finger should then be individually wrapped with Xeroform or fine mesh gauze. Moist gauze over the inner dressing will help soak up blood and exudate. Mesh grafts result in good function and also minimize the risk of hematoma formation. If the mesh is barely opened, the cosmetic defect is minimal. Sheet grafts are feasible with very early excisions or grafting on granulation tissue, but are less practical for the greater than 5-day old burn because of the profuse punctate bleeding that inevitably develops. One can anticipate a longer operative procedure if sheet grafts are to be used because of need to more completely stop all bleeding. A compression dressing should be applied over the gauze dressing to control bleeding and to minimize edema. A hand splint is then placed with the fingers and thumb maintained in the functional position. An alternative solution is traction using pins through the wrist and digits. Motion should begin in 3 to 4 days; therefore pin placement may be more appropriate for the fourth degree burn for which immobilization and joint fixation is required for a much longer period of time. Fingertips should remain exposed no matter what technique is used to observe circulation. Postoperative management also requires a physical or occupational therapist with considerable expertise to maximize the benefits of the early wound closure. If therapy is not optimal, function will be impaired even though the wound is closed.

## Back

### Massive Deep Burn

It is often difficult to distinguish a deep dermal back burn from a full-thickness injury unless char is present. The skin of the back is quite thick and a significant amount of dermis may remain. Excision to fascia is therefore not indicated unless there is no doubt that the wound is third degree, especially in the presence of limited donor sites. Back excision is a lower priority than chest, abdomen, or legs. The procedure is more difficult because the potentially unstable patient must be positioned on his side or prone. This position change can lead to an accentuation of cardiopulmonary instability. Vascular catheters, tubes, etc., are also likely to be dislodged. In addition, the massively edematous patient is difficult to maintain positioned without utilizing the services of several assistants. It is not necessary and can be dangerous to place the patient prone during excision. Three quarters of the back can be excised and grafted with the patient in the lateral position. The remainder of the burn can be excised 2 to 3 days later with the other side up. It is a big advantage performing the procedure on the patient's bed because dressings can be placed ahead of time beneath plastic sheets and the patient rolled directly back to the supine position, which minimizes shifting of the grafts. If the excision is carried to the fascia or muscle, a 3 to 1 mesh can be used followed by a skin substitute (or moist antibiotic soaked dressings). If the deep back burn is not excised and grafted early, paring down of the eschar is indicated to improve penetration of the topical agents. Viable tissue should not be exposed unless a skin substitute is to be used because the viable dermis can result in desiccation. The patient can be positioned from supine to side to side postoperatively to avoid continued constant pressure on the grafts. The prone position is not necessary. A circumferential compression dressing should be applied, changing the gauze once or twice daily, depending on the amount of drainage. Drainage can be considerable with the excised and grafted area in the dependent position.

*Moderate Burn*

The third degree burn can be excised with placement of 3 to 1 mesh using remaining donors for higher priority areas. The deep dermal burn should not be excised until sufficient donors are available for coverage and other priority areas have been closed. It is possible that a significant amount of remaining dermis is still present, which can lead to primary healing of at least a portion of the back. A thin layer of epidermis will restore an antibacterial barrier and decrease inflammation. The area may break down later at a time when donor sites are again available. Dressing and positioning is the same as previously described.

*Small Burn*

The deep back burn should be tangentially excised and covered with 1.5 to 1 mesh grafts.

## Buttocks

The buttock is one of the more difficult if not the most difficult area to manage. A small burn can be tangentially excised and grafted with 1.5 to 1 mesh. Although there is a fascial plane laterally, fatty fibrous tissue is encountered medially and inferiorly. An endpoint is often difficult to find with full-thickness burns. Leaving behind remaining necrotic fat is of major concern. A skin substitute such as biobrane can be placed over the graft, sutured to the medial extent of the excision, stretched, and sutured to the lateral extent. This approach will help protect the grafts from stool or infected anal exudate. With a large body burn, the buttocks are not a top priority for early grafting. However, parring down the eschar is necessary to decrease burn wound sepsis.

Mafenide is a useful agent on deep burns because the eschar separation can be delayed for up to several weeks, improving patient comfort and allowing some time for other areas to be covered. It is usually not necessary to perform a colostomy with buttock burns. Stools in the perioperative period can usually be controlled by use of a no-residue diet or parenteral nutrition along with constipating agents such as codeine or opiates. By 4 to 5 days, the wound covered with 1.5 to 1 mesh is usually revascularized and more resistant to infection.

## Perineum

The perineum is usually not treated with early excision because of difficulties of the excision itself, especially an endpoint, as well as considerable difficulty maintaining a graft in place. After deep perineal, scrotal, and penis burns heal with topical antibiotics and dressing changes via contraction.

# DECISION-MAKING WITH EARLY BURN EXCISION

## Chest, Abdomen
1. First priority for fascial excision with massive burn
2. Use mesh grafts and skin substitute
3. Taper skin edges
4. Place small sheet grafts over areas of central line use
5. Use tangential excision for smaller burns with 1.5 to 1 mesh grafts
6. Do procedure on patient's bed, placing circumferential dressing prior to procedure

## Back
1. Third or fourth priority for early fascial excision
2. May heal because skin is quite thick
3. Tangential excision for small to moderate burn;

## Lower Extremity
1. Second priority with massive burn to excise to fascia
2. Do one leg (18% total body surface) per operation
3. Can use tourniquet
4. Leave some soft tissue over popliteal fossa and anterior tibia; try to spare patent veins
5. Tangential excision preferred if donor sites available
6. Splint knee and elevate legs; do not need skeletal traction
7. Maintain compression to control edema

## Upper Extremity
1. Third or fourth priority for fascia excision with massive burn
2. Can use tourniquet
3. Leave some soft tissue over elbow and wrist
4. Spare patent veins and watch for nerve injury
5. Tangential excision for small to moderate burns using 1.5 to 1 mesh and sheets over joints
6. Splint elbow and elevate arms; do not need skeletal traction
7. Maintain compression to control edema

## Neck
1. Later priority unless immediate access for tracheostomy needed
2. Can perform tracheostomy through a skin graft within hours to days
3. Use 1.5 to 1 mesh or sheet graft

## Breast
1. Spare areola and breast tissue with early excision in young patient
2. Remove if charred
3. Remove in elderly patient with large third degree chest burn
4. Ideal approach is tangential excision and sheet grafts

## Perineum
1. Not good area for early excision
2. Treat with topical antibiotics while waiting for spontaneous healing

## Buttocks
1. Difficult for for fascial excision
2. Tangential excision 1.5 to 1 mesh if possible
3. Colostomy usually not needed

## Axilla
1. Use tangential excision approach to avoid leaving large axillary defect
2. May need to wait for granulating bed
3. Cover with 1.5 to 1 mesh or sheet
4. Need to maintain arm in abduction postoperatively

## Foot
1. Low priority in massive burn
2. High priority in Small burns for early Tangential excision
3. Burns of soles: Debulk eschar and await spontaneous healing in most cases

## Hand
1. Not top priority with massive burn
2. Top priority with small to moderate burn
3. Approach is early tangential excision sparing dorsal veins if they are patent
4. Cover with 1.5 to 1 mesh or sheet
5. Compression dressing and splint for 3 to 4 days, then begin motion
6. Exception is fourth degree burn that is treated more conservatively; usually need flap coverage for amputation

145

SECTION 3

# Inflammation-Infection Phase (7 Days to Wound Closure)

Management of this phase of a large burn injury is the most complicated of all the phases. The generalized effects of inflammation after all organ functions and magnify any preexisting organ dysfunction, in particular cardiopulmonary dysfunction. The altered metabolism, as a result of the inflammatory response, is very complex and requires a working knowledge of metabolism and nutrition in order to provide adequate care. The remaining wound is now colonized with bacteria and wound sepsis is of prominent concern. Continued alterations in the wound flora, through the use of topical and systemic antibiotics, will lead to increasing numbers of resistant organisms, further complicating the control of infection. Infection, whether lung or wound, becomes increasingly difficult to diagnose due to the continued presence of a hyperdynamic state. Multisystem organ failure (MSOF), if it is to occur, will be seen during this period. Prevention is the only real mode of management because mortality approaches 100% in the burn patient. As with the discussion of the other phases, the section will include chapters on pulmonary abnormalities, hemodynamic stability, which includes a discussion of metabolism and nutrition, and management of the burn wound itself. In addition, a chapter on sepsis has been added because of the high risk of this process developing during this period.

# 9
# Pulmonary Abnormalities

Pulmonary problems remain a major cause of morbidity and mortality during this phase. Pulmonary failure and pulmonary sepsis exceed burn wound sepsis as a cause of mortality. There are three major processes occurring during this period that will be discussed.

- Nosocomial Pneumonia
- Hypermetabolism-Induced Respiratory Fatigue (Power Failure)
- Adult Respiratory Distress Syndrome (Low Pressure Pulmonary Edema)
- Common Pitfalls
- Summary of Pulmonary Problems

These three processes are closely interrelated. The burn patient is very prone to infection, particularly after a smoke-inhalation injury. The hypermetabolic state produces a marked increase in oxygen needs and carbon dioxide production. The increased work demands on the lung as a gas-exchanging organ can exceed the adequacy of lung function. Adult respiratory distress syndrome (ARDS) is a severe complication of the sepsis process, which is very difficult to reverse in the burn patient.

## NOSOCOMIAL PNEUMONIA

### Pathophysiology

The term "nosocomial pneumonia" refers to the pneumonia that develops in the hospital with no evidence of lung infection present on admission, i.e., it is hospital-acquired. Although another form of nosocomial infection, namely, wound infection, is more common, the mortality rate for pneumonia is much higher. Burn patients with a combination of inhalation injury and a major body burn have the greatest risk of pneumonia, with a rate exceeding 50%. The high incidence is due to the presence of virulent organisms in the intensive care unit environment and the immunosuppressed state of the burn patient. The major events occurring in the majority of nosocomial lung infections are:

- Colonization of the naso-oropharynx by pathogens

Aspiration of infected tracheobronchial secretions
Impairment of systemic or local (lung) defense mechanisms

## *Colonization*

Colonization or bacterial overgrowth of the oro- and nasopharynx with potential pathogens occurs in about 50% of critically burned patients. Nearly 100% of major burn patients with a major respiratory problem have colonized their oropharynx with pathogens. There are a number of routes and events by which colonization occurs.

*Transmission of pathogens on the hands of hospital personnel* is a major cause. Up to 50% of personnel have been shown to carry either gram-negative bacilli or *Staphyloccus aureus* on their hands. Compulsive hand washing has been shown to decrease this route of transmission markedly.

*Endogenous organisms from the patient's burn wound* are a major source of bacteria, eventually being transmitted to the oropharynx. The oropharyngeal organisms will, in turn, contaminate the burn wound.

*Endogenous organisms from the patient's gastrointestinal tract* is also a common source. Transmission by hands or by retrograde movement of organisms from stomach to oropharynx are two important routes. The routine neutralization of gastric acidity can increase the pathogen content in the stomach. The presence of a nasogastric tube can assist in the transmission of the stomach bacteria to the oropharynx. The necessity to avoid gastric distention in this patient makes this route of transmission difficult to eliminate. Sucrafate is a good alternative to antacids and an $H_2$ blocker. This agent protects by increasing mucosal blood flow but does not block acid production.

*Reservoirs of pathogens in the burn unit or intensive care unit* are well-known sources. Aerosol nebulizers, ventilator tubing, etc., are potential sources because of the moist environment. Recent introduction of more disposable equipment and unit dose packaging of aerosols has decreased the incidence of this route of contamination.

*Administration of broad-spectrum antibiotics* will reduce the normal oral flora, which usually helps inhibit pathogen growth and increase colonization.

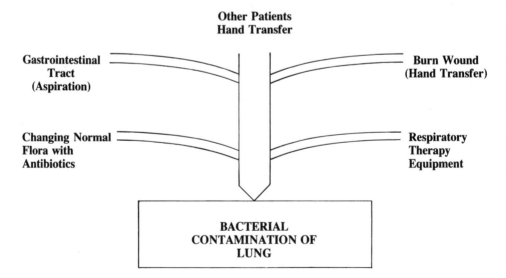

## Tracheobronchial Aspiration

Aspiration of infected secretions is the next step following colonization. Aspiration is potentiated by sedation or any process that impairs normal clearance of oral secretions, e.g., a nasogastric tube. Pooled contaminated secretions present above the cuff of an endotracheal tube can readily be aspirated into the tracheobronchial tree. Suctioning of the oropharynx before cuff deflation or extubation is, of course, mandatory. The endotracheal tube (or tracheostomy) itself increases the potential for aspiration of secretions because the glottis and vocal cords cannot be effectively closed and secretions can track down both the inside and outside of tube. The *causes of tracheobronchial aspiration* are as follows:

> Pharmacologic impairment to clearance of secretions, e.g., sedation, anesthesia, paralysis
>
> Anatomic impairment to clearance of secretions, e.g., oropharyngeal edema, trauma, nasogastric tube, endotracheal tube, oral airway, etc.
>
> Direct contamination of lower airways by catheters, lavage fluid, or deflation of cuff on endotracheal tube

## Impairment of Lung Defenses

Altered lung host defenses can dramatically increase the potential for lung infection as a result of the aspiration of bacteria (Table 9-1). The altered defenses that are most prominent in the process of lung infection will be described.

**Impaired Cough.** Impairment of this reflex is a common occurrence in the burn patient. A decrease in the state of consciousness markedly suppresses both the initiation of the reflex and the quality of the cough. This will be the case with the need for narcotics for pain control and during recovery from anesthesia. The ability to take a large inspiration, necessary for an adequate cough, will be impaired by a chest burn and also by muscle weakness from catabolism. The presence of an endotracheal tube, although maintaining an adequate airway, can decrease the ability to generate a sufficient propulsive force to

**Table 9-1** Altered Host Defenses That Result in Pneumonia

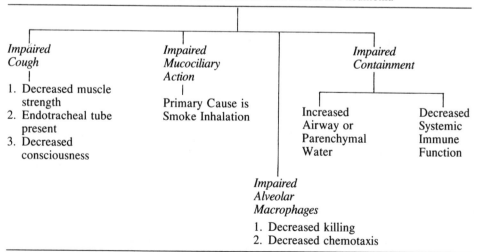

clear secretions effectively. Any aspirated, infected oral secretions will then have the opportunity to proliferate. Thus, the *factors required for adequate cough* are:

> Near-maximum inspiration
>
> Epiglottic closure and cord apposition
>
> Forceful contraction of intercostal and abdominal muscles, generating a large intrathoracic pressure gradient
>
> Opening of epiglottis and cords with forceful expulsion of air

**Impairment of Mucociliary Action.** The airways are lined with ciliated mucous-coated epithelia that beat toward the pharynx, thereby assisting in the continued clearance of particles and microorganisms. This is particularly useful in the smaller airways, which are less effectively cleared by coughing. The ciliary action is directly injured by heat and chemicals in inhaled smoke.

**Impairment of Alveolar Macrophage Function.** Bacteria or particles deposited in the alveoli are rapidly phagocytized by the alveolar macrophage, which destroys them by direct killing via oxygen radical release. Chemoattractants are released from the macrophage, which attract neutrophils to assist in the containment process. The microorganism-laden macrophages are cleared via the mucociliary system or may also migrate through the interstitial space to be cleared by the lymphatics, thus entering the regional lymph nodes and systemic circulation.

A number of factors in the burn patient will impair macrophage function. Inhalation anesthetics, inhalation injury, malnutrition, anemia, and hypoxia will impair macrophage function, thereby increasing the risk of lung infection.

**Impairment of Containment.** The postburn *immunodeficiency state* involving both the cellular and humoral component of resistance will impair the ability of the lung defenses to contain infection. Another major factor that impairs the containment process is *increased lung water*. The movement of edema fluid allows a rapid spread of bacteria to uninvolved areas both as a vehicle for carrying bacteria and as an impairment of the sequestration and containment process.

## Diagnosis

The early precise diagnoses of the pneumonia is often very difficult (Table 9-2). The pros and cons of the usual methods will be discussed.

Table 9-2  Criteria for Diagnosing Pneumonia

| Clinical Signs | Differential Diagnosis |
| --- | --- |
| Fever, leukocytosis | Nonpulmonary infection |
|  | Burn wound, inflammation |
| Pulmonary infiltrate | Inhalation-induced inflammation |
|  | Postoperative atelectasis |
|  | Aspiration |
| Purulent sputum | Oropharyngeal colonization |

## Clinical Diagnosis

The usual criteria for diagnosing pneumonia are fever, leukocytosis, purulent sputum, new or increasing infiltrates on radiographs, and pathogens growing from the sputum.

These criteria are of much less value in the burn patient where other sources of infection and burn inflammation can initiate a sepsis syndrome. For example, approximately 75% of intensive care unit patients have a colonized upper airway, usually with gram-negative organisms. The purulent sputum may simply be aspirated oropharyngeal secretions. Pulmonary infiltrates are also a common finding in the postburn patient. Approximately 30% of new infiltrates in the surgical intensive care unit patient turn out not to be pneumonia. Based on these facts, clinical criteria alone are not sufficiently accurate to allow a precise diagnosis of the presence or absence of nosocomial pneumonia (Table 9-3).

**Table 9-3** Diagnosis of Nosocomial Pneumonia

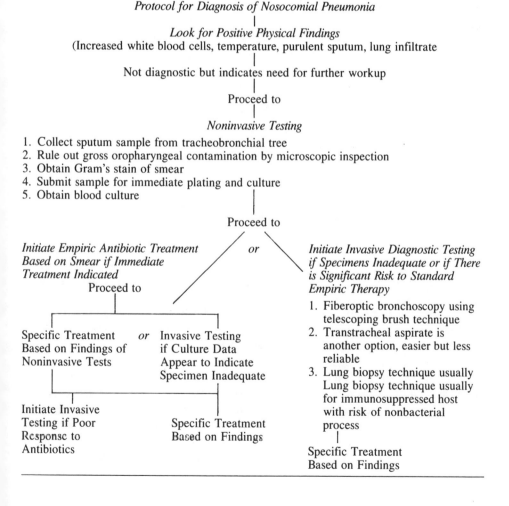

## Examination of Sputum

Examination of expectorated sputum remains the most common method of detecting a respiratory tract infection. Although reliable in about half of the patients, there is clear discrepancy in the other 50% between the culture data of sputum versus cultures obtained from the lower respiratory tract by more invasive means. The major reason is contamination of sputum by organisms colonizing the upper airways. This is most evident in the patient with an endotracheal tube in place. The *criteria for obtaining an adequate sputum sample* are:

1. Sputum expectorated after deep cough
2. More than 25 leukocytes per low-power field
3. Only occasional squamous cells present
4. Presence of alveolar macrophages

The other difficulty relates to the handling of the specimens. Some organisms, such as *Streptococcus pneumoniae* (pneumococcus) and *Haemophilus influenzae* are rapid growing and will overgrow a mixed culture, especially if there is a delay in plating. If the patient is on antibiotics, growth of the etiologic pathogen may be suppressed in culture. In addition, the antibiotics will lead to further pharyngeal colonization and specimen contamination. The presence of large numbers of squamous cells indicates the sample is more likely to be from the oropharynx rather than the lung. The *causes of error in sputum analysis* are:

Colonization of oropharynx
Collection of saliva rather than deep sample
Delay in plating sputum sample
Antibiotic use prior to sample collection

## Transtracheal: Bronchoscopic Aspirates

Transtracheal aspiration is done by passing a small catheter into the lungs through the thyroid membrane in an attempt to obtain lung secretions expected to be uncontaminated with oral flora. This technique has been shown to be much more reliable as far as diagnosing the true pathogen in the lung infection rather than standard sputum analysis. This technique, however, cannot be utilized in the intubated patient. Complications of the method are usually minor, including some bleeding, but severe complications have been reported and the method cannot be considered innocuous.

Bronchoscopic sampling is another method used to try to bypass contamination by the upper airway. Unfortunately, some contamination is inevitable, due simply to passage of the bronchoscope through the upper airway. A technique of much greater sensitivity is the tube within a tube. Contamination of a protected catheter brush is prevented by a distal biodegradeable plug that is not ejected until the catheter reaches the deep area of the lung to be sampled. The brush is then advanced beyond the distal orifice of the scope, the sample taken, and the brush retracted. The technique, known as plugged telescoping catheter, has substantially improved the sensitivity and specificity of results obtained both for sputum smear and bacteriologic evaluation. Bronchoscopy, however, is not without risk. Hypoxemia and bronchospasm can occur if proper precautions are not taken.

*Blood Cultures*

If another source of infection can be ruled out, a positive blood culture in the presence of the pneumonic infiltrate provides an accurate diagnosis of the etiologic agent. Bacteremia, however, is not that common an event with pneumonia.

## Prevention and Treatment

Since eradication of an established pneumonia in the burn patient is very difficult, prevention is of primary importance.

Preventive measures focus in four areas:

- Improving systemic defenses
- Improving local lung defenses
- Minimizing oropharyngeal colonization
- Minimizing tracheobronchial aspiration

*Improving Systemic Host Defenses*

Maintaining adequate oxygen delivery to the burn wound and other tissue at risk for infection is necessary by optimizing blood volume, hemoglobin, and cardiac output. Nutritional status, both adequate calories and protein, using the correct mix of nutrients must be maintained. In addition, underlying chronic diseases that are also immunosuppressive, such as diabetes, must be kept in as good a control as possible.

*Improving Local Lung Defenses*

Maintaining an adequate cough mechanism is of utmost importance in the patient at risk for pneumonia, particularly in the absence of positive-pressure support, since there is a greater risk of hypoventilation and atelectasis. Analgesics and sedation must be used carefully. It is necessary to provide adequate pain relief, especially if splinting due to a chest wall burn is present. In addition, adequate sleep is required to maintain muscle activity. Oversedation and analgesia are, of course, counterproductive unless mechanical ventilatory support is being provided.

An endotracheal tube, although adequate for maintenance of a patent and protected airway, impairs the ability to clear thick secretions by coughing. It is very difficult to propel secretions the length of the tube. If continued intubation is expected to be necessary for many weeks, conversion to a tracheostomy performed in the first 7 to 10 days will greatly assist the clearance of secretions. The tracheostomy should not be placed through burned tissue. If the neck is burned, early excision and grafting of the neck area is indicated, and the subsequent tracheostomy can be performed through the skin graft in 24 to 48 hours.

Chest wall muscle mass must be maintained. Adequate nutrition and oxygen delivery are obvious requirements. The use of intermittent mandatory ventilation (IMV) or continuous positive airway pressure (CPAP) systems when ventilatory assist is needed will allow for sufficient chest wall exercise to avoid atrophy.

The cough reflex alone will be insufficient to maintain small airway patency. Frequent position changes, hyperinflation, and postural drainage will be necessary to move the small and moderate airway secretions to the proximal airways so that cough clearance can occur. Ambulation is the ideal approach. The intubated, ventilated patient with a lung injury who cannot ambulate is best managed using side-to-side position change. The side-to-side rotating bed is ideal for this purpose because the need for pushing on the painful burn areas to move the patient is eliminated.

Beside improved mucus clearance, maintaining local containment of the infection is needed by avoiding increased lung water.

### Minimizing Risk of Oropharyngeal Colonization

Decreasing the potential cross-contamination of bacteria from personnel or equipment to the patients airway will certainly decrease the risk of colonization with a virulent resistant hospital organism. Avoiding unnecessary use of broad-spectrum antibiotics will also decrease risks. Thus, the risk-reduction methods are:

> Minimize personnel or equipment transfer of bacteria with compulsive handwashing and surveillance for bacterial reservoirs
>
> Avoid inappropriate use of broad-spectrum antibiotics

### Minimize Risk of Tracheobronchial Aspiration

Once oropharyngeal colonization occurs, the risks of aspirating the infected secretions should be minimized. Positioning with the head elevated will decrease orofacial edema and improve secretion clearance. Transfer of bacteria from the upper to the lower airway by way of endotracheal tubes and suction catheters needs to be controlled by careful aseptic technique.

## HYPERMETABOLISM-INDUCED RESPIRATORY FATIGUE (POWER FAILURE)

### Pathophysiology

The increase in oxygen consumption and carbon dioxide production during this period will require increased gas exchange relative to that seen in the previous periods. A 50 to 100% increase in carbon dioxide production will be seen with burns in excess of 50% total body surface. In addition, the severe catabolism, initiated by the inflammatory response, can lead to not only extremity weakness, but also weakness of the chest wall muscle. Chronic pain and anxiety will lead to sleep deprivation and fatigue. Common causes of impaired oxygenation during this period are heart failure leading to lung edema and hypoventilation-induced atelectasis as fatigue develops. The major problem during this period is, however, usually not hypoxemia but rather hypercapnia because carbon dioxide removal is directly dependent on alveolar minute ventilation. A doubling of carbon dioxide production means a doubling of alveolar ventilation to maintain a normal $PaCO_2$. Increased ventilation means increased work of breathing, especially if a decrease in compliance or an increase in dead space is also present. Large tidal volumes are necessary to maintain adequate alveolar ventilation because small tidal volumes ventilate little more than airway dead space. Increased tidal volumes require an increased inspiratory force and the added work must be sustained 24 hours a day. If fatigue develops, impaired clearance of secretions will also occur, which can lead to *nosocomial pneumonia* as well as hypercapnia.

A common period during which the "power failure" syndrome occurs is in the perioperative period. Underestimation of the increased ventilatory needs can lead to hypercapnia during the anesthesia period. The immediate postoperative period is the most vulnerable time because oxygen consumption and carbon dioxide production return to preoperative values nearly immediately after the anesthetic has been turned off. However, the return of chest wall muscle and diaphragm muscle function can lag for several hours after the anesthesia period. The patient is often assumed to be ventilating adequately if a minute ventilation of 5 to 6 L is being generated. This volume, however, is often inadequate for the carbon dioxide production. The resulting hypercapnia is difficult to correct in view of the need to increase alveolar ventilation even further. An increase in arterial carbon dioxide tension produces an intense catechol release, anxiety, and a further increase in oxygen demands and carbon dioxide production. An additional increase, however, in carbon dioxide will also be produced if an excess amount of carbohydrate is infused. The respiratory quotient for carbohydrate burned for energy is 1.0 and for excess carbohydrate conversion to fat the value approaches 8.0.

## Diagnosis

Dyspnea occurs if the ability adequately to remove the carbon dioxide is impaired and hypercarbia develops. Fatigue develops if lung mechanics are not adequate to clear carbon dioxide with a reasonable work effort, i.e., if the dead space ventilation to tidal volume ratio ($V_D/V_T$) is increased or more work per breath is required:

Alveolar ventilation = total ventilation − dead space ventilation

If dead space remains constant but tidal volume decreases due to fatigue, a further increase in rate will be required, which leads to more fatigue. Fatigue with its effects on impaired cough, and a decrease in tidal volume, is often subtle, with the first clear evidence being a deterioration in blood gases or a new infiltrate on radiographs. Two processes should be assessed to make the correct diagnoses and plan the correct therapy.

### Mechanical Problems

The first step in evaluating hypercapnia is to determine whether the patient is actually achieving the appropriate tidal volume and minute ventilation. This determination is particularly important for the patient on a ventilator. Loss of a portion of the tidal volume through compression loss in the ventilator tubing or abnormalities in endotracheal tube and ventilator function are common problems. An air leak must also be considered.

### Increased Carbon Dioxide Production or Increased Dead Space

If mechanical factors are not present, the remaining differential diagnosis includes: an increase in carbon dioxide production, and an increase in dead space ventilation, $V_D/V_T$.

**Table 9-4** Mechanism of Power Failure

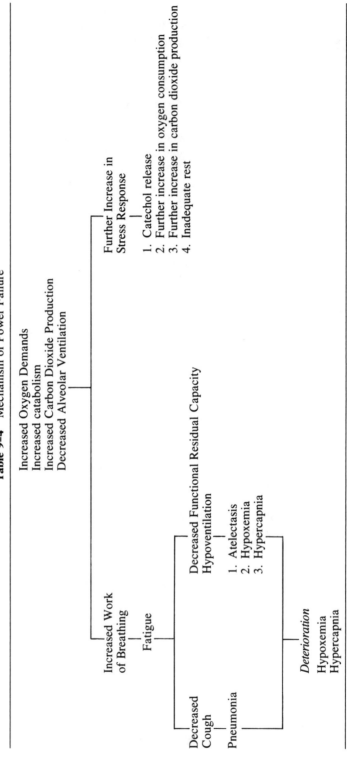

Increased dead space can be due to a decrease in regional lung perfusion relative to ventilation, often due to lung overexpansion. Vascular occlusion from pulmonary emboli must also be considered. The distinction can be made by directly measuring carbon dioxide production and then calculating $V_D/V_T$. Thus, diagnosis includes:

> Assessing tidal volume, vital capacity, inspiratory force
>
> Measuring carbon dioxide production; $V_D/V_T$, respiratory quotient

Serial measurements of tidal volume, vital capacity, and inspiratory force will allow one to detect early deterioration. In addition, the measurements of carbon dioxide production will allow one to determine whether the production is in excess of that predicted for the burn size alone. Oxygen consumption can also be measured directly using available spirometric techniques or the Fick method and the respiratory quotient directly calculated.

## Treatment

Protection of the lung against processes that will impair function is the best form of support. Controlling edema and infection while maintaining nutrition and adequate rest as well as chest wall exercise are key components. Excess carbon dioxide production should be controlled by avoiding excess carbohydrate calories and controlling excessive hyperthermia. The nutrient mix should be well controlled in order to avoid too few or too many calories. Fatigue and early evidence of respiratory compromise should be treated with assisted ventilatory support. An increase in $V_D/V_T$ due to low blood volume or excessive positive end-expiratory pressure (PEEP) can be in part corrected by volume loading.

Partial ventilatory support via a tracheostomy may be useful, especially if the anticipated problem will last several weeks, as is the case with a large body burn. Adequate rest must be assured as well as control of pain and anxiety, which can lead to a further increase in catechols and resulting hypermetabolism. The patient receiving an anesthetic must be accurately evaluated preoperatively to determine intraoperative ventilatory needs. In addition, added ventilatory support should be provided in the early postoperative period until the patient can resume sufficient spontaneous ventilation.

## ADULT RESPIRATORY DISTRESS SYNDROME (LOW PRESSURE PULMONARY EDEMA)

ARDS is the name given to the clinical manifestation of a number of indirect lung injury states characterized by dyspnea, severe hypoxemia, and decreased lung compliance with radiographic evidence of diffuse bilateral pulmonary infiltrates. Alveolar consolidation with fluid, protein, and inflammatory cells in the presence of a normal capillary or wedge pressure is also a characteristic finding, i.e., low pressure pulmonary edema. The altered permeability results in a rapid movement of fluid from plasma to interstitial space with even a normal capillary (wedge) pressure. The causes and differential diagnosis of ARDS are given in Table 9-5.

Table 9-5  Causes and Differential Diagnosis of ARDS

| Causes | Differential Diagnosis |
|---|---|
| Sepsis: Endotoxin | High-pressure edema |
| Tissue inflammation; necrosis | Focal atelectasis |
| Non-lung trauma; fractures, burns | Direct lung injury |
| Disseminated intravascular coagulation, fat emboli; massive transfusion | Aspiration pneumonia |
|  | Nosocomial pneumonia |
|  | Inhalation injury |

## Pathophysiology and Diagnosis

The lung damage is the result of a systemic process initiated by burn tissue, infection, or inflammation rather than a direct lung injury. However, the term "ARDS" is commonly but inappropriately used to describe direct lung injury processes, such as an inhalation injury. There are probably several distinct ARDS states, each with a different cause. Although the pathophysiology may be extremely complex and the etiologic agents varied, the presenting signs and symptoms for the ARDS states are nearly identical. The hypoxemia produced is characteristically refractory to an increase in fractional inspired oxygen, indicating increased shunting. In addition, the degree of shunt is not directly correlated with the degree of increased water content, as is the case with cardiogenic edema.

There is definitely a significant ventilatory impairment or airways component to the disease process not related to water. There is a decrease in dynamic compliance and functional residual capacity resulting in increased ventilation to perfusion mismatch, probably due to mediator-induced bronchoconstriction. The pathophysiologic abnormalities produced by this inflammatory process can be divided into four phases (Table 9-6).

### Phase One

In the *first, or initial, phase* dyspnea and tachypnea are noted, with a relatively normal arterial oxygen tension and a hyperventilation-induced respiratory alkalosis. Lung findings are absent on physical examination or radiographs. The prodome is mediator-induced. Initial treatment should focus on finding the source of the lung response, i.e., a septic focus, necrotic tissue, an area of inflammation. Pulmonary emboli need to be considered as well.

### Phase Two

The *second phase,* usually beginning within 12 to 24 hours of the early symptoms, is characterized by physiologic and pathologic evidence of lung injury. Initial parenchymal changes are patchy and not homogenous, appearing initially in the dependent lung field. Hypoxemia is now evident, along with continuing dyspnea. An increasing shunt fraction or venous admixture is primarily responsible, since little effect is noted by increasing the fractional inspired oxygen. The dynamic and static compliance decreases modestly, as does functional residual capacity, reflecting the stiff lung. Minor auscultatory findings are present that consist mostly of signs of early patchy consolidation.

**Table 9-6** ARDS (Low Pressure Pulmonary Edema)

*Cause*
Systemic infection, inflammation, trauma
Altering pulmonary circulation and airways

*Phase 1 (Early Changes)*

| *Radiographic Changes* | *Clinical Findings* | *Physiologic Change* |
|---|---|---|
| Normal Radiograph | Dyspnea, tachypnea | Mild pulmonary hypertension |
| | Normal chest examination | Increased airways resistance |
| | | Some ventilation/perfusion mismatch |
| | | Mild hypoxemia |

With Progression (12 to 24 Hours)

*Phase 2 (Onset Parenchymal Changes)*

| | | |
|---|---|---|
| Patchy alveolar infiltrates beginning in dependent lung | Dyspnea, tachypnea, cyanosis, tachycardia, course rales | Increased lung permeability |
| No cuffs (unless a component of high pressure edema is present) | | Increasing shunt, dead space |
| | | Progressive decrease compliance |
| | | Increased work of breathing |
| Normal heart size | | Increasing minute ventilation |

With Progression (2 to 7 Days)

*Phase 3 (Acute Respiratory Failure)*

| | | |
|---|---|---|
| Diffuse alveolar infiltrates | Tachypnea, tachycardia, hyperdynamic state | Progression of impaired gas |
| Air bronchograms | Sepsis syndrome | Increasing shunt fraction |
| Decreased lung volume | Signs of consolidation | Increased minute ventilation |
| | | Decreased static compliance and impaired tissue oxygenation |
| | | Decreased alveolar oxygen gradient |
| | | Lactic acidosis |

With Progression (Beyond 10 Days)

*Phase 4 (Pulmonary Fibrosis)*

| | | |
|---|---|---|
| Persistent diffuse infiltrates | Symptoms as above | Pneumonia |
| Superimposed new pneumonic infiltrates | Recurrent sepsis | Progressive restrictive lung disease |
| Recurrent pneumothorax | | |
| Normal heart | | |

Early pathogenic findings consist of interstitial edema, focal hemorrhage, and atelectasis, with pulmonary microvascular congestion. This progresses to intra-alveolar edema and hemorrhage with severe congestion and atelectasis. Hyaline membranes are seen in the alveoli. The mechanism of the acute injury process is not totally defined, but the initiating event is an injury to the circulatory side of the alveolar capillary membrane. At this stage, the ARDS process is reversible if the initiating factor is controlled.

*Phase Three*

Progression to *phase three* is manifested by the onset of acute respiratory failure, as previously outlined, necessitating mechanical ventilation. The lungs become more diffusely involved and more stiff. The shunt fraction increases as a result of patchy atelectasis from surfactant denaturation and focal alveolar consolidation due to increased permeability. The increase in carbon dioxide production during this postburn period can also lead to hypercapnia when the lung is damaged. A hyperdynamic state frequently evolves with an increase in cardiac output, evidence of lactic acidosis, and a characteristic decrease in oxygen extraction from hemoglobin. The impairment in the ability of tissues to increase the extraction of oxygen from hemoglobin, in order to compensate for increased oxygen needs, is a characteristic of the sepsis syndrome when ARDS is present. The mechanism may be related to impaired metabolic function of the lung, which normally removes vasodilator agents released from inflammation.

*Phase Four*

The *fourth phase* is one of progressive pulmonary fibrosis and recurrent pneumonias. Areas of lung infection become evident due to impaired bacterial clearance. Areas of the lung become relatively acellular, being replaced by fibrous tissue. The process becomes much less reversible at this stage.

The progression of single organ lung failure to a multisystem failure (with liver, gastrointestinal tract, and kidney dysfunction) commonly occurs with late ARDS. Further lung insults need to be avoided if the fibrosis is to resolve. Mortality rate is more than 90%, once burn patients enter this phase.

## Treatment

Mortality rate of ARDS caused by burn inflammation and infection is extremely high. The major reason for the lethal nature of the process is that resolution will not occur until the initiating process is removed. The wound, especially in the large burn, cannot be readily excised and closed at this stage of the postburn process. The most important early tretament is prevention, i.e., early removal of as much of the potential source as is feasible.

*Phases 1 and 2*

Treatment, once the disease evolves, is aimed at preventing progression while an attempt is made to delete the source. If the patient clearly has evidence of a rapidly progressing process approaching the criteria for acute respiratory failure, then endotracheal intubation and positive-pressure breathing will be necessary. Fluid overload should be avoided at this stage while assuring adequate maintenance of tissue perfusion. However, the increase in lung capillary permeability results in a rapid progression of the edema process with even small increases in capillary hydrostatic pressure. Blood volume can be well maintained with blood and colloid in combination with the necessary crystalloid used to replace water and electrolyte losses. A pulmonary artery catheter is advantageous during this early period because a clinical assessment of volume status is frequently misleading.

## Phases 3 and 4

Positive-pressure ventilation will be required to support gas exchange and decrease the shunt fraction with the onset of acute respiratory failure (see Section 7). A pulmonary artery catheter will be required at least during the initial course to assure that an optimum cardiac output is maintained during the positive airway pressure while avoiding a large increase in wedge pressure, which results in more edema. The optimum PEEP is that value that best accomplishes this goal (best PEEP). A very finely balanced treatment regimen is required to allow for successful resolution of ARDS. Of course, elimination of the initial cause is essential. Besides this component, an adequate oxygen delivery must be provided to systemic tissues. Aggressive diuresis may well improve arterial oxygen pressure but can lead to an overall deterioration in the state of perfusion. Lactic acidosis means the delivery system is inadequate. Excessive oxygen demands caused by pain, anxiety, excessive muscle activity, or hyperthermia should be controlled. These same components will also increase carbon dioxide production, which in turn requires an increase in minute ventilation.

Close monitoring for the onset of nosocomial pneumonia is necessary because local lung and systemic immune defenses will be impaired. Appropriate antibiotic therapy needs to be initiated early in the course of any acute lung infection in order to avoid the perpetuation of the acute ARDS process into one of chronic inflammation and fibrosis.

## ARDS TREATMENT SUMMARY

Phase 1
1. Administer oxygen: maintain oxygen saturation more than 90%
2. Determine and delete source of lung response
3. Maintain perfusion but avoid volume overload

Phase 2
1. Administer oxygen: maintain oxygen saturation more than 90%
2. May need positive airway pressure (PEEP, CPAP)
3. Avoid volume overload (consider pulmonary artery catheter)

Phase 3
1. Requires positive pressure ventilation; add PEEP
2. Needs pulmonary artery catheter
3. Adjust PEEP, tidal volume to improve static compliance and arterial oxygen tension but not impair oxygen delivery
4. Maintain wedge pressure below 15 mmHg, preferably 10 to 12 mmHg.
5. Maintain blood volume and hemoglobin

6. Avoid overhydration but be careful of diuretics
7. Maintain close surveillance for nosocomial pneumonia

Phase 4
1. As above
2. Minimize barotrauma (may need muscle paralysis)
3. Avoid excess oxygen consumption and carbon dioxide production
4. Must maintain lungs as infection-free as possible to minimize stimulus to progression of lung injury

## COMMON PITFALLS

### Underestimation of Risks for Pneumonia

Once resuscitation is completed and the patient has become stabilized and is beginning to be more active, there is a tendency to be lulled into complacency regarding pulmonary support. The patient remains at high risk for pneumonia for several weeks.

### Underestimation of Increased Ventilatory Requirements in Perioperative Period

Maintenance of a "normal" minute ventilation in the perioperative period is not adequate in a patient generating up to twice the normal amount of carbon dioxide. Hypercapnia in the intraoperative or early postoperative period with its resultant massive catecholamine release can almost always be avoided by maintaining preoperative ventilatory needs in the intra- and postoperative period.

### Underestimation of the Workload of Breathing During the Hypermetabolic State

A two- to threefold increase in minute ventilation is a substantial work load. Ventilatory assist may be needed and should be initiated before respiratory deterioration.

### Underutilization of the Tracheostomy

Although a tracheostomy is usually not indicated in the first several days and is contraindicated through burn tissue, its use for chronic respiratory support is very advantageous. A tracheostomy through a nonburn or excised and grafted skin can improve pulmonary toilet, improve rehabilitation efforts by physical therapy, and will improve comfort.

# PREVENTION AND TREATMENT

## Nosocomial Pneumonia

*Maintain Cough*
1. Controlled analgesia and sedation
2. Maintain chest wall muscle mass (nutrition and exercise)
3. Repositioning and chest physical therapy
4. Avoid lung edema
5. Consider tracheostomy at 7 to 10 days if long-term support anticipated

*Minimize Oropharyngeal Colonization*
1. Compulsive hand washing
2. Surveillance for possible bacterial reservoirs
3. Avoid inappropriate antibiotic use

*Improving Systemic Host Defenses*
1. Early removal of burn tissue
2. Nutrition
3. Maintain adequate oxygen delivery to tissues

*Minimize Risk of Tracheobronchial Aspiration*
1. Head elevation
2. Aseptic suction techniques

*Antibiotic Therapy*
1. Initiate with evidence of bacterial infection in airways

## PREVENTION AND TREATMENT OF POWER FAILURE

### (Relative Hypoventilation)

Maintain Nutrition
Aggressive Pulmonary Toilet

*Mechanical Problems*

1. Maintain adequate rest (consider partial mechanical assist, IMV or CPAP) especially in the perioperative period
2. Avoid increasing $V_D/V_T$ (adequate blood volume low mean airway pressure)

*Excessive Carbon Dioxide Production*

1. Control excess carbohydrate
2. Control temperature
3. Avoid excess anxiety or pain

# SUMMARY OF PULMONARY PROBLEMS

## Prevention and Treatment

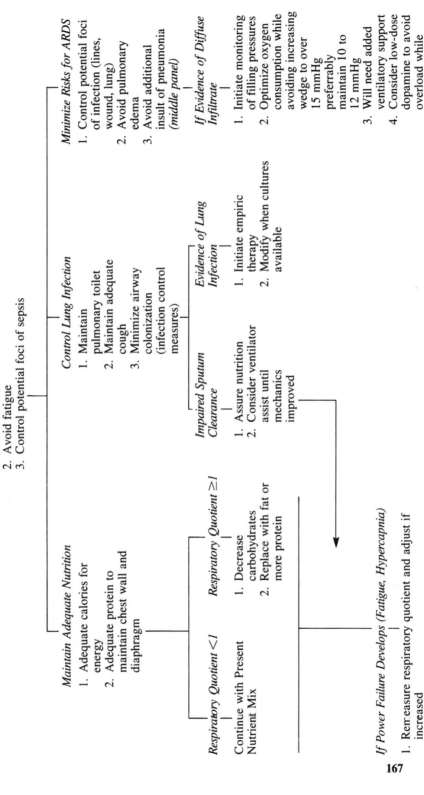

# 10

# Hemodynamic and Metabolic Support

The onset of the hypermetabolic state and infection along with continued fluid and protein losses make this a challenging time to maintain hemodynamic stability. A good understanding of burn-induced metabolic and physiologic changes is necessary in order to determine what type of fluid, electrolyte, and nutrient is required. The following general areas will be discussed:

> Pathophysiology of the Postburn Hypermetabolic State
> > Fluid, Protein, and Red Blood Cell Losses
> > Hypermetabolic State
>
> Practical Approach to Management
> > Type of Volume Replacement
> > Provide Adequate Nutrition to Meet the Increased Tissue Demands

Chapter 21 on Nutritional Support includes a discussion of the use of parenteral and enteral nutrition.

## PATHOPHYSIOLOGY OF POSTBURN HYPERMETABOLISM

### Fluid, Protein, Red Blood Cell Losses

Fluid, protein, and red blood cell losses during this period are primarily those from evaporation and losses due to wound debridement. Processes to be discussed include:

> Evaporative water losses
> Urine output
> Wound care losses (blood)
> Protein stores
> Electrolyte shifts

## Evaporative Water Loss

Evaporative water losses remain increased until the wound is closed. Even after closure, evaporative losses through skin-grafted wound are much higher than normal skin. The standard formula for assisting in estimating losses can still be used:

Evaporative water loss ml/hr = (25 + % total body surface burn) × $m^2$ body surface area

However, water losses from the soft eschar or the debriding wound with granulation tissues are considerably greater than from the earlier thick dry eschar because surface blood flow is now much higher. Wound losses are comparable to those expected from a pan of water of equal surface area at the same environmental temperature. Donor sites, although usually occluded, are an added source of loss. Losses are further increased by the invariable increase in body temperature accompanying this period.

## Urine Output

The hypermetabolic state and the resulting increased solute load from both catabolism and anabolism, in the large burn produce an obligate increase in urinary output, characteristically an output 2 to 2.5 L/day, with a specific gravity of more than 1.020. The additional 1 to 1.5 L of urine loss, over that seen in normal man, needs to be considered when assessing fluid needs. Hyperglycemia, especially with the use of nutritional support, can dramatically increase urine output leading to an inappropriate diuresis relative to the true status of the extracellular fluid.

## Wound Losses (Blood)

The friable vascularized wound tends to be a source of constant blood loss even with very gentle daily care. Frequent blood sampling also is a source of continued loss. The lack of red blood cell production (until the wound is closed) and the continued dialy losses cause a constant need for blood replacement. Losses from wound excisions during the early part of this period with wound hypervascularity can be massive.

## Protein Stores

Protein losses from wound exudation and from bleeding persist until wound closure. Albumin production by the liver is markedly decreased during the hypermetabolic state in favor of acute-phase protein synthesis. Therefore albumin losses are not compensated for by adequate new albumin synthesis and hypoalbuminemia will persist despite adequate nutritional support.

## Electrolyte Shifts

As with the previous time period, electrolyte abnormalities are quite common. Replacement of water alone often leads to hyponatremia if gastrointestinal losses are increased, e.g., tube feeding diarrhea. Addition of excess salt in the presence of large evaporative water losses, in turn, can lead to hypernatremia. Potassium abnormalities are common, particularly with the onset of nutritional support. Calcium, magnesium, and phosphate abnormalities are also common and must be monitored.

Of particular concern is the initial loss of water and electrolytes from the gastrointestinal tract with the onset of enteral feedings. Diarrhea is particularly common when the gut has not been used for the first week. Mucosal atrophy and decreased surface area for absorption will occur very rapidly after burn if initial nutrients are not able to be provided. The majority of calories and nutrients for protein synthesis to the gut, itself, is derived from enteral not parenteral feedings.

## Hypermetabolic State

Beginning at day 5 or 6, there is a gradual increase in metabolic rate from a normal of 35 to 40 cal/m$^2$/hr (25 cal/kg/day) to levels up to 2 to 2.5 times this value at about 10 days. The increase in metabolic rate after burns is far in excess of that seen after any other severe injury, including sepsis. The magnitude of increase is directly related to burn size. Young patients appear to generate a higher postburn metabolic rate than do elderly patients.

The hypermetabolic state is characterized by increased oxygen consumption, increased heat production, increased body temperature, and increased protein catabolism. Body temperature increases from a normal of 98°F (37°C) to 100 to 101°F (38 to 38.5°C). This process is believed to be due to a resetting of the hypothalamic temperature center due to the altered hormonal environment. A current hypothesis as to the increased temperature is interleukin-1 or tumor necrosis factor, released from the wound, which triggers prostaglandin $E_2$ production in the hypothalamus. Thus the *major metabolic abnormalities after burn injury* are:

1. A sustained increase in body temperature
2. A marked increase in glucose demands and therefore a marked stimulus to liver gluconeogenesis
3. Rapid skeletal muscle breakdown caused by a demand for amino acid substrate both for use as a direct energy source, for gluconeogenesis, and for use by the liver for acute-phase protein production
4. Increased ureagenesis
5. The stimulation of the liver to produce large quantities of acute-phase proteins
6. Lack of ketosis indicating fat is not the major caloric source: Ketones, however, are still used as a calorie source

Table 10-1 Metabolic Rate and Core Temperature in Normal Persons and Burn Patients at "Preferred" Ambient Temperatures

|  | Comfort Temperature (°C) | Core Temperature (°C) | Metabolic Rate (Kcal/m$^2$/hr) |
|---|---|---|---|
| Normal persons (n = 5) | 28.6 ± 0.7 | 36.9 ± 0.1 | 34.1 ± 0.8 |
| Burn patients (n = 7) (37% body surface area burn) | 31.5 ± 0.7 | 38.1 ± 0.4 | 63.9 ± 5.7 |

Endotoxin can also cause the increased temperature by the same hypothalmic effect. Excess heat loss will certainly accentuate the stress response.

The stimulus for gluconeogenesis and the hyperglycemia characteristic of the hypermetabolic state appear to be caused by a number of efferent mediators released as a result of afferent stimuli (Table 10-2). Plasma levels of catecholamines, cortisol, glucagon, and growth hormone are all increased postburn. It appears that the burn response is a result of the interaction between all these hormones. Urinary cathecholamine excretion is increased in proportion to the severity of injury and the metabolic rate. Insulin levels are also elevated, but the high levels of anti-insulin hormones appear to impair glucose transport into cells, particularly into skeletal muscle. The decrease in tissue responsiveness to insulin may result in the necessity for exogenous insulin supplementation. In the early postburn period, levels of thyroxine are normal, but serum levels of triiodothyronine are decreased. Thyroid hormone, however, does not appear to play a key role in this process because burn thyroidectomized animals reach the same increase in oxygen consumption as those with an intact thyroid.

The result of the afferent and efferent stimuli is a marked requirement for calories and a rapid loss of body nitrogen. Much of the glucose generated by the liver is utilized anaerobically by the burn wound generating lactate, which is then transported back to the liver for gluconeogenesis. Lactate is rapidly cleared so that plasma levels are usually not increased unless sepsis or hypovolemia is also present. The increased blood flow to the wound supports the increased nutrient demands of the wound. Fat is also utilized for calories, as is evident by the fact that the respiratory quotient of the burn patient is about 0.8.

Although the afferent and efferent mediators are responsible for the characteristics of this hyperdynamic state, there is clear evidence of a central nervous system modulation of the response. The afferent signal can be accentuated by the brain, particularly in the presence of excessive pain. High-dose narcotic infusions or general anesthesia can substantially attentuate the response. The wound and wound mediators initiate the response, but the manner and degree to which the wound controls the process is not well understood. The metabolic rate will return to normal once the wound is closed and the inflammation resolves. Immediate closure of the wound postburn would be expected to attenuate the response. As yet, this has not been verified by any human study.

The local mediator- and endocrine-induced hypermetabolic state leads to major physiologic changes. Cardiac output increases to levels two- to threefold above normal. Oxygen consumption increases from a normal value of about 125 ml/M$^2$/min to values approaching 300 ml/M$^2$/min. Carbon dioxide production can also reach values more than

**Table 10-2**

Afferent (Wound) Mediators
   Prostanoids, oxygen radicals, lipid peroxides
   Macrophage factor
     Interleukin-1
     Tumor necrosis factor
Endotoxin; bacterial by-products
Efferent (hormonal) mediators
   Catecholamines, cortisol
   Glucagon, growth hormone

two times normal. Urine output will remain 1 to 2 ml/kg/hr as long as an increased solute load is present. Pulse rate again increases, as was seen in the initial hypoxemia phase, but now systemic vascular resistance is decreased. Systemic hypertension is relatively common, particularly in patients with a relatively noncompliant vascular tree. Heart failure may well occur in patients with an impaired myocardium during this period if the increased cardiac work demands cannot be met by an increase in myocardial blood flow. In summary, the *physiologic effects of hypermetabolism* are:

    Increased cardiac output

    Increased oxygen consumption

    Increased carbon dioxide production

    Decreased systemic vascular resistance

The full-thickness burn wound that is not yet closed begins to develop granulation tissue with sloughing of the outer eschar. Increased pain is evident. The added stress of continued pain can result in an accentuation of the hypermetabolism, as can an increase in anxiety level. The mechanism is an accentuated release of catecholamines.

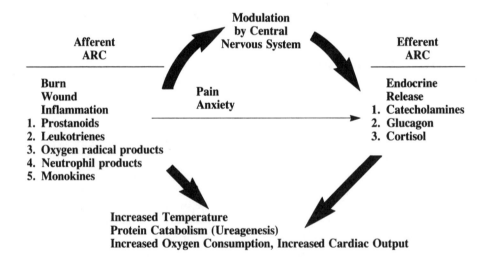

## PRACTICAL APPROACH TO MANAGEMENT

### Type of Fluid Replacement

Free water losses must be accurately replaced, especially after the extra fluid reservoir found in initial burn edema has been resorbed. This reservoir is usually close to dry after the first 7 to 10 days. Electrolyte abnormalities usually relate to the increased metabolic rate and nutritional support. Potassium and phosphate replacement are especially important. The extra water losses allow for the use of more dilute solutions of nutrients and often the use of peripheral veins instead of central veins to supplement enteral feeding. It is preferable to maintain a serum albumin above 2.5 g/dl, especially if lipids are used as a major nutrient source to allow for adequate binding of free fatty acids to avoid hypoproteinemia-induced tissue edema. Although a hematocrit of less than 30 may be sufficient for a young patient after nonburn trauma, the tissue oxygen needs of a major burn are considerably greater and therefore severe anemia is less well tolerated.

## Provide Adequate Nutrition to Meet the Increased Tissue Demands

It is expected that nutritional support is started in the early postresuscitation period so that demands are met during this period of increasing metabolic activity. The first requirement is an estimation of energy needs followed by an organized approach at nutrient delivery tailoring the carbohydrate, protein, and fat to the individual patients needs. More specific information on nutritional support can be found in Section 7.

### Estimation of Energy Requirements

The objective of nutritional support is to provide the necessary calories for the required energy needs. The energy required is dependent on *energy expenditure,* which is divided into three components: basal metabolic rate, muscle activity, and stress-induced energy needs.

"Basal metabolic rate" is the term describing the energy required to maintain cell integrity in the resting state and at thermoneutrality. The latter term means an ambient temperature usually close to 80°F (28°C) where heat loss and the need for increased heat production to maintain body temperature are minimal. Environmental temperature in a normal adult below 65°F or above 85°F will increase sympathetic activity and in turn increase caloric needs. The basal metabolic rate for an adult has been defined by direct calorimetry. Body size is a principal factor and the value is therefore normalized to $m^2$ body surface. Other variables include age and, to a lesser extent, sex. A large portion of this energy goes into heat production maintaining body temperature.

Activity level relates to the energy utilized by muscles for average daily activity. In the patient in the intensive care unit, this activity is usually quite limited and is usually considered to be no more than an additional 25% of the basal metabolic rate. Excessive muscle activity, e.g., from "fighting the ventilator," from an excessive work of breathing, or as a result of a combative disoriented state, will markedly increase the energy expenditure. Sedation or, if necessary, muscle paralysis may be needed to control this component.

The third component, namely, stress-induced energy needs, includes the *"stress factor,"* which defines the hypermetabolism induced by the burn that is present (Table 10-3). The stress factor is a multiple of the basal metabolic rate (normalized to 1.0). The value takes into consideration the type of size of burn injury present and the average metabolic response seen with this degree of injury.

Caloric requirements can be measured directly using *direct calorimetry techniques.* These are, however, impractical for the intensive care unit. Since more than 95% of energy generated requires oxygen, there is a direct proportion between *oxygen consumption* and *metabolic rate.* The increase in oxygen consumption compared with normal can be

**Table 10-3** Stress-Induced Energy Needs

| Burn Size (%Total Body Surface) | Stress Factor |
|---|---|
| 10 | 1.25 |
| 20 | 1.5 |
| 30 | 1.7 |
| 40 | 1.85 |
| 50 | 2.0 |
| 60-100 | 2.1 |

used to calculate the increase in metabolic rate. An estimation of caloric needs is based on the following simple formula:

Energy requirements = basal metabolic rate × 1.25 (activity) × stress factor

If the activity level is markedly increased or additional stress, e.g., severe pain, is present, metabolic rate can be further increased.

## *Assessment of Nutrients Required (Amounts of Carbohydrates, Fat, and Protein)*

Carbohydrate is the preferred fuel for most tissues, but there is a clear limit to the amount that will be used, especially in the hypermetabolic or septic patient. Current recommendations are that carbohydrate infusion not exceed 5 to 7 mg/kg/min, or approximately 1800 to 2200 carbohydrate calories per day. Excess carbohydrate will only result in fat formation, which is energy requiring rather than energy producing and the respiratory quotient approaches 8 for this process, leading to a marked increase in carbon dioxide production.

Approximately 60% of estimated nonprotein calorie requirements needs to be given as glucose in order to spare the nitrogen effectively. Fat can be used as a calorie source for the remaining 40% of nonprotein calories. Monitoring of triglyceride levels is necessary to avoid exceeding a value of 250 mg/dl, 4 hours after cessation of the lipid infusion. Lipid clearance is not impaired in the majority of burn patients; in fact, lipid utilization may well be increased. The respiratory quotient for fat is 0.7; therefore less carbon dioxide is produced per calorie utilized.

Protein (nitrogen) requirements are calculated in a number of fashions. A standard estimate of 1.5 to 2 g of protein per kg body weight can be used for all major burns. A more specific quantitative estimate is that based on the appropriate calorie to nitrogen ratio to be used. A 150:1 calorie to nitrogen ratio has been the standard used for a number of years. Recent data in burn patients would indicate that a 100:1 ratio may be preferable. This is based on the findings that a protein-rich diet is more effective in reversing the immune deficiencies seen the postburn period. Noninjured man normally consumes a diet with a ratio of about 250:1. In order to avoid the added protein from being utilized as substitute for gluconeogenesis, sufficient glucose must also be infused.

## Provision of Necessary Vitamins and Trace Elements

A number of vitamins are lost in increased quantities in the burn patient both because of loss in wound secretions and with increased metabolism. The vitamins A and C are of particular concern because they are essential for healing. Vitamin A should be given in a daily dose of 10,000 to 25,000 U and vitamin C in a daily dose of about 1 g. Zinc, a trace element required for healing, is also lost in increased amounts. Replacement is usually 220 mg $ZnSO_4$ twice daily given orally or 45 mg daily given parenterally. The vitamin B complex is also essential with doses for burn being 5 to 10 times the recommended daily allowance. The specific added needs of the other trace minerals is not well defined.

## Route of Administration of Nutrition

Nutritional support is best managed during this period by the enteral route, usually through a combination of a balanced tube feeding and voluntary intake. Parenteral supplementation through a peripheral vein may be necessary in the very large burn patient. Parenteral hyperalimentation through a central vein is occasionally required if, for some reason, the gastrointestinal tract is not functioning adequately, as sometimes occurs with the patient on a ventilator or the patient with significant sepsis.

Since there is a large obligate fluid requirement, with large body surface burns, the majority of the calorie and protein requirements can be infused through a peripheral vein. Enteral feedings utilizing a nasogastric feeding tube can usually be initiated within 4 to 5 days after burn. The limiting factor to success, at least initially, is again the osmolarity of the solutions. Isosmolar solutions are reasonably well tolerated if begun slowly. Many of these standard solutions have a caloric density of 1 cal/cc but are low in protein (calorie to nitrogen ratio, being more than 200:1). Solutions with a higher protein content tend to be hyperosmolar, leading more frequently to diarrhea. Specific information on tube feeding can be found in the Section 7.

## SUMMARY OF HEMODYNAMIC AND METABOLIC SUPPORT

*Restore and Maintain Adequate Oxygen Delivery*

1. Replace red blood cell losses to maintain hematocrit more than 30
2. Maintain serum albumin 2.5 g/dl or higher
3. Maintain cardiac index approximately 1.5 to 2.0 times normal
4. If lactic acidosis is present, increase oxygen delivery
5. Keep arterial oxygen saturation more than 90%

*Maintain Fluid and Electrolyte Balance*

1. Replace increased water losses (evaporative and urinary)
2. Replace electrolyte losses (especially increased gastrointestinal, diarrhea, nitrogen losses)
3. Replace extracellular, which shift into cells with nutrition (especially $K^+$, $PO_4^-$)

*Maintain Nutrition*

1. Determine calorie needs based on % total body surface burn and kilogram of body weight (basal metabolic rate × activity (1.25) × burn stress factor)
2. Give 1.5 to 2 g protein/Kg body weight (100:1 calorie to nitrogen ratio)
3. Readjust needs as wound heals or is grafted

*Avoid Excess Stress*

1. Avoid excess temperature (>102°F) for sustained periods
2. Avoid excess heat loss
3. Avoid excess pain, anxiety
4. Assure adequate rest

## Route

1. Begin parenteral on day 2 to 3; peripheral solution
2. Begin enteral as soon as possible
3. Use enteral as primary for tube feeding
4. Supplement: Peripheral or central solution depending on fluid needs and intravenous access
5. Change intravenous catheter frequently
6. See Section 7 for specifics

## Type of Calories

### Carbohydrate (3.3 cal/g)

1. Give no more than 5-7 mg/kg/day
2. Should equal more than 50% of total nonprotein calories
3. Supplement with insulin if needed
4. Assess respiratory quotient if excess carbohydrate is being considered
5. If respiratory quotient 1.0 or higher decrease carbohydrate and increase fat or protein (glucose intolerance common with added sepsis)

### Fat (10 cal/g)

1. Should equal or be less than 50% of total nonprotein calories
2. Give no more than 2 g/kg/day
3. Make sure clearance is adequate triglyceride less than 250 mg/dl

### Protein (4 cal/g)

1. Should equal about 15 to 20% of total calculated calories
2. Check nitrogen balance

## Supplements

1. Vitamin A 10,000 U every day
2. Vitamin C 1 g every day
3. Zinc sulfate 220 mg orally twice daily or 45 mg
4. Vitamin B complex 10 times recommended daily allowance

# Summary of Hemodynamic and Metabolic Changes

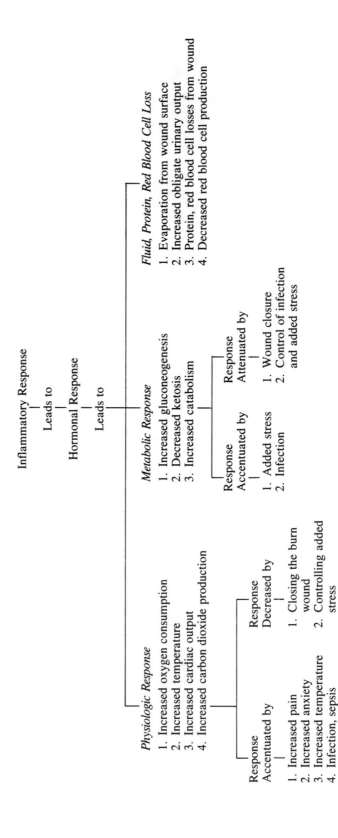

Inflammatory Response
|
Leads to
|
Hormonal Response
|
Leads to

*Physiologic Response*
1. Increased oxygen consumption
2. Increased temperature
3. Increased cardiac output
4. Increased carbon dioxide production

Response Accentuated by
1. Increased pain
2. Increased anxiety
3. Increased temperature
4. Infection, sepsis
5. Wound manipulation

Response Decreased by
1. Closing the burn wound
2. Controlling added stress

*Metabolic Response*
1. Increased gluconeogenesis
2. Decreased ketosis
3. Increased catabolism

Response Accentuated by
1. Added stress
2. Infection

Response Attenuated by
1. Wound closure
2. Control of infection and added stress

*Fluid, Protein, Red Blood Cell Loss*
1. Evaporation from wound surface
2. Increased obligate urinary output
3. Protein, red blood cell losses from wound
4. Decreased red blood cell production

# 11
# Management of the Burn Wound

The wound during this period has changed considerably from the wound during the first several days. The superficial burn is rapidly healing, the deep second degree burn is beginning to debride and become much more uncomfortable and prone to infection. The full-thickness burn is now colonized and revascularized and the eschar is beginning to separate. The deep burn, which is now inflamed, hyperemic, and colonized (or infected) with bacteria, must be managed much more gently than in the prior phases. Bacteremia and endotoxemia will occur with any vigorous wound manipulation. Antibiotic-resistant organisms also become more common. During this phase, surgical procedures on the wound are most safely performed after a granulation tissue bed has developed. After 7 to 10 days, fascial excision is no longer feasible and tangential excision of thick eschar down to a viable base has the increased risks of disseminating infection and increased blood loss. A much safer procedure is the tangential excision of a thin layer of granulation tissue on a clean granulating wound followed by immediate application of skin grafts. The specific wound changes will be discussed, as will the approaches to wound management.

## GENERAL SECTIONS

    Pathophysiologic Changes in the Burn Wound
    Practical Approach to Treatment
        Daily Burn Care
        Surgical Management
        Pitfalls in Management

## PATHOPHYSIOLOGIC CHANGES IN THE BURN WOUND

### Superficial Second Degree Burn

The superficial to mid second degree burn begins to reepithelialize rapidly during this period, since the necessary and wound healing elements have arrived in the first postburn week. Healing is primarily from wound surface up, not from encroachment by the wound edge. The wound base usually does not have sufficient time to develop significant fibrosis and collagen deposition so that the wound remains quite pliable. The wound is at relatively low risk for infection unless blood flow is somehow impaired as, e.g., with a burn on an ischemic leg or in a diabetic. The new epidermis is initially relatively thin but is anchored quite firmly to the underlying dermis by remaining rete pegs. Blistering, however, can occur with minor trauma in the first several weeks. The wound hyperemia often takes several weeks to resolve. Heat and evaporative losses will also be increased above that for normal skin for several weeks until normal autoregulation of skin blood flow returns. Significant scarring with this depth of burn is usually minimal because the wound heals before extensive wound collagen deposition. However, oil gland function is impaired for several weeks to months and the skin tends to become dry and scaly for several weeks. Some discomfort persists, especially with stretching or with exposure to extremes of temperature. Autoregulation of skin blood flow remains impaired for several weeks, thereby decreasing the tolerance to heat or cold. Repigmentation of dark skin may require several months.

## Deep Second Degree Burn

The relatively thick eschar of a deep dermal burn begins slowly to separate from the underlying viable dermis. Inflammatory mediators, proteases, etc., are released in increased quantities once blood flow is increased. The wound inflammation, along with loss of heat from the open surface, maintains the hypermetabolic state. Infection markedly accentuates the local inflammation and the systemic hypermetabolism. With eschar separation, heat and evaporative water loss and pain increase. The friable tissue bleeds readily with minor tissue trauma. Hemostasis can usually be controlled by pressure alone. The eschar usually separates in a nonuniform fashion due to regional differences in burn depth and blood supply. Frequently, the actual depth of the injury cannot be discerned until the eschar has been removed and the amount of or lack of remaining dermis is noted. Fibroblasts and myofibroblasts begin to populate the wound base at the 2- to 3-week period, replacing inflammatory cells. A significant amount of wound exudate usually develops on the surface, especially if topical antibiotics are used. The exudate is made up of inflammatory cells and necrotic debris. Extensive angiogenesis at the wound base leads to a marked increase in wound vascularity. The granulation tissue is composed of a dense network of capillaries in which is interspersed fibrous tissue. The wound becomes an active metabolic organ using large amounts of oxygen and nutrients. Lactate is also produced in large amounts by the wound, even in the presence of adequate molecular oxygen. Small islands of remaining epidermal cells begin to hypertrophy, forming little mounds or buds that are also innervated and are extremely painful to mechanical stimulation. The previously relatively anesthetic deep second degree burn now becomes much more uncomfortable. In addition, regenerating exposed nerve endings and an increasing mast cell population, releasing histamine, produce ongoing irritation and severe pruritus.

Infection remains a significant problem during this period and wound conversion can still occur several weeks after injury, especially if systemic sepsis and hypoperfusion develop. Pyrogens are released as well as bacteria with each wound manipulation, resulting in a continued febrile response as well as additional transient fever spikes.

Conversion to a full-thickness injury can occur with infection, hypoperfusion, or desiccation. Epithelialization, which can take 8 to 12 weeks for completion, occurs by proliferation of remaining epithelial cells in skin appendages and also migration from the wound edge. The end result is a thin layer of epidermis that is poorly fixed to underlying dermis or scar. The epidermal layer is extremely friable for several months, with blistering and subsequent epidermal loss being quite common. Surface heat and water losses remain increased over that seen with normal skin. The wound is also very susceptible to infection and subsequent loss of the new skin. The local infection is often produced by *Staphylococcus aureus*. Small cysts, from obstructed sebaceous glands, occur over the next weeks to months, again with a *S. aureus* superinfection. The scar tissue continues to increase and the wound becomes quite nonpliable due both to scar thickening and wound contraction. Impaired motion is a major problem if the wound crosses a joint.

## Third Degree Burn

The full-thickness burn becomes inflamed, revascularizes, and becomes colonized (or infected) in a similar fashion to the deep second degree burn. However, the underlying fat frequently takes longer to develop sufficient blood supply for adequate immune defenses. The healing rate is impaired by the presence of a thick wound eschar. The rate of subsequent new tissue formation is in direct proportion to the amount of oxygen and nutrients delivered to the tissues. The wound inflammatory response will also lead to

**Table 11-1** Open Wound Beyond 7 to 10 Days

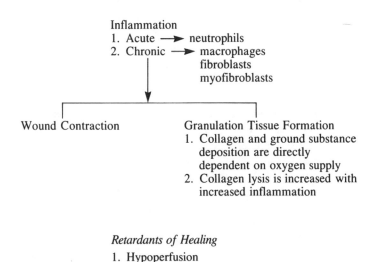

dissolution of the overlying eschar as proteases are released from the wound leukocytes. The loss of eschar integrity and the increased wound vascularity increase the surface evaporation and heat losses. Blood loss can be significant with even minor wound manipulations. The risk of invasive infection increases as poorly vascularized fat or other subeschar tissue is exposed to a high bacterial content in the overlying necrotic eschar. Pockets of infection and purulence often develop during this period in the subeschar space. These local infections are often the source of the systemic bacteremias and endotoxemias that occur with wound manipulation. Pyrogen release from the wound probably due to stimulation of wound macrophages will occur with or without infection. As the eschar is removed, the wound base develops a superficial layer of granulation tissue. Vascular granulation tissue is more resistant to surface infection than fat. However, the granulation tissue needs adequate oxygen and blood flow for its continued presence and a low flow state will lead to rapid dissolution of the new tissue. A purulent exudate present on the wound surface will also impair new growth so that the rate of lysis exceeds the rate of new tissue formation. The wound with the new layer of granulation tissue is much more painful than in the first 7 to 10 days when a thick eschar was still present (Color plate 13, page 316). The hypermetabolic state will persist as long as the wound remains open.

## Wound Contracture and Scar Production

During the first 6 days, wound inflammation has begun and the various components of healing have been initiated, as described in Section 2. In superficial burns, epidermal regeneration will be relatively rapid, if the wound environment is optimized. The injured dermal elements are usually covered by new epithelium within 2 weeks. The hyperplasia of dermal fibroblasts then begins to resolve, and healing is complete with only modest amounts of collagen deposited. The wound usually becomes relatively pliable with time and minimal wound contraction is seen. Cosmetically, the superficial second degree burn, which heals in 2 weeks, results in minimal to no long-term scarring.

The histology of the wound, however, changes dramatically if it has not been closed by 2 weeks, as would be the case with a nongrafted deep dermal or full-thickness burn. Fibroblasts and macrophages become the predominant cells. Large numbers of myofibroblasts also enter the wound. These are modified fibroblasts that also have some of the contractile properties of smooth muscle. Microfilament bundles can be seen in their cytoplasm, lined parallel to each other and parallel with the direction of contraction. Cells are linked together via extracellular extensions that allow transmission of the contractile forces. This results in a synchronized contractile process similar to that in smooth muscle. Myofibroblasts compose over three fourths of the cells in granulating wounds and in hypertrophic scar the number of cells correlating with the rate of wound contraction. Besides leading to contraction, these cells continue to deposit large quantities of collagen and glycosaminoglycans. Mast cells are also present in this very active wound. These cells degranulate, releasing not only more mucopolysaccharides into the wound, providing a matrix for more collagen deposition, but also histamine, which results in the hyperemia. Closure of this wound by reepithelialization or grafting does not eliminate the stimulus for ongoing scar formation. Angiogenesis continues, as does mucopolysaccharide and collagen production. A marked increase in the proteoglycan content of chrondroitin sulfate A can be seen as well. This substance, which is usually found in firm tissues such as cartilage, produces a harder, less pliable wound. As myofibroblasts contract, thereby shortening the scar, the deposition of the mucopolysaccharides and ground substances results in fusion of the collagen fibers in the contracted site. The process of wound contraction will lead to joint contractures.

Collagenase is also released by inflammatory cells. Synthesis of new and lysis of old collagen are ongoing processes. Any exaggeration of lysis or retardation of synthesis will lead to dissolution of the new tissue. Rapid dissolution of the newly found granulation tissue occurs with wound infection as a result of the exaggerated wound inflammation and the release of neutrophil proteases. In addition, any hypoperfusion of the wound, especially that caused by systemic sepsis, will lead to rapid disappearance of the new granulation tissue and collagen deposition ceases and lysis persists.

## PRACTICAL APPROACH TO TREATMENT

### Daily Burn Care

The objectives of daily burn care are to optimize the rate of wound healing while minimizing the systemic complications of the wound. The wound care plan should be sufficiently flexible so that the care plan can be altered with changes in the wound.

#### *Standard Principles*

Standard principles basically hold for all wounds. *First,* adequate hemodynamic monitoring must be provided. *Second,* bacterial cross-contamination must be minimized. Clean areas, e.g., new grafts, donor sites, etc., and healing burns should be managed separately from contaminated wounds or areas with a high bacterial content, such as the rectum and perineum. *Third,* the wound should be managed gently. Vigorous surface care during this phase can lead to bacteremias. *Fourth,* hypothermia must be avoided. The room should be adequately warmed, as should the wash solutions. Total body exposure at one time leads to a greater heat loss than if individual body parts are sequentially managed. *Finally,* adequate pain control needs to be provided, which is best done with the use of analgesics given as a pretreatment and supplemented as needed intravenously. Use of antipyretics just before burn care will also attenuate the subsequent pyrogen response.

#### *Superficial to Mid Second Degree Burn*

If the wound is being managed with a synthetic skin substitute, then continued daily inspection is necessary to look for both evidence of spontaneous wound closure and also of focal areas of infection, especially beneath any synthetic skin substitute. In the latter case, an exudate is usually present beneath the skin substitute, which impairs adherence. The skin substitute should be removed in these areas and a topical agent applied. Areas managed by a grease gauze and an agent such as bacitracin usually require fewer dressing changes at this stage of healing. If the grease gauze is dry and adherent, only the outer soft gauze dressing needs to be changed. Areas initially treated with water-soluble agents such as silver sulfadiazine can usually be switched to a grease gauze at this stage. The advantage to this change is that the wound dressings need to be changed less frequently, which means less pain. In addition, wound healing, in particular epithelialization, is improved with an occlusive adherent dressing and retarded with most water-soluble, cream-based topical antibiotics. The wound should be protected from mechanical trauma, once reepithelialized, to avoid blistering and skin loss. The rapid removal of adherent dressings can often lead to debridement of the new epithelium. It may be better to leave an adherent dressing in place, applying topical agents if necessary on the surface of the dressing, rather than to peel off both dressing and epidermis. Skin moisturizers such as a lanolin-based cream should be gently applied two to three times daily to avoid drying and cracking of healed skin.

### Deep Second Degree Burn

A surgical approach requiring both excision of eschar and grafting at this time is more complicated than in the earlier period due to increased blood loss from the marked increase in wound blood flow. When the eschar has been gradually removed with daily debridements and natural separation, a clean vascularized wound base develops that will provide a base upon which to graft. The determination as to whether a burn is deep second or third degree often cannot be made until 14 to 21 days after injury when the eschar is totally removed, revealing remaining dermal elements or granulation tissue. Cream-based topical antibiotics under gauze dressings, changed twice a day, remain the primary mode of treatment during this period. Silver sulfadiazine is the agent of first choice. However, bacterial resistance can develop in 10 to 14 days, at which point a different agent should be used, at least temporarily to control wound bacterial growth. Povidone-iodine, gentamicin, and nitrofurazone are all agents that are useful for a wound if only a thin eschar is present. Mafenide should be reserved for the wound with an invasive infection. A light chlorhexidine wash on the wound surface with forceps removal of only loose eschar is indicated. Any vigorous debridement or scrubbing will not only lead to bleeding and severe pain, but also to an excessive release of wound pyrogens and bacterial by-products.

Monitoring of surface bacteria along with the appearance of the wound is helpful in determining whether a change in the topical agent is required. Quantitative biopsy often is not feasible or unreliable if the eschar is quite thin. Systemic antibiotics should be added if there is evidence of wound infection and conversion to a deeper injury. Once epithelialization on the clean wound begins, a more occlusive dressing such as a grease gauze changed once a day or a synthetic skin substitute can be used to increase healing and minimize trauma to the thin epidermal covering. Of paramount importance is the maintenance of adequate wound blood flow and oxygen delivery. Hypertrophic scarring can be decreased by the use of pressure applied to the surface initially by elastic dressings and later by fitted pressure garments. This technique will be discussed in more detail in the next section.

### Third Degree Burn

As with the deep second degree burn, excision and grafting of the third degree burn is more complicated and dangerous during this period. The eschar is now much more vascular and also colonized with bacteria. The twice a day use of topically applied antibiotics to control wound colonization along with removal of loose tissue is the usual nonsurgical approach. Again, vigorous wound manipulation is contraindicated. Quantitative biopsies of the eschar are useful to diagnose invasive infection and the need for the addition of systemic antibiotics or for a change in the topical antibiotic. A change in the topical agent used is dependent on the adequacy of the control of burn wound bacteria. Unroofing of any pockets of suspected purulence below the eschar is necessary to avoid invasive infection. Loose eschar should be removed from the wound to decrease bacterial content and also to decrease the surface exudate and inflammation, which can injure the new tissue being formed. Sharp dissection should not be continued into viable tissue beneath the eschar to avoid a large blood loss and the possibility of bacteremia. Hypertrophic granulation tissue will continue to develop until the wound is surgically closed. Wound contraction will decrease some of the wound surface but at the expense of mobility and function.

## Surgical Management

As with the prior period, the surgical management of the burn wound during this period is complicated by both wound- and anesthesia-related problems. The patient is now much more hypermetabolic, and maintenance of anesthesia can be quite complex. Both anesthesia and surgical techniques will be discussed in this section.

### Anesthesia

It is well known that the skeletal muscle neuromuscular receptors are more sensitive to depolarizing muscle relaxants beginning 4 to 5 days after burn injury, which results in release of large amounts of $K^+$ and potentially fatal hyperkalemia during muscle fasciculations. A depolarizing agent is therefore contraindicated and a nondepolarizing agent is used when paralysis is indicated. The choice of agents depends on concerns over the degree of increased sympathetic discharge present in some agents compared with others.

Patients requiring endotracheal intubation may require an awake intubation if residual facial edema or burns make gas induction more difficult. Securing the tube is also quite difficult and usually requires tying the tube in place around the head. The *important components of anesthesia management* are:

1. Manner of airway maintenance and approaches to intubation
2. Providing increased ventilatory needs
3. Choice of agent
4. Approach to monitoring
5. Maintenance of temperature and hemodynamic stability

Choice of agent is similar to that for the postresuscitation period. Ventilatory requirements are markedly increased during this period. Residual lung injury from smoke inhalation or restrictive chest wall dysfunction from chest wall burn will markedly compound the problem. The preoperative ventilatory requirements need to be accurately determined. The anesthesiologist must also recognize the restrictive component to ventilation caused by a chest wall burn, healed or grafted. Chest wall compliance will be significantly decreased. Use of a muscle relaxant may dramatically compromise the patient's ability to return to an adequate minute ventilation in the early postoperative period. In addition, setting the tidal volume too high on positive-pressure ventilation will markedly increase mean airway pressure and lead to hemodynamic instability.

Positive end-expiratory pressure (PEEP) is often required to decrease airway collapse and shunt, especially in patients with unstable airways seen after smoke inhalation. A ventilator capable of maintaining PEEP and of delivering a sufficient minute ventilation (often exceeding 20 L) may not be available in the standard operating room and modifications may be required before beginning the case. In addition, these same increased ventilatory needs must be provided during transport to and from the operating room. In fact, rates of oxygen consumption and carbon dioxide production are often markedly increased immediately postoperatively, due to inflammatory mediator release with wound manipulation as well as any shivering or increased pain.

Adequacy of cardiopulmonary monitoring is of major importance in these potentially very unstable patients. The lack of sites for invasive monitoring and even for noninvasive monitoring will require the ingenuity of the anesthesiologist. Needle electrocardiographic electrodes and the use of pulse oximetry and end tidal carbon dioxide can solve some of the access problems. Prior knowledge of the patient's ventilatory and hemodynamic status and maintaining preoperative values are mandatory. Assessment of blood loss requires frequent communication between surgeon and anesthesiologist. Blood loss should be replaced with blood products and crystalloid should be given to replace evaporative losses, not blood losses. As described in the prior section, blood and blood products should be present in the room before starting a major case. The need for a warm operating room (at least 80°F), using heating blankets and warm fluids, etc., are all standard requirements. As with earlier surgical procedures, the operating time should be limited to 2 hours in large burns, especially in patients who have any significant cardiopulmonary instability.

## Surgical Procedures

The four wound procedures commonly performed during the inflammation-infection period are:

1. *Skin grafting of a previously excised but not grafted wound* (usually covered with a skin substitute after initial excision)
2. *Skin grafting of the deep dermal or full-thickness burn* in which remaining eschar has been removed by daily care and the wound surface is now not infected and is covered with *a layer of granulation tissue*
3. *Excision* of remaining eschar *and skin grafting of the* moderately sized, *noninfected burn*
4. *Excision* but not grafting *of the infected burn* eschar to control infection.

All procedures should be performed using the same guidelines as outlined in the prior section, namely, limiting time and blood loss and careful immobilization of the grafted area. The patient must be hemodynamically stable before surgery. Perioperative antibiotics are indicated, the antibiotic being determined by preoperative wound culture. A first generation cephalosporin is usually preferred, if no specific organism is noted, as reasonable coverage for *S. aureus* and the more common gram-negative bacteria. *S. aureus* is the most common organism affecting the skin graft and donor site. The wounds, with the exception of the wound protected by a synthetic skin, are gently painted with povidone-iodine solution. The burn wound itself cannot be scrubbed at this stage.

## Grafting of the Early Excised Burn

The areas excised early, but not grafted, are covered with skin substitutes. The skin substitutes are then removed in the operating room in a sterile field and the clean wound bed grafted, usually with meshed skin graft. The wound bed must be closely inspected to assure that there are not remaining areas of necrotic tissue requiring further excision. Further debridement may be needed. Blood loss is usually minimal, with the loss coming primarily from donor sites. Usually the wound bed has vascularized sufficiently (if a several day period has elapsed since the excision) to use a 3 to 1 mesh, if donor sites are limited, and expect a good graft take. A 0.010 to 0.012 inch thickness graft is preferred. A thicker graft can be used for areas such as hands, feet, and over joints. If there are limited donors or if a donor site is being reused, a thinner graft 0.008 to 0.010 is used. Meshed grafts are used to allow egress of blood and to cover more area (exception is the face and neck). The grafts are held in place by tapes, staples, or often simply by grease gauze or moistened fine mesh gauze. A layer of gauze moistened with a dilute antibiotic solution (e.g., bacitracin-neomycin) is then placed over the fine mesh or Xeroform, followed by a layer of dry gauze and a elastic dressing. We prefer to remove the outer dressings, down to Xeroform, fine mesh, or the skin substitute on the following day to remove any blood or exudate in the wound, which may accentuate bacterial growth, also checking for hematomas or shifting of the graft. Dressings are changed daily in a similar manner. The inner dressing, in direct contact with the graft, is usually not removed for 4 to 5 days or longer on wide-meshed grafts, if no exudate or clot has formed.

## Skin Grafting on Noninfected Granulation Tissue

The deep second or third degree burn, not previously excised, is usually treated with twice daily dressing changes until the majority of the remaining eschar has been gently removed and a vascularized bed has developed. The deep dermal burn often has areas of granulation tissue along with areas covered by a very thin layer of friable epidermis. It is necessary to scrape the wound base gently or excise the layer of granulation tissue until punctate bleeding is seen. It is not necessary or advantageous to excise much below the granulation tissue. Not only is profuse bleeding encountered in the wound excised much below granulation tissue, but reexposure of fat prevents the use of wide-meshed grafts. Diffuse small vessel bleeding from the excised granulation tissue bed is best controlled by immediate application of the split-thickness skin graft followed by pressure. This approach often works as well or better than topical thrombin, epinephrine, or other applied agents.

Split-thickness grafts should be harvested first so that ready application is possible. Bleeding from donor sites, especially reuse donors, should be controlled before beginning the wound excision unless there are two teams working. Blood loss from reuse donor sites can be massive. The type of graft depends, in large part, on donor site availability. Sheet grafts give the best cosmetic result and should be used on the face and neck. Mesh grafts can be used for most other areas. The mesh allows any residual bleeding to be vented into the dressings rather than accumulating beneath the graft. Since the wound base is much more vascular with granulation tissue than the exposed fat or fascia of the early excised third degree wound, a 3 to 1 mesh can be used if necessary because of limited donors. A layer of gauze moistened with antibiotic solution followed by dry gauze and an elastic wrap or a skin substitute and dry gauze with an elastic wrap are the choices for wound dressing.

*Eschar Excision and Grafting of the Uninfected Burn*

Excision of retained eschar is much more difficult after inflammation and neovascularization have developed. An infected wound, i.e., greater than $10^5$ organisms per gram eschar, should not be excised and grafted because graft take will predictably be unsatisfactory. The excision of the noninfected burn should not exceed a total surface area of 10% and preferably less. A wound bed free of eschar is essential. Inspection is often complicated by the profuse bleeding present. Pressure to the wound bed between inspections will help to avoid placement of grafts on nonviable tissue. Expect profuse bleeding when removing eschar to good tissue. Manipulation of inflammatory tissue can result in considerable toxicity in the early postoperative period. Expect an accentuation of the hyperdynamic state in the immediate postoperative period. Often a high temperature, tachycardia, and increased rate of oxygen consumption develops 1 to 2 hours after the procedure as a result of the wound manipulation. Blood loss should not exceed 50% of blood volume (i.e., approximately 5 U in the 70 kg patient). The wound dressings are managed in a similar fashion to that described for the early excised wound.

*Donor Sites*

The skin grafts are removed in the same fashion as described in the prior section, with thickness depending on surface covered, donor site availability, and thickness of the patients donor skin. A reuse of donor sites will be required during this period with large burns. The thickness of reuse donors should be no greater than 0.012 inch. The wound surface of the reused donor will bleed profusely and more attention to immediate hemostasis with placement of fine mesh or a grease gauze and application of pressure is required for several minutes. Skin substitutes are less useful with reuse donor sites because of the difficulty of obtaining a dry enough wound.

*Excision of the Infected Wound*

Normally the wound is debrided very conservatively during this period because of risks of bacteremia and bleeding. The exception is the patient with an invasive subeschar infection that must be unroofed. Tangentially excising eschar to but not into viable tissue will sufficiently unroof and debulk the eschar to allow better penetration of topical agents. One or two applications of mafenide before excision or subeschar injection of systemic antibiotics will decrease the wound bacterial load, minimizing the risks of disseminating infection. An attempt should not be made to excise down to a clean bed and graft unless the wound is very small and the patient is very stable. Expect a postoperative temperature spike and a picture of sepsis, at least transiently.

## Pitfalls in Management

*Underestimation of Ventilatory Needs During Anesthesia*

Unless the measurement has been obtained preoperatively, it is common to underestimate the minute ventilation, needs of the hypermetabolic patient. Characteristically, the patient's own tidal volume and rate increase to compensate for the increased carbon dioxide production. Once the anesthesiologist assumes control, this two- to threefold increase in minute ventilation must be maintained. Hypercapnia is a potent stimulus to the sympathetic nervous system. Extreme agitation, hyperpnea, tachycardia, etc., will develop intraoperatively and immediately postoperatively, if arterial carbon dioxide tension is allowed to increase. In addition, it is difficult enough for the patient to remove the carbon dioxide continually being produced, much less to correct a hypercapnic state.

## *Underestimation of the Blood Loss That Occurs with Excision During This Time Period*

The burn wound is extremely vascular at this stage and even normal skin blood flow is increased in the major burn due to the high cardiac output. The blood loss with excision can be immense, and the small subsurface capillaries now look like arterioles. One has to recognize this fact before embarking on a procedure, the extent of which may be in excess of that which is safe.

## *Underestimation of the Effect of Debridement of Infected Tissue*

Drainage of an abscess beneath the eschar is very appropriate and necessary. However, cutting through infected tissue is comparable to cutting through a phlegmon anywhere. There is a significant risk of bacteremia or endotoxemia, or both. The benefits of any vigorous wound manipulation at this stage of the wound must be weighed against risks.

## SUMMARY OF PATHOPHYSIOLOGIC CHANGES IN THE BURN WOUND BEGINNING AT 7 DAYS

### All Wounds Develop Inflammation

*Superficial to Mid Second Degree*

*7 to 21 Days*
1. Local hyperemia, inflammation pain
2. Rapid reepithelialization
3. Infection-low risk
4. Itching due to mast cell degranulation and injured nerves
5. New skin prone to mechanical trauma

*After Reepithelialization*
1. Minimal long-term scarring
2. Some wound contraction (less pliable skin) which relaxes after 2 to 4 more weeks
3. Decreased tolerance to changing temperature for several weeks to months, until skin thickens
4. New skin fairly durable

*Deep Second Degree Burn*

*7 Days Until Healed or Grafted*
1. Local hyperemia, inflammation with eschar separation
2. Wound colonization with moderate risk for invasive infection
3. Manipulation-induced bacteremia and endotoxemia and mediator absorption
4. Increased pain, heat loss
5. Slow reepithelialization with poor quality skin
6. Wound conversion with sepsis
7. Wound contraction prominent

*After Reepithelialization*
1. Blistering common with focal surface breakdown
2. Itching prominent
3. Skin nonpliable

*Third Degree Burn*

*7 Days Until Grafting*
1. Local hyperemia, inflammation with eschar separation
2. Wound colonization with high risk for invasive infection
3. Manipulation-induced bacteremia, endotoxemia, and mediator absorption
4. Increased pain, heat loss, and blood loss with wound care
5. Granulation tissue develops as eschar is removed
6. Wound contraction prominent

# SUMMARY OF DAILY BURN CARE

## General Principles

1. Maintain adequate perfusion with assurance by adequate monitoring
2. Minimize bacterial cross-contamination. do clean and dirty areas separately
3. Do not vigorously manipulate the wound
4. Avoid hypothermia: warm room, warm solutions minimize exposure
5. Use adequate premedication for pain, anxiety, antipyretics

### *Superficial to Mid Second Degree*

*7 to 21 Days*

1. Use of occlusive dressings, temporary adherent skin substitutes, or grease gauze
2. Switch from cream-based to less macerating agents
3. Be careful not to debride new epithelium with dressing change
4. Protect healing wound from mechanical trauma

*After reepithelialization*

1. Use of sunscreens
2. Avoid temperature extremes

### *Deep Second Degree*

*7 Days Until Wound Closure*

1. Continue cream-based topical antibiotics twice daily until eschar removed
2. Switch topical agents if no longer effective in controlling colonization
3. Avoid debriding new epithelium with dressing changes
4. Protect from mechanical trauma

*After Healing (or Grafting)*

1. Use skin moisturizers
2. Avoid temperature extremes
3. Will need pressure garments to control hypertrophic scarring

### *Third Degree Burn*

*7 Days Until Grafting*

1. Continue cream-based topical agents twice daily
2. Switch when bacterial resistance evident
3. Switch to less macerating agent when clean granulating wound present
4. Proceed to surgical mode

# SUMMARY OF SURGICAL APPROACHES TO THE BURN WOUND

## General Principles

1. The patient must be hemodynamically stable before surgery
2. Operative time should be limited to 2 hours in the major burn patient
3. Blood loss should not exceed 50% of one blood volume
4. Body temperature should be maintained by warm room; expose only operative areas
5. Perioperative antibiotics

### Grafting the previously excised wound

1. Remove protective covering of excised wound (usually a skin substitute)
2. Remove any foci of nonviable tissue
3. Obtain split-thickness grafts, mesh as needed based on availability
4. Apply split-thickness skin graft immediately and cover with fine mesh or grease gauze. Apply layer of moist antibiotic soaked gauze, or use synthetic or biologic skin substitute
5. Immobilize grafted area

Postoperative Care (24 to 48 Hours)

1. Change outer gauze dressing (down to the layer directly covering the graft) daily to remove blood, exudate
2. Remove innermost layer 4 to 5 days postgraft (or later if wide mesh grafts used)

### Grafting on Clean Granulation Tissue

1. Wash donors and paint wound areas with chlorhexidine or povidone iodine
2. Obtain split-thickness skin graft and stop bleeding
3. Tangentially excise the layer of granulation tissue until punctate bleeding is noted
4. Directly apply grafts: usually use meshed grafts except face, neck
5. Dress and immobilize grafted area as described on the left panel

Postoperative care (See left panel)

### Excising the Infected Wound

1. Unroof areas of possible infection
2. Remove eschar down to viable tissue
3. Do not cut into viable vascularized tissue
4. Do not graft infected wound bed
5. Follow with daily dressing procedures to allow granulation tissue formation

### Excision and grafting of the uninfected burn

1. Biopsy full-thickness eschar to assure wound not infected; (i.e., $10^5$ organisms/g)
2. Wash donors but paint wound, do not scrub
3. Obtain grafts, control donor site bleeding, mesh grafts
4. Limit excised area to less than 10% total body surface (usually 5 of 6%)
5. Apply pressure, can use topical thrombin, but early application of split-thickness skin graft controls bleeding nicely
6. Dress and immobilize as described in left panel. Consider use of frequent application of dilute antibiotic solution if fatty tissue or a wide mesh is used.

Postoperative care (See left panel)

# 12

# Infection and Sepsis

Sepsis is the leading cause of morbidity and mortality during this postburn period. The reasons for increased infection are:

   Loss of the skin *barrier* to microbial invasion
   Presence of invasive catheters and tubes
   Severe *immunosuppression* caused by burn injury

The burn wound, oral and pulmonary secretions, and perineal and anal regions are the major sources of microorganisms. The burn wound, lung, and intravascular catheters are the primary sites of infection.

## PATHOPHYSIOLOGY

### Definition and Etiology of Sepsis

Sepsis can be defined as the systemic response to dividing and invading microorganisms of all types, that is, gram positive, gram negative bacteria, fungi, and viruses. In addition, the same systemic response can be seen with severe inflammatory processes not induced by bacteria as, for example, the necrotic burn. The response is a host-related phenomena rather than related to the type of insult. Since many inflammatory processes in the surgical intensive care unit are either initiated by or subsequently involved with a microorganism, there has been a tendency to equate sepsis with infection.

Any stimulus that activates a severe inflammatory reaction can produce a picture of sepsis. Microorganisms play a dominant role in the burn patient. However, in only 50% of cases of sepsis syndrome is there documented bacteremia. Circulating endotoxin will also produce the same response.

The sepsis syndrome often looks very much like the postburn hypermetabolic state and can be characterized initially by fever, leukocytosis, tachycardia, and a hyperdynamic state reflected by increased cardiac output, decreased vascular resistance, and increased oxygen consumption. Evidence of impaired tissue oxygenation is, however, also present. This evidence would include lactic acidosis or hypotension not seen with hypermetabolism alone. There is considerable variability in the initial sepsis symptom complex. A combination of a decrease in systemic vascular resistance (SVR) with decreased cardiac output and oxygen consumption or increased SVR with an increased cardiac output and oxygen consumption can be seen. The process will progress if uncorrected to either an

**Table 12-1** Hyperdynamic Sepsis State

| Clinical Findings | Laboratory Findings | Physiologic Changes |
|---|---|---|
| Increased temperature, chills<br>Warm dry skin<br>Tachycardia, tachypnea<br>Blood pressure probably low to normal<br>Mental changes<br>Urine variable | White blood cells increased<br>Hyperglycemia<br>Metabolic acidosis<br>(Lactate 1.5 to 2 mM/L) | Increased rate of oxygen and carbon dioxide consumption<br>Arteriovenous oxygen difference: Normal to low<br>Wedge pressure: Normal to low<br>Cardiac output: Increased<br>Systemic vascular resistance decreased |

acute hypodynamic state in which shock is the principal characteristic or a multisystem organ failure state (Tables 12-1, 12-2).

Autonomic discharge of catecholamines and the release of a number of factors, including interleukin-1 and tumor necrosis factor, from the activated macrophage and neutrophil appear to be the important initiators of the systemic response. The initiating products appear to trigger the release of a wide variety of inflammatory mediators. Oxygen radicals and proteases released from activated inflammatory cells cause not only damage to bacteria but to local tissues as well. Further tissue injury, in turn, accentuates the inflammatory response. The complement fragment, C5a, released locally or systemically during complement activation, is a potent neutrophil attractant, as is leukotriene $B_4$. In addition, C5a increases the adherence of the neutrophil to local vascular endothelium with the result that, when activated, the released tissue destructive factors alter local capillary permeability leading to edema. Adult respiratory distress syndrome (ARDS) is initiated by this process.

**Table 12-2** Hypodynamic Septic State (Shock)

| Clinical Findings | Laboratory Findings | Physiologic Changes |
|---|---|---|
| Temperature increased or decreased<br>Skin cool<br>Tachycardia, tachypnea<br>Hypotension<br>Obtundation<br>Oliguria | White blood cells high or low<br>Left shift present<br>Hyper- or hypoglycemia<br>Metabolic acidosis<br>(lactate >2 mM/L)<br>Thrombocytopenia<br>Disseminated intravascular coagulation decreased fibrinogen | Decreased rate of oxygen consumption<br>Arteriovenous oxygen difference: low<br>Wedge pressure-variable<br>Cardiac output inadequate<br>Systemic vascular resistance variable |

## Hemodynamic Response

A generalized vasodilation often occurs initially, which appears to be a response to the inflammatory, hypermetabolic state. Vascular capacitance increases as does oxygen consumption, cardiac output, and heart rate. The arteriovenous oxygen (A-VO$_2$) difference is initially unchanged or only slightly increased from normal. With progression of the process, there occurs a marked abnormality in tissue oxygenation due to a combination of impaired flow, an impaired pump, and increased demands.

### *Maldistribution of Blood Flow*

There is a *maldistribution of tissue blood flow* caused by the inflammatory response to infection or injured tissue. A venodilation leading to increased venous capacitance is characteristic, as is a low systemic vascular resistance. A rapid transit time or bypass of capillary blood flow occurs in some tissues. In other tissues, normal or decreased blood flow may be evident due, for example, to the effect of increased thromboxane. The increased blood flow to some tissues beyond the oxygen needs and the relative bypass of other tissue beds is, in part, responsible for the narrowed arterial to venous oxygen difference. Also, the rapid transit time may impair adequate oxygen unloading. Oxygen delivery becomes the determining factor in oxygen consumption because the extraction of further oxygen from arterial blood becomes hampered.

Systemic hypotension develops if the increased venous capacity is not compensated for by an increased blood volume. In addition, microembolization and microvascular thrombosis results due to intravascular activation of coagulation and leukocyte aggregation. If the impaired blood flow is not corrected, the decreased perfusion to vital organs will lead to severe tissue damage. Oliguria is often present. However, urine output may actually increase in early sepsis due to the redistribution of intrarenal blood flow to the medulla and away from the cortex, impairing the concentrating ability of the kidney. Progression of the hemodynamic changes will lead to a more characteristic picture of hypovolemic shock and a change from a hyperdynamic to a hypodynamic state.

### *Direct Microvascular Damage*

The release of mediators results in direct microvascular endothelial cell damage and microvascular occlusion. Intravascular complement activation occurs with release of the complement component C5a, which is a potent stimulus of leukocyte aggregation and adherence to vascular endothelial cells. Capillary occlusion with aggregates of neutrophils can result. A local mediator release occurs, causing endothelial cell damage, increased permeability, and loss of intravascular fluid and protein into the interstitium. In addition, the sepsis stimulus (or activated complement itself) activates intravascular coagulation with further microembolization and local tissue capillary thrombosis, resulting in a further impairment to perfusion. The effects are most evident in the lung, leading to ARDS. The damage, however, is reversible if the inflammatory stimulus can be controlled. A systemic capillary leak is a later finding, usually seen after protracted sepsis or inadequate treatment of a low flow state. The increased fluid needs seen in early sepsis are due primarily to the blood flow maldistribution abnormalities.

## Oxygen Demands

The other cause (besides decreased perfusion) of impaired tissue oxygenation is inflammatory mediator and stress hormone-induced *increased tissue oxygen demands*. Metabolic abnormalities will increase thermogenesis and lead to a marked hypermetabolic state. Demands will exceed that provided by a normal oxygen delivery, especially with the added problem of blood flow maldistribution. The compensatory increase in cardiac index is essential to avoid progressive tissue ischemia. A relative anaerobic state develops because oxygen delivery is inadequate, now leading to the development of a progressive *lactic acidosis*. If the process is not rapidly reversed, septic shock will develop. If the hemodynamic instability is treated by volume replacement but the inflammatory focus persists, shock can be avoided but instead a multisystem organ failure syndrome (MSOF) can develop. Once initiated, MSOF appears to be self-perpetuating and extremely difficult to reverse. At a late point in the disease, all adaptive mechanisms will fail and cell death will result. This process is usually heralded by a decreasing A-VO$_2$ difference and decreasing oxygen consumption.

## Myocardial Changes

Due to the vascular dilation with peripheral pooling, a decrease in preload is evident. In addition, there is an impairment in left ventricular compliance due to: (1) pulmonary hypertension-induced right ventricular dilation; and (2) direct sepsis effects on the myocardium. This process will result in the need for increased preload for the same cardiac output.

There appears to be a relative depression in left ventricular contractility in severe sepsis characterized by a decreased response to alpha- and beta-receptor stimulation. The defect may only become evident with attempted pharmacologic increases in cardiac output. There is also a significant decrease in afterload in the hyperdynamic state, but with progression to a hypodynamic state, SVR will again increase. This potentially deleterious factor then becomes quite important with regard to cardiac performance.

## Metabolic Response

Metabolic responses to sepsis result in marked changes from normal. The changes are similar to the hypermetabolic state from burns alone. However, the glucose intolerance and catabolism can become more exaggerated. Hyperglycemia and glucose intolerance in the presence of stimulated gluconeogenesis are common characteristics.

With progression of sepsis, less glucose is utilized and more protein is burned. Fat is also used if infused, but fat mobilization with sepsis is not very efficient. The liver must function adequately to be able to metabolize the increased amounts of amino acids released from muscle as well as produce the acute-phase proteins, clotting factors, etc., which are required to maintain homeostasis and immune function.

In early stages of sepsis, oxygen delivery appears to be the limiting factor to providing metabolic needs. If the process progresses to a preterminal state, a marked impairment in cell function results. There is an uncoupling of adenosine triphosphate synthesis. Triglyceride clearance decreases, impairing the burning of fat, whereas lactate production and amino acid oxidation increases. Nutrients, in particular glucose, are less effectively utilized and there develops a preference for branched chain amino acids as fuel, which leads to further protein breakdown. Less oxygen is now being utilized as the process progresses from the hyperdynamic to the hypodynamic state or MSOF. Whether this response is due to a problem of inadequate delivery or reflects faulty cell machinery remains unclear. Maintenance of oxygen delivery and adequate nutrients to the cell, however, are essential to restore cell integrity.

## Sites of Sepsis

The most common sites of infection in the burn patient are lung, the burn wound, and vascular catheters. Intra-abdominal sites are well described but clearly much less common. The assessment of the burn wound has been described as the assessment of the lung.

The high risk of intravascular lines cannot be overemphasized. Although a positive blood culture is evidence of septicemia, lack of a positive blood culture does not rule out an infected line. The elevation in temperature can occur 1 to 2 hours after the actual bacteremia because there is an inevitable lag time between bacteremia (endotoxemia) and the hypothalamic response to the released pyrogens. A strict infection policy on vascular catheters is required. Diagnosis is often that of a high index of suspicion. Proof is often that of defervescence of the septic episode after removal of the catheter. Three blood cultures, each obtained 3 to 5 minutes apart, is the recommended approach. Intra-abdominal processes, in particular acalculous cholecystitis, are uncommon but are a well-recognized source of sepsis in the severe burn patient. Pancreatitis, with superimposed infection, is another potential cause of intra-abdominal sepsis.

A source that is now considered to be a likely one for producing the "sepsis syndrome" is a leak of endotoxin and bacteria from the gastrointestinal tract, which results from a combination of mucosal atrophy from lack of enteral feeding, a hypermetabolic state leading to visceral protein catabolism, and additional stresses, such as hypovolemia or another source of sepsis. Bacterial translocation, i.e., movement of enteric organisms to mesenteric lymph nodes across the gut mucosa and loss of the gastrointestinal barrier to macromolecules, have been experimentally identified after burn injury (Table 12-3).

## PRACTICAL APPROACH TO TREATMENT

### Fluid Treatment

#### Restoration of Preload

The primary treatment of the inadequte tissue oxygenation in sepsis syndrome is to increase preload. Restoration of an adequate blood volume is of primary importance. With successful volume restoration, the degree of lactic acidosis should decrease. The appropriate fluid regimen used in the septic patient is that which restores and maintains optimal tissue perfusion (usually reflected in maximum oxygen consumption) while

Table 12-3   Most Common Causes of Sepsis in Burn Patient

Most common
1. Lung: Pneumonia, bronchitis
   Diagnosis: Adequate sputum sample
              Chest radiograph
2. Burn: Invasive wound infection
   Diagnosis: Wound biopsy-quantitative bacteriology
              Subeschar abscess pockets
3. Intravenous catheter: Catheter sepsis, suppurative thrombophlebitis
   Diagnosis: Catheter tip culture
              Vein exploration
4. Pyelonephritis
   Diagnosis: Urine with white blood cell casts

Other possible causes
1. Gut leak of endotoxin or bacteria
   Diagnosis: Nonavailable at present
2. Cholecystitis
   Diagnosis: Ultrasound
              Dimethyl iminodiacetic acid scan showing duct obstruction
3. Bowel perforation
   Diagnosis: Plain films of abdomen
              Physical examination
4. Other gastrointestinal sources, abscess, pancreatitis, etc.

minimizing the complications and cost of the fluid infusion. The secondary goal is to minimize the complications. In summary, the *goals of volume resuscitation* are:

Primary:   Restore optimum tissue perfusion

Secondary:   Minimize complications of fluid infusion, namely, edema, allergic reactions, transmission of disease, coagulation disorders

Both crystalloid and colloid solutions are effective in restoring circulatory volume, the major difference being the increased quantities required with crystalloid and the subsequent tissue edema. Crystalloid alone may accomplish the first goal but will certainly result in more edema. Nonprotein colloids, such as dextran, are also very effective if not given in excess of safe amounts. Fresh frozen plasma should be reserved for treatment of a coagulopathy in view of the concern over transmission of disease. Since in early sepsis the problem is not increased vascular permeability but vasodilation and blood flow redistribution, colloid remains intravascular and is thus more effective at restoring blood volume than isotonic crystalloid.

It would appear that the most appropriate regimen is to use isotonic crystalloid to initiate resuscitation, i.e., 2 to 3 L fluid challenge then add colloid and blood to maintain blood volume and oxygen transport better while minimizing the edema process.

### Assessment of Adequacy of Preload

Because the endpoint of resuscitation with sepsis is much more difficult to assess using clinical criteria, information obtained by a pulmonary artery catheter is frequently required. The required increase in cardiac output and oxygen transport is usually about twice the normal value in order to maintain oxygen consumption at about 1.5 times normal, which is a good initial estimate of needs in the septic patient. The elevation in filling pressures required to generate the necessary cardiac output depends in large part on the effect of the septic state on left ventricular function. Fluid challenges should therefore be used to determine the response of increasing filling pressures and cardiac output, in other words to define the Starling curve for the patient.

It may be necessary to increase pulmonary wedge pressure to above the normal 10 to 12 mmHg to optimize left ventricular function. An impairment in ventricular compliance from, e.g., positive end-expiratory pressure (PEEP), may necessitate a filling pressure to 15 mmHg and sometimes greater to obtain the optimum left ventricular end-diastolic volume. Even higher filling pressures may be necessary with severe pulmonary hypertension, i.e., mean pulmonary artery pressure exceeding 25 mmHg. Although volume loading may improve output, the lungs may be severely compromised in the process, especially if ARDS is present. Under these circumstances, an inotrope is added when wedge pressure reaches 15 mmHg (or sooner if edema is developing at a lower wedge pressure).

### Assessment of Adequacy of Perfusion

Reversal of lactic acidosis is biochemical evidence of improved perfusion. Clinical parameters are more difficult to assess. Blood pressure may be on the low side of normal with a wide pulse pressure in view of the decrease in SVR. Tachycardia may also persist in the presence of a septic focus. Urine output can initially be increased even in the case of impaired perfusion as a result of an altered blood flow distribution to the kidney. This, however, will lead to oliguria if the septic low flow state persists. A blood pressure sufficient to maintain organ perfusion must be maintained. The value for mean pressure must exceed 80 mmHg and systolic pressure should be 90 or greater. Thus, the parameters for *optimum tissue perfusion* are:

> Cardiac index 4 to 4.5 L/min/m$^2$
> Oxygen consumption 1.5 times normal
> No lactic acidosis; base deficit <3
> Urine output >0.5 cc/kg/hr
> Pulse <120 beats/min
> Mean blood pressure of >80 mmHg

## Antibiotic Therapy

### Empiric Therapy for Sepsis Without a Clearly Defined Organism or Source of Infection

Empiric antibodies should be started if the presumed infection is a greater immediate risk to the patient than the antibiotic therapy to be initiated. The antibiotic regimen can be appropriately altered once culture data and more definitive data from diagnostic studies becomes available. The *risks of empiric therapy* are:

1. Breakdown of colonization resistance (capacity of normal flora to resist local colonization with pathogens)

2. Malabsorption due to altered gastrointestinal flora
3. Intrinsic antibiotic toxicity
4. Hypersensitivity reactions

Combined antibiotic therapy, usually with a first generation cephalosporin and an aminoglycoside, is at present the most effective initial management of the septic patient.

### Antibiotic Modification When Culture Data Are Available

Combined therapy is the most effective initial therapy. As a general rule, once an organism that is considered to be the cause of the sepsis is isolated, the antibiotic should be changed to a single drug or drug combination most effective for that specific bacteria as well as least toxic and least expensive. Regular monitoring of drug levels, particularly aminoglycosides, is necessary to maintain adequate bacterial killing while minimizing toxicity.

### Antibiotic Dosage

Appropriate antibiotic dosing is a crucial aspect of management. The burn patient because of the hypermetabolic state as well as the loss of antibiotics with body fluids from the wound itself generally requires a larger total antibiotic dose and also increased frequency of doses to maintain adequate levels. The increased requirements are well documented for the aminoglycosides. A lower dose will, of course, be needed if renal impairment is present. Monitoring antibiotic levels is the only valid approach to the use of systemic antibiotics in the major burn patient.

### Candida and Other Fungi

Because of the immunocompromised nature of the burn patient as well as the use of topical and systemic antibiotics, the finding of fungi in the lung and wound as well as on the intravenous catheter, especially *Candida albicans,* is relatively common. The prodome is often more subtle than with other microorganisms, with patients appearing more chronically ill and just "not doing well" as opposed to the often dramatic shaking chill seen with gram-negative organisms or high fever seen with *Staphylococcus aureus.* Diagnosing Candida sepsis versus Candida (or other fungi) colonization becomes more difficult than just identifying the organism. Detecting a Candida bacteremia is diagnostic of sepsis but, as with other organisms, is not seen in more than 50% of cases of invasive Candida infection. Quantitative wound biopsy or frozen section analysis can also be diagnostic. Inspection of the retina should be done to look for Candida lesions. The current recommendation is for initiation of amphotericin.

## Surgical Management

As with any form of sepsis, the removal or control of the septic focus is of primary importance. *Burn wound sepsis* was discussed in the preceding chapter. Mafenide is the agent of choice for topical management of wound infection, if the wound is not massive in size and the carbonic anhydrase inhibitor effect can be tolerated. Debridement should be gently performed to unroof pockets of infection and allow for better local wound and topical antibiotic care. Large excisions are often poorly tolerated during this period because of dissemination of infection and of blood loss. *Catheter sepsis* is assumed to be present if an invasive line is in place and the patient is septic. Invasive catheters should be changed to a new site with the first evidence of sepsis. If this approach is not feasible, then the line can be changed over a wire, the old catheter tip cultured and bacteriology checked in 12 to 24 hours. If bacteria grow from the tip, the line should be moved to a new site. Septic thrombophlebitis should also always be considered, especially in the presence of repeatedly positive blood cultures. A tender peripheral vein or vein with overlying induration should be inspected via a cutdown. If there is any question of purulence, the vein should be surgically removed. The endpoint is an area of normal nonclotted vein. Central veins cannot be readily removed and usually do not become directly involved in a closed space abscess. However, a soft tissue abscess in proximity to the vein can occur, for example, in the subclavicular area or in the neck. Any small local induration should lead to, at least, a limited local exploration, looking for a deeper abscess. *Acalculous cholecystitis* is common in the burn patient, especially if enteral feeding has not been initiated for a long time. Treatment is surgical, namely, cholecystectomy. Cholecystostomy is an alternative therapy. Other intra-abdominal sources are also possible, as with any critically ill patient, and the surgical treatment is identical to that for a nonburn patient.

## Pharmacologic Support of Circulation

### Inotropic Support

Inotropic support will be required if volume loading is not sufficient to maintain the goals of resuscitation. Dopamine is the preferred inotrope. Isoproterenol worsens the hypotension of sepsis. Dopamine is probably superior to dobutamine except in patients with high filling pressures where dobutamine is better. If another inotrope is being used in addition to dopamine, in particular one with alpha effects, the dopamine can be infused at renal doses to maximize renal blood flow. Low-dose dopamine (1–3 µg/kg/min) can then neutralize the renal vasoconstrictor effects of, e.g., epinephrine or norepinephrine.

### Increasing Systemic Vascular Resistance

The alpha adrenergic receptor appears to be down-regulated with sepsis, whereas circulating vasodilators are increased, making pharmacologic control of the decrease in SVR difficult. In general, pure alpha agonists such as norepinephrine are not particularly successful. In addition, increasing the SVR by vasoconstriction can further impair perfusion. There is no particular advantage to increasing SVR by vasoconstriction unless hypotension is refractory to a combination of volume loading and inotropic support. The role of these agents should be short term to restore coronary and cerebral perfusion. The exception would be refractory hypotension; i.e., mean arterial pressure less than 60 mmHg. However, under these circumstances in sepsis, there is no evidence that increasing SVR by an alpha agonist will improve long-term survival.

### Afterload Reduction

If SVR is usually low, as in early sepsis, afterload reduction is not necessary and contraindicated until volume infusion has restored preload. If SVR is increased or preload has been restored and blood pressure is now adequate, a further reduction in SVR will frequently result in a further increase in oxygen transport. Nitroprusside would be advantageous in this condition because this agent works primarily on the arterial side of the circulation, i.e., the resistance vessels. Nitroglycerin is more advantageous in cases of volume overload and systemic hypertension because both arterial and venous capacitance are increased, thereby decreasing both the increased preload and afterload.

## Use of Diuretics

Loop diuretics are indicated for the management of an oliguric state only after adequate preload has been restored and inotropic support has been initiated to restore renal perfusion. The premature use of a diuretic can result in a further decrease in perfusion. Also, one loses a useful parameter for monitoring the adequacy of perfusion.

## Mediator Inhibitors

Current information indicates that corticosteroids are of no benefit and, in fact, are deleterious in the patient with sepsis, except in the patient with adrenal insufficiency. Increased endogenous opiates are increased in stress states such as sepsis and are known to lead to hypotension. Naloxone is the most commonly used agent, which has endorphin-blocking properties. The major side effect is, of course, reversal of any of the analgesic effects of administered narcotics, a problem of some concern in the surgical patient. Current use of naloxone is in the shock state of sepsis in which blood pressure cannot be maintained with fluids or inotropes. A transient increase in pressure is seen with naloxone doses of 0.01 mg/kg. If an increase in pressure is not seen, the dose is increased to 0.1 mg/kg. The dose can be repeated if necessary in 15 to 30 minutes. Side effects have been reported, including pulmonary edema and seizure activity, usually in those patients also receiving opiates or anesthetics. Side effects have been reported, including pulmonary edema and seizure activity, usually in those patients also receiving opiates or anesthetics. Side effects are minimal in the absence of these other agents.

Prostaglandin and leukotriene inhibitors as well as oxygen radical scavengers, at present, have not been sufficiently studied in man to recommend their use.

## Nutritional Support

The nutritional requirements are increased in the septic state, but the demands are not necessarily additive to the already increased needs of the burn patient unless the burn is relatively modest in size, i.e., less than 30%. Burns larger than 30% total body surface cause an increase in nutrient needs of 50% or greater from baseline, which is comparable to the metabolic increase seen with sepsis. In the septic burn patient, who is already receiving 1.5 to 2 times normal caloric and nutritional needs, an impairment in glucose utilization is often seen. In this case, some glucose calories can be replaced with added protein or fat calories. An increased branch chain amino acid solution is a more ready source of fuel in the glucose intolerant patient. Increased branch chains are also more appropriate than standard amino acid solutions in the patient with liver dysfunction. The same rules should be followed for nutrition as described from the nonseptic burn patient, including control of excessive stress levels.

# SUMMARY OF HEMODYNAMIC RESPONSE TO SEPSIS

## Focus of Infection Tissue Necrosis

*Mediator Activation and Systemic Release*
1. Complement activation products
2. Arachidonic acid metabolites
3. Vasodilators, vasoconstrictors
4. Monokines

*Peripheral Vascular Effects*
1. Maldistribution of blood flow
2. Increased oxygen consumption
3. Tissue hypoxia-lactic acidosis
4. Decreased sensitivity to alpha agonists
5. Mediator-induced endothelial damage with resulting capillary leak, pulmonary and systemic

*Myocardial effects*
1. Decreased preload
2. Depressed ejection fraction and stroke work (masked due to decrease in systemic vascular resistance)
3. Decreased sensitivity to beta agonists

Impaired Tissue Perfusion

If the Process Continues,
One or More of the Following Occurs

*Severe Decreased Systemic Vascular Resistance*

Hypotension, which is often refractory to alpha agonist or volume

*Multiorgan Dysfunction (Several Week Time Course)*

1. Pulmonary failure often first event
2. Liver failure
3. Renal failure
4. Gastrointestinal Failure

*Severe Myocardial Dysfunction*

Low cardiac output increasingly refractory to volume or beta agonist

Decreasing Oxygen Consumption
Cell Hypoxia and Death

# SUMMARY OF NUTRITIONAL SUPPORT IN SEPSIS

## Remove or Control Source of Sepsis

Provide Total Calories: 1.5 to 2.0 Times the Normal 35 to 40 cal/kg/day
Provide Protein: 1.5 to 2.0 g/kg/day
Calorie: Nitrogen Ratio, 100:1

### Nonprotein Calories

**Fat**

Fat Infusion up to 50% of Nonprotein Calories, Depending on Clearance (Triglycerides Should Be less than 250 mg/dl) and on Glucose Tolerance

**Carbohydrate**

Use Carbohydrates for more than 50% of Total (Do Not Exceed 5 mg/kg/min)

If Hyperglycemia, Add Insulin

If Hyperglycemia Persists on Moderate Amounts of Insulin or if Respiratory Quotient Approaches or Exceeds 1.0, Then Decrease Carbohydrates and Increase Fat to 50% of nonprotein calories

### Protein

1. Need to provide 15 to 20% of total calories as protein
2. Need to provide sufficient protein for positive nitrogen balance
3. Expect increase in blood urea nitrogen due to increased ureogenesis

# SUMMARY OF TREATMENT OF INFECTION COMPONENT

Identify Presence of Sepsis
Identify Source and Organisms
History, Physical, Laboratory, Cultures, (Blood Three Times, Sputum, etc.

**Source Unknown**

*Begin Empiric Therapy*
First Gen Cephalosporin Plus Aminoglycoside

*Culture Data Available*
1. Modify when organisms defined
2. Monitor levels closely

**Source Known**

*Begin Most Appropriate Empiric Therapy for the Particular Source*

*Culture Data Available*
Modify as described and monitor levels

*Burn Wound or Infected Vein*
1. Oxacillin or cefazolin plus aminoglycoside
2. Add anti-Pseudomonas penicillin if suspect Pseudomonas; alternative third generation cephalosporin
3. Add vancomycin if suspect resistant Staphylococcus aureus
4. Consider Candida (or other fungi) and need for amphotericin

Surgical Removal if at All Possible as Soon as Possible

# SUMMARY OF TREATMENT OF HEMODYNAMIC COMPONENT OF SEPSIS SYNDROME

Maintain Oxygen Saturation more than 90%
Fluid Challenge
Crystalloid 7 to 10 ml/kg or Colloid 3-5 ml/kg

## *Condition Deteriorates or Minimal Improvement*

1. Consider need for added pulmonary support
2. Increase monitoring pulmonary artery catheter arterial line
3. Continue volume loading to isotonic crystalloid (2 to 3 L) and add colloid to improve hemodynamics
4. Maintain cardiac index (more than 4.5 young) (more than 3.0 elderly)
5. Maintain oxygen delivery about 1.5 × normal value
6. May need to maintain hematocrit >30 to include oxygen delivery
7. May need to increase wedge pressure up to 15 mmHg

### *Patient Not Adequately Responding to Fluid Alone*

1. Add inotropic support, dopamine (first choice), dobutamine in wedge pressure greater than 20
2. Consider increasing preload

### *Patient Responds*

1. Continue with treatment of infection and metabolic component
2. Remove invasive monitors as soon as process resolves

*Systolic Blood Pressure Less Than 90*
*Mean Arterial Pressure Less Than 60*

1. Add alpha agonist, dopamine or add epinephrine or norepinephrine
2. If use norepinephrine, also use low-dose dopamine
3. If hypotension persists add nalaxone, 0.01 mg/kg

*Systolic Blood Pressure Greater Than 100*
*Mean Arterial Pressure Greater Than 80*

Consider adding nitroprusside to decrease systemic vascular resistance and improve oxygen delivery but avoiding hypotension

## *Clear Improvement in Hemodynamics and Lung Function Stable*

1. Continue increased fluids
   Use isotonic crystalloid
   Add colloid at this point to maintain albumin greater than 2.5 g/dl
2. Continue close clinical monitoring: vital signs, urine, blood gases, acid-base equilibrium
3. Assure adequate perfusion for patient needs
4. Continue with treatment of infection and metabolic component

SECTION 4

# Rehabilitation and Wound Remodeling Phase

Rehabilitation means to return to a functional state. This process is particularly difficult in the burn patient because of the more chronic nature of the healing process and the permanent nature of the burn scar. The rehabilitation phase basically begins on the day of admission. A primary objective of the initial care is to not only restore cardiopulmonary stability, but also to minimize the musculoskeletal dysfunction caused by the overlying skin burn. A wound can be "successfully" closed and severe musculoskeletal function can still develop.

*The principles of rehabilitation are:* to maintain and restore function to the affected area; control scarring and wound contractures; restore the whole patient to functional activity; to provide the psychologic support needed to accept the cosmetic and functional abnormalities.

This section will focus on basic concepts of rehabilitation. Late reconstruction (i.e., after initial wound closure) is an important component of the long-range rehabilitation goals. However, this area is sufficiently complex, both technically and in decision-making, that it is not covered in this book. This aspect of care is initiated months to years after initial wound coverage.

# 13
# Rehabilitation and Wound Remodeling

## BURN EDEMA AND ESCHAR RIGIDITY

The initial massive edema that develops beneath the eschar and the nonpliable nature of the eschar itself will markedly impair muscle and joint motion. The edema-induced stiffness lasts a sufficient time (7 to 10 days) for a beginning contracture to develop if correct position is not maintained. The burn eschar is very noncompliant compared with normal skin. In addition, the skin shrinks when burned due to loss of water and cell substances. The eschar becomes very rigid, with muscle and joint motion being dependent on stretching of contiguous nonburned or more superficially burned skin. The eschar may remain in place for extended periods of time, depending on the approach to grafting and the availability of donor sites. It is important to recognize the functional limitations produced. Joint stiffness and muscle atrophy can result.

## FUNCTIONAL IMPAIRMENT FROM PAIN AND RESTRICTED ACTIVITY

Stretching of the burn wound will initiate pain. The position of comfort is invariably the position that minimizes stretch. Continued flexion or adduction at large joints often develops as well as hyperextension of the metacarpophalangeal joints. A particularly disabling process with a third degree hand burn is pressure necrosis of the central slip of the digital extensor tendon at the proximal interphalangeal joint. This is caused by the exaggerated flexion at the joint when the metacarpophalangeal joint is hyperextended. The *most common position abnormalities* are:

1. Adduction of shoulders
2. Flexion at elbows, wrists, neck, interphalangeal joints
3. Hyperextension of feet and metacarpophalangeal joints

In addition to pain, severe limitations of motion are placed on the patient as a result of monitoring devices, ventilator tubing, etc. The forced immobility is sometimes necessary if the patient is in a life-threatening situation with cardiopulmonary instability. However, the lack of motion is often more for convenience for both patient and medical care providers. Inactivity in the nonburned patient is often well tolerated and minimal to no permanent sequelae. The burn patient, however, will lose the battle against the contracting wound. What begins as a voluntary immobility rapidly evolves into an intrinsic defect. Another form of restraint is that initiated after early skin grafting (and later reconstructive procedures). Although it would be ideal to immobilize the graft for 7 to 10 days, as may be done in a nonburn patient, this time period in the burn wound can result in significant tissue rigidity and muscle atrophy leading to a major loss of motion. A much briefer period of immobility is used.

The next three pathophysiologic processes are potentiated by lack of motion whatever the cause.

## HYPERTROPHIC SCAR AND CONTRACTURE FORMATION

As previously described, the natural course of the wound that remains open for more than 3 weeks is the deposition of dense scar. Complete epithelialization before 3 weeks usually leads to only minimal scarring, although some patients will produce incredible amounts of scar for relatively superficial injuries. Wound contraction develops. This is produced by the contractile myofibroblasts and the deposition of ground substance and collagen. The end result is a shortened noncompliant wound that, if it crosses a joint, will result in a contracture. The most common contractures are essentially identical to the most common position abnormalities produced with inadequate motion:

1. Flexion: elbows, wrists, neck, interphalangeal joints
2. Adduction: shoulder
3. Extension: feet, metacarpophalangeal joints

The second process is hypertrophic scar formation (Color plate 14, page 317). Continued scar deposition in the reepithelialized wound results in a raised, hyperemic pruritic wound that produces functional impairment due to rigidity and pain as well as a severe cosmetic abnormality. Severe discomfort results. Pain with any scar movement retards activity and continued itching leads to scratching and skin breakdown. Superficial infection of the skin breakdown can then result. The scar often splits with exercise, especially if it becomes dry. The open wound increases pain and risk of infection. Keloid formation is the exaggerated form of this process. Delay in wound closure correlates best with this process. Wounds requiring more than 4 weeks to heal are at highest risk. Grafted wounds develop much less hypertrophic scarring than the deep dermal burn that heals spontaneously. Both the contracture and hypertrophic scarring process peak between 3 and 6 months after injury, frequently long after the patient has been discharged.

**Contracture formation and hypertrophic scarring peak 3 to 6 months after injury and partially resolve at 12 to 18 months.**

It is crucial that the care providers recognize the delayed onset so that precautionary measures can be taken. The hypertrophic scar begins to decrease with time as collagen lysis begins to exceed the rate of deposition. The latter begins to decrease as the inflammatory process diminishes. Between 12 and 18 months, a softening and flattening of the scar can be seen along with a loss of scar hyperemia. The presence of any hyperemia indicates that active scar turnover is still present. The lack of hyperemia is a good sign that the scar is now mature and will remain in its present state. Although the scar may relax, the underlying tissues can become permanently foreshortened and joint ankylosis develops.

## MUSCLE LOSS FROM CATABOLISM, INACTIVITY

Inactivity of muscle leads to rapid atrophy, as is evident from the muscle loss seen with a casted fracture or the generalized loss seen in the head-injured or spinal cord-injured patient. The muscle catabolism seen in the burn patient will markedly accentuate the muscle loss caused by any degree of inactivity. The first muscles to decrease in size and strength are the proximal thigh muscles. These muscles of ambulation are essential to preserve. Restoration of muscle mass requires a continuing increase in workload, a feat that will be severely hampered by any contractures or hypertrophic scarring. It is clearly more efficient to maintain muscle mass than to try and rebuild muscle, especially in the elderly patient where increased workload will be hampered by lack of cardiopulmonary reserve.

## HETEROTOPIC CALCIFICATION AND OSSIFICATION

Deposition of calcium and phosphate into soft tissues is called heterotopic calcification. Deposition of these minerals to produce bone is called ossification. This process can occur in the ligaments and capsule around a joint or in tissues distant from the joint. Heterotopic calcification or, less commonly, ossification can be seen in 1 to 3% of burn patients. The process is most commonly seen in patients with major burns, with the area of calcification involving a joint with an overlying burn. The degree of confinement and immobility appears to correlate directly with the degree of calcium deposition. There are usually no measureable changes in serum calcium phosphorus or alkaline phosphatase. The mechanism remains unknown, but immobility and hypermetabolism with rapid tissue turnover are clearly involved. Both *Staphylococcus aureus* and β-hemolytic streptococci are frequently found in the wound; however, infection does not appear to be a prerequisite. Forceful range of motion with bleeding into the joint can also occur.

The process usually appears 3 to 6 months after injury. The earliest sign of calcification is loss of range of motion. Increased pain on attempted motion is also found. X-ray evidence of calcium deposition usually post dates initial symptoms by at least a week. Bone scanning is the most reliable method to follow the motivation process of new ossification. The most common joint involved is the elbow followed by the shoulder.

## TEMPERATURE REGULATION

The thin-grafted or healed skin is more prone to heat loss than normal skin even years after injury. The loss is most prevalent with the increase in blood flow to the wound. With scar maturation, wound blood flow decreases, as does the potential for heat loss. Autoregulation of the microcirculation is impaired, especially in the early period (several months), limiting the ability to vasoconstrict and vasodilate in response to changes in environmental temperature. With large, deep body burns, the sweat gland apparatus is also destroyed. Sweating is an important mechanism for eliminating body heat. Increased heat generation by pyrogens or by exercise is therefore more difficult to dissipate rapidly. In addition, hypothermia can readily develop as well. Intolerance to temperature extremes will be a continued problem for large body burns once discharged.

## DRYING AND SKIN BREAKDOWN OF THE HEALED BURN

The grafted or healed burn is not only thin but devoid of oil glands. Skin becomes very dry and prone to cracking, with development of secondary infection. The hypertrophic scar is particularly prone to this process. The dry skin markedly impairs flexibility, which, in turn, impairs motion. The formation of blisters and skin breakdown from minor trauma, especially in healed wounds, is due to both the lack of rete pegs anchoring epidermis as well as edema in the wound from the increased blood flow.

## BEHAVIORAL DISTURBANCES

It is well recognized that many burn patients have preexisting psychologic problems that frequently are, at least in part, responsible for the burn. Alcohol and drug abuse are common components. The injury itself, however, will also result in major psychosocial problems. Anger and depression are common emotions manifested during the initial hospitalization, which carry into the rehabilitation period. Both types of emotional behavior can markedly impair rehabilitation efforts. Regression to an earlier stage of dependence is one of the most characteristic postburn disturbances. Regression to a childlike behavior allows the patient to escape the reality of the situation. Refusal to cooperate with care and abusive behavior toward the medical staff are commonly seen. The behavior pattern is an attempt at a defense mechanism and should not be considered an abnormal response. Sleep deprivation accentuates all the potential emotional problems. Drugs used to assist in patient care can often exaggerate behavioral disorders. Sedation in the elderly can lead to disorientation. Although narcotics are needed for pain management for long time periods, a dependency on these drugs is not as common as one might anticipate unless, of course, there was a prior dependency or a personality disorder that increased the risk of a drug dependency.

Often, the behavior disorder becomes most manifest after initial discharge when the patient leaves a very structured hospital environment and enters a less defined family and social environment. Support systems that are present in the burn unit may not be adequately provided in the home environment. Psychologic problems will markedly impair physical rehabilitation efforts, and patient motivation and cooperation are essential. The physical rehabilitation program, which was well organized at the time of discharge, then disintegrates, leading to the loss rather than a continued functional gain.

# 14

# Treatment

There are six key components to the rehabilitation efforts that are aimed at minimizing disability. The total plan requires all of its parts to be effective. Each part is dependent on special expertise. Therefore, an integrated team approach is absolutely essential.

## EARLY WOUND CLOSURE

Early wound excision will help minimize short-term and long-term functional loss by removing the nonpliable eschar and eliminating the wound pain, which will occur as the eschar separates and granulation tissue develops. Even with deep burns, pain develops after eschar separation, which occurs beginning at the end of the first burn week. A split-thickness skin graft, although more elastic than eschar, does not have normal elasticity and wound stiffness will still be present, which must be counterbalanced with aggressive therapy and splinting.

There are two aspects of early grafting, however, that can hamper general function. The first is the pain and discomfort caused by the new skin donor sites. With an aggressive approach to early wound closure, large donor site areas are usually present that limit range of motion to nonburn areas and can markedly impair ambulation. The use of skin substitutes can decrease the donor site pain and improve mobility. The second problem is the need for immobilization of the grafted area to allow for neovascularization (graft take). This time period should be as short as possible. Usually 3 to 5 days is adequate if grafts are placed on residual dermis or fascia. Grafts on fatty tissue take 5 to 7 days to revascularize and therefore require a longer period of immobility. Superficial second degree burns and donor sites can be closed using temporary skin substitutes. These products improve function by decreasing pain and increasing flexibility.

## EXERCISE: ACTIVE AND PASSIVE

The next three treatment modalities are closely linked and should be perceived as a single treatment. An assessment of the burn areas as to current and potential later limitations of motion is made as soon as feasible after injury. This should be done immediately in the first 24 hours after the small to moderate burn and usually during the first 24 to 48 hours in the large burn. Supervised motion of burned areas should begin as soon as possible. The *goals of exercise* are:

>   Maintain normal joint range
>   Maintain strength and endurance
>   Promote functional independence

Functional independence is the long-range goal but progressive independence is needed throughout the burn course. Exercise must be accomplished by proper positioning and splinting to avoid loss of the gains in between active sessions.

There are a number of *exercise techniques* used that are chosen based on the magnitude of injury and progress of the patient:

>   Active: Patient achieves range
>   Resistance added with progress
>   Self-exercise program initiated
>   Active assistive: Assistance is given with weights, pulleys, etc.
>   Allows stretch that exceeds strength
>   Passive: Used in critically ill
>   Used often with anesthesia to increase range
>   Resistive: Use of weights, etc., to increase strength and endurance
>   Stretching: Addition of slow continued force to active or passive range of motion to restore position
>   Use in conjunction with splints
>   Endurance: Combination of above plus techniques, such as stationary bicycle
>   Ambulation: Improves range, strength, endurance, and independence

Active and passive motion is assisted by the use of hydrotherapy. The warm water relaxes the patient and the local muscles. A daily hydrotherapy session is ideal to begin motion in previously immobilized joints.

Muscle activity should be performed each day, usually beginning with shorter time periods, 3 to 5 minutes every several hours, evolving into longer periods, 25 to 30 minutes twice daily. The initial shorter period will assist in maintaining joint motion, whereas the longer periods are aimed at improving muscle strength. Increased muscle action will more rapidly resolve tissue edema. Activity also tends to stimulate appetite as well as to improve self-image with a feeling of progress. Weight lifting and isometric exercises added to range of motion can usually begin in 2 to 3 weeks postinjury. Early exercise for hand should emphasize active finger range of motion, particularly flexion of the metacarpophalangeal joints, extension of the interphalangeal joints, and thumb abduction and opposition. Wrist exercises should emphasize extension and ulnar deviation, since flexion and radial deviation is the most common abnormality. Forearm supination and pronation is performed with the elbow close to the side to prevent the shoulder from substituting for the forearm motion. Elbow extension should be emphasized because flexion is usually easier. Shoulder abduction and external rotation should be emphasized. Riding a stationary bicycle is an excellent means of strengthening the lower extremities while improving cardiopulmonary reserve. The organized activity plan must be consistently maintained and considered to be an essential component of care, even in the massively burned patient. Two elements are key to the success of this program. One is control of pain and anxiety and the other is motivation. These components are clearly interrelated and require a team effort with the involvement of all care providers. Premedication before exercise is important. Biofeedback techniques are also very beneficial, although difficult to learn.

Exercise tolerance is closely monitored using the criteria of pulse, blood pressure, respiration, fatigue, pain, and electrocardiography as monitors. Pain is probably the most difficult criteria to monitor because it is the most subjective. The exercise plan must be integrated into the other day's activities, especially burn care, sleep, and nutrition. All components are essential and none should be minimized as to importance. Exercise and nutrition can be combined by fabricating simple devices to allow the patient to feed himself. This approach also increases independence and improves the patients self-image. Progress is a key factor in maintaining patient cooperation and enthusiasm. Seeing progress is very important. Simple techniques, like marking the floor where the last attempt at ambulation stopped or the wall at the height of the last stretch, will show progress as well as set the day's goals. Careful supervision is required in cases in which a joint has been immobilized for a long period or muscle atrophy has eliminated joint protection by muscle tone. Heterotopic calcification is a process particularly difficult to treat once it has formed because movement will be very painful and forced movement may exaggerate the local inflammatory process. Early mobilization of the injured areas and ambulation appears to be the best approach to prevention.

## POSITIONING

Although exercise is a very effective factor in preventing loss of function, the patient will invariably resume the position of comfort between exercise sessions. This position will then lead to contractures (Table 14-1).

## SPLINTING

Splints are required to maintain position in areas not amenable to positioning techniques or in the postgrafting period to allow graft take. Splints are frequently required for burns

Table 14-1  Positioning of Burn Areas During Rest

| Burn Area | Position During Rest |
|---|---|
| Neck | Maintain pillow or rolled towel beneath neck to maintain extension |
| Arms | Maintain shoulder abducted 80 to 90°, elbows fully extended, and wrists extended 30 to 40°. Use pillows and bedside tables to accomplish position. Wrist extension will relax tendons in fingers |
| Hand | Maintain elevated with metacarpophalangeal in 90° flexion, the fingers separated with interphalangeal joints in midflexion, and with the thumb in a position of midabduction |
| Trunk, hips | Maintain hip abducted 20° and knee extension. Placing prone for short periods will help hip extension |
| Foot | Neutral ankle position with heel padding |

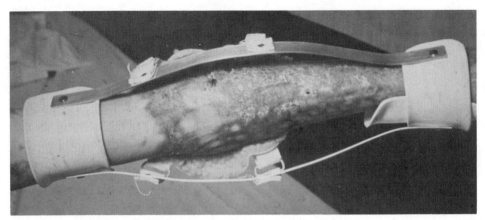

**Figure 13–1.** Splinting technique for elbow.

of the neck in addition to positioning, especially at night or when fatigue develops. Splints for elbows are also frequently necessary (Fig. 13-1). The most common area requiring a splint is the burned wrist and hand (Fig. 13-2). Wrist flexion is a common abnormality that also affects hand and finger function. For the wrist, a splint over the wound dressing should be applied beginning in the proximal forearm and stopping at the palmer crease, extending the wrist 20° to 40°. The burned hand requires a splint that maintains wrist extension while maintaining the metacarpophalangeal joint at 80° to 90° flexion and the interphalangeal joint fully extended. The thumb should be abducted and opposed. Splints are also frequently required to maintain the foot in neutral, overcoming the more powerful pull of the extensors. Thermoplastic materials are used to make many of the splints. These

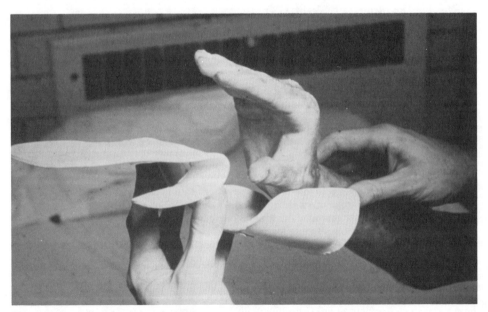

**Figure 13–2.** Splinting technique for hand.

material becomes pliable (at 160° to 170°F) in hot water and cool rapidly at room temperature. Splints can therefore be molded and readjusted as edema resolves or as gains are made.

Splints should be worn at night and during periods of extended inactivity. There are many variations of splinting techniques with dynamic splinting, i.e., addition of a pull, usually by elastics, adding a component of exercise. These techniques require a well-trained therapist because major complications can result with improper splints. Pressure necrosis is one of the most common complications.

## PRESSURE GARMENTS AND SKIN CARE

Constant pressure of 25 to 30 mmHg on the hypertrophic scar reduces the hypertrophy and hyperemia. The initial reduction is due to the decrease in wound edema and wound blood flow. The long-term effect appears to be a reduction in collagen and ground substance deposition also due to the decrease in blood flow and in available tissue oxygen. Within several weeks of continuous pressure, i.e., 22 to 23 hours/day, there is a measurable reduction in wound chondroitin sulfate and myofibroblasts. The pressure garments also improve venous return, which is of particular importance if the venous system was compromised by a deep burn or excision to fascia. Areas such as the eyes, nose, and mouth and anterior chest usually do not receive adequate pressure because of their contour. In these cases, a mold of the contour can be fitted and a garment placed over the mold, which now provides the pressure. A number of custom-made pressure inserts can be made to fit any area. Garments are used once the wound is closed. The garment should be worn for several hours in the beginning and advanced to about 22 hours of each day. The pressure needs to be applied until the scar is matured, as is evident from lack of hyperemia. This process takes 12 to 18 months. Potential problems occur if the fitting is not perfect or rapid weight gain makes the fit too tight. Wound erosions can develop, necessitating removing of the garments until healing has occurred.

The skin must also be constantly lubricated to avoid drying and cracking (Table 14-2). Skin moisturizers, usually lanolin based, need to be applied several times a day. A

**Table 14-2** Skin Care

| Problem | Treatment |
| --- | --- |
| Skin surface blistering and breakdown | 1. Avoid shearing with poor fitting compression garments, splints, or clothing<br>2. Use lubricating lotions<br>3. Use nonadherent dressing<br>4. Use mild soaps |
| Pigmentation | 1. Wear pressure garments<br>2. Avoid direct sunlight until scar matures, skin thickened<br>3. Use heavy sunscreen, hats, etc. |
| Itching | 1. Antihistamines, hydrocortisone cream may be useful<br>2. Use nonirritating skin lubricants<br>3. Avoid temperature extremes that will induce sweating |
| Impaired thermoregulation | 1. Avoid temperature extremes<br>2. Wear loose fitting clothing appropriate for the season |

special lubricant is required if pressure garments are used, which does not harm the fabric. Prolonged exposure to direct sunlight should be avoided until the scar has matured or the skin thickened. Temperature and humidity extremes need to be avoided, especially after large burns. The patient and employer must be instructed in the prevention of hyper- or hypothermia. Increased humidity is poorly tolerated in the summer if sweat glands have been destroyed. An air conditioner and dehumidifier in the home or at work is often necessary. The dry air indoors in cold weather leads to rapidly drying of skin. A humidifier is often helpful in the home. Many of these early problems resolve with time (12 to 24 months).

## PSYCHOSOCIAL SUPPORT

Management requires first and foremost a recognition of the problems by the medical staff. In addition, lack of adequate communication and preparation of the patient by the staff, to procedures and to prospects for outcome, will accentuate fear and deepen emotional problems. Because of the potential problems related to regression and dependence, the patient must be strongly encouraged and, in essence, required to be as independent as possible. This patient independence must be maintained by the family as well. Independence first requires a form of daily structure wherein the patient has some control. Thus, the *approach to psychosocial support* requires:

>  Maintaining good communication with patient
>  Avoiding unnecessary anxiety due to the unknown
>  Encouraging patient independence
>  Maintaining organized daily plan
>  Avoiding sleep deprivation
>  Providing adequate sedation, analgesia
>  Providing psychosocial assistance to patient, family, and staff

The patient should know the schedule and have some input, especially as to the timing of events, i.e., the schedule should have some flexibility. The goals may need to be maintained more by the staff, at least initially. Sleep deprivation must be avoided and adequate sedation and analgesia provided. Because of the close interaction of patient and staff over a long time period, it is often difficult for staff to remain objective. In addition, the family is often severely stressed due to the time course as well as the magnitude of injury. A psychiatrist or psychologist and a social worker are key members of the burn team. They must become involved very early in the treatment and not be used only when extreme difficulties arise, since preventive measures are much more effective than treatment modalities.

## COMMON PITFALLS IN MANAGEMENT

### Underestimating the Loss of Function from Immobility

It is very easy to interpret the progress of the burn wound but a concerted effort needs to be made to maintain musculoskeletal function during the process of wound healing and grafting.

## Excessive Immobilization After Skin Grafting

Maximum immobilization should be 5 days, with some motion of the grafted area beginning by 3 to 4 days if excision is to fascia or dermis. Waiting 7 to 10 days will result in considerable loss of motion and require even more work to resume motion that was present before surgery.

## Underestimating the Hypertrophic Scar Formation Occurring After Discharge

The burn patient often has the least amount of scar tissue present on initial discharge, especially in the healed deep dermal burn. Hypertrophic scarring usually peaks several months after burn. Plans must be made before loss of function and onset of pain, itching, etc., by early use of pressure garments. Garments should be used on burns not healing within 3 weeks.

# REHABILITATION SUMMARY
## Prior to Wound Closure

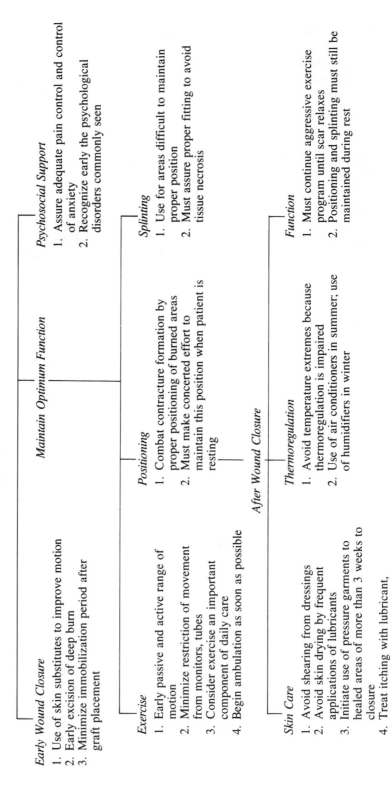

*Early Wound Closure*
1. Use of skin substitutes to improve motion
2. Early excision of deep burn
3. Minimize immobilization period after graft placement

*Exercise*
1. Early passive and active range of motion
2. Minimize restriction of movement from monitors, tubes
3. Consider exercise an important component of daily care
4. Begin ambulation as soon as possible

*Skin Care*
1. Avoid shearing from dressings
2. Avoid skin drying by frequent applications of lubricants
3. Initiate use of pressure garments to healed areas of more than 3 weeks to closure
4. Treat itching with lubricant, antihistamine
5. Avoid direct sunlight

*Maintain Optimum Function*

*Psychosocial Support*
1. Assure adequate pain control and control of anxiety
2. Recognize early the psychological disorders commonly seen

*Positioning*
1. Combat contracture formation by proper positioning of burned areas
2. Must make concerted effort to maintain this position when patient is resting

*Splinting*
1. Use for areas difficult to maintain proper position
2. Must assure proper fitting to avoid tissue necrosis

*After Wound Closure*

*Thermoregulation*
1. Avoid temperature extremes because thermoregulation is impaired
2. Use of air conditioners in summer; use of humidifiers in winter

*Function*
1. Must continue aggressive exercise program until scar relaxes
2. Positioning and splinting must still be maintained during rest

SECTION 5

# Electrical Burns

Electrical burn injuries account for less than 5% of admissions to major burn centers. However, the injury is much more complex than a skin burn and the morbidity and mortality rate is considerably higher. The mortality rate changes from 3 to 15%, with about 1,000 deaths attributed to electrical current in the United States each year. More than 90% of injuries occur in males, most between ages 20 and 34 years. There are three components to the usual high tension electrical injury, and these are covered in the following chapter. Additional chapters cover low voltage oral burns and lightning injury.

# 15

# High Tension Electrical Burns

## GENERAL PRINCIPLES

In order to understand electrical current injury, familiarity with the terminology is necessary.

### Terminology

*Voltage* (electrical or energy potential) is the electromotive force generated by the power source.

*Amperage* (intensity) the amount of current flowing, per unit time.

*Resistance* to flow is described in *ohms*

$$\text{Resistance} = \frac{\text{Voltage}}{\text{Amperage}} \qquad \text{Amperage} = \frac{\text{Voltage}}{\text{Resistance}}$$

*Household current* = 110 to 220 volts

*Residential power lines* = 5000 to 10,000 volts

*High tension wire* = up to 100,000 volts

The electrical current produces heat when it meets a resistance to flow. This process is defined by Joules law with the heat production defined in terms of Joules (J):

$J = IRT$
where I = amperage, R = resistance, and T = contact time.

Electrical current produces tissue damage in two ways:

> *Local generation of heat during passage of current*
> *Direct tissue damage by the current*

The degree of tissue injury is dependent on the:

> Voltage of the source
> Amperage of current passing through the tissues

Resistance of tissues traversed by current
Duration of contact
Pathway of the current
Type of current: alternating (AC) or direct (DC)

## Voltage and Amperage

Electrical injuries are classified into low voltage (less than 500 volts) and high voltage (usually greater than 1,000 volts). Low-voltage injuries occur characteristically in a home or residential environment. Electrocutions in bathtubs and by electric hair dryers are the most common causes of low-voltage deaths. High-voltage injuries characteristically occur in an outdoor environment near power sources and lines. Electrical current can arc (jump) 1 inch from a power source or line for every 10,000 volts being carried, so that a person does not actually have to touch the source to sustain injury.

The severity of injury to tissues is dependent on the amperage, i.e., the actual amount of current passing through the tissues (Table 15-1). It is impossible to know the amperage because of the variability of resistance and exposure time at the accident, but one can infer amperage from the voltage of the source, at least as to high or low. A low-voltage source is capable of producing major cardiopulmonary complications and death if a sufficient current passes across the chest to initiate ventricular fibrillation.

A high-tension source is usually required to produce the tissue necrosis characteristically seen along the path of the current. The damage is caused by both heat production and direct current damage. The initial resistance to flow of current, namely, skin or clothing, is overcome by the heat generated from the high voltage, and subsequent tissue necrosis occurs with continued contact. A dry hand may have sufficient resistance to avoid passage of current from a low-voltage source over a short time period. However, the generation of several thousand degrees at the contact site with a high-tension source will lead to an immediate local coagulation and disruption of the electrical barrier. The current can now pass more readily through the tissues with a high water content because water is an excellent conductor. Local tissue damage at the contact site can be seen with low voltage as well, again due to local heat generation. A good example is the oral burn seen in children biting on an electric cord.

Besides heat injury, there is also tissue damage from the current itself. The

**Table 15-1** Effect of Current on Severity of Injury

| Current in Milliamps | Effect |
|---|---|
| High tension source, 5000 or more | Severe tissue destruction from heat and coagulation Cardiopulmonary failure |
| Household source | |
| 60 | Cardiac fibrillation |
| 30 | Respiratory muscle tetany: suffocation |
| 5 | Pain |

mechanism of tissue damage is complex and not completely defined. There is clearly an injury to nerves, blood vessels, and muscle from the current itself, damaging the cells. Endothelial cell injury due either to heat or current will result in loss of protection against local clotting and microvascular thrombosis, and tissue devascularization will result.

## Resistance

The resistance of tissues to passage of current is in large part dependent on water content, water being a good conductor. Tissue resistance in decreasing order from high to low is *bone, fat, tendon, skin, muscle, vessels, nerve*. However, with high-voltage injuries, the current readily passes through all tissues indiscriminately. Skin resistance is also dependent on skin moisture content. A moist hand has a resistance to passage of current 10 to 100 times lower than a dry hand. Heat produced as the current passes is proportional to tissue resistance (heat = $amp^2 \times R$). Local heat generated along bone from a high voltage source can be of sufficient degree, i.e., more than 1000°C, to cause bone destruction and total coagulation necrosis of surrounding tissues. Similarly, the heat produced as current enters and exits the body leads to coagulation necrosis of the skin and underlying tissues.

## Pathway of Current

The pathway of current can be somewhat unpredictable, but, in general, current passes from a point of entry through the body to a grounded site, i.e., a site of lower resistance to flow compared with air, which is a poor conductor. Extremely high voltage sources usually exit in multiple areas in an explosive fashion. Current passing from hand to hand or hand to thorax has a high risk of producing cardiac fibrillation compared with hand to foot passage. Passage through the head is likely to cause an initial respiratory arrest and subsequent severe neurologic impairment.

## Type of Current

Most household current is AC. A low-voltage AC is more dangerous than DC of the same voltage because of the production of muscle tetany. The tetany that is due to rapid depolarization and repolarization impedes attempts at escape from the source of electricity. High-voltage AC injuries are also more severe than DC, although both will lead to devastating injuries.

## Duration of Current

The severity of injury is also directly proportional to the duration of current flow. However, even extremely brief exposures to high amperage will produce massive tissue damage.

## PATHOPHYSIOLOGY OF HIGH-TENSION INJURY

A vast array of injuries result from the electrical damage (Table 15-2). These will be discussed more specifically in subsequent sections with specific emphasis being placed on the tissue necrosis.

### Cutaneous Injury (Entrance and Exit)

The determination that a current injury to underlying tissue may be present is the finding of entrance and exit sites. Their presence is pathognomonic of an electrical injury beneath the skin.

The heat generated at the skin surface is dependent on the local resistance, which in the dry hand can be sufficient to generate heat in excess of 1000°C with high-voltage sources. This will lead to local mummification at the entrance. The skin appearance at the site of contact is that of a well-defined charred wound that is depressed due to loss of tissue bulk (Color plate 15, page 317). The latter is due to evaporation of local water content by the high temperature. The wound may sometimes appear like a typical deep flame burn, except in this case the injury extends well below the dermis. The arc burn (later section) is basically a thermal burn caused by the intense heat generated from the high-tension current arcing from the wire.

Tissue appearance at the site of current exit varies considerably. With moderate exposures, the appearance is often that of small skin ulcerations with a depressed center and heaped up edges (Color plate 16, page 318). Look for the exit site where the patient was believed to be grounded. With passage of a large current, multiple exit sites are frequently seen along the route of the current. The appearance is often that which would be expected from an explosion, since pieces of cutaneous tissue are often absent, having been blown out by the immense energy of the exiting current.

*Remember: The exit wound is a deep wound and the magnitude of injury can easily be underestimated by the appearance on the surface.*

### Muscle Necrosis

Electrical burns more closely resemble a crush injury than they do a thermal burn. The damage below the skin where the current passes is usually far greater than the appearance

**Table 15-2** Common Complications

| | |
|---|---|
| Ventricular fibrillation | Muscle necrosis |
| Other rhythm abnormalities | Fractures |
| Respiratory arrest | Hemolysis |
| Seizures/coma | Renal failure |
| Mental changes | Hemorrhage |
| Hypertension | Limb loss |
| Retinal detachment | Anemia |
| Cataract (delayed) | Paresis/paralysis and other neurologic (delayed) |

of the overlying skin would indicate. The immediate damage to these tissues is caused by the heat destruction of cells, which is usually patchy in distribution along the course of the current. The second process is that of devascularization caused by injured blood vessels that progressively thrombose over a period of several days. The third process is that of compartment syndrome with pressure necrosis especially prominent in nervous tissue and muscle enveloped by a nonyielding fascial covering. The fourth process is that of tissue infection. Thus:

Immediate damage:  Heat and current cell death
Delayed damage:   Pressure necrosis
                  Progressive devascularization
                  Infection

There will be some immediate tissue death from heat coagulation. Dead muscle has a pale pink to white appearance due to release of myoglobin content. The dead muscle is noncontractile and is often found near the entrance and exit areas as well as *along the bone* where the heat released by the high bone resistor is the greatest. Local blood vessels in the area are thrombosed. The immediate necrosis *does not* follow the anatomic division of muscles but is very uneven, reflecting the uneven nature of the current passage. Muscle irreparably damaged but not immediately coagulated often cannot be readily distinguished from normal muscle in the first several hours after injury. Progressive necrosis is usually evident over the next 4 to 5 days. It is very common to find dead muscle in the presence of excellent local blood supply, indicating that the muscle damage is not totally vascular in origin and that the temperature required to produce muscle cell death is less than that required to coagulate a blood vessel.

Within minutes to hours of injury, the damaged but still perfused muscles begin to swell. The finite boundaries of the fascial envelope causes a rapid increase in tissue pressure, which, when exceeding the 20 to 25 mmHg microvascular hydrostatic pressure, produces further local tissue ischemia and local compressure nerve injury. A tissue pressure exceeding 30 mmHg is clearly abnormal and must be decreased to avoid further damage. Edema increases over the ensuing 24 to 48 hours.

Vascular thrombosis can occur immediately and over the ensuing 3 to 4 days due to initial current-induced vessel damage. The progressive devascularization results in a further loss of muscle tissue. The combination of endothelial cell damage and weakening of the vessel wall can lead not only to local thrombosis, but also local tissue hemorrhage.

The combination of these processes, the uneven nature of the necrosis, and, in particular, the damage to muscles and nerves closest to bone results in severe functional impairment and a high rate of amputation (30 to 40%). Muscle atrophy and replacement of injured muscle by fibrous tissue is another cause of subsequent dysfunction.

## Cardiovascular Injury

*Immediate cardiac arrest* is the most common cause of death after electrical injury. The process is due to both the direct alteration of rhythm by the current, leading to fibrillation or to the depression of respiration and subsequent hypoxia. Both brain and chest wall muscle changes will occur, leading to impaired ventilation. Hand to hand passage of a high voltage current has a reported immediate mortality of 60%. The initial cardiac arrhythmia is often reversible and cardiac resuscitation should be initiated at the scene. Current-induced myocardial necrosis is rare, although myocardial infarction can occur. The most common electrocardiographic changes seen other than fibrillation are sinus tachycardia and nonspecific ST-T wave changes.

*Systemic hypertension* is quite common with high voltage, possibly due to a massive and sustained release of catecholamines.

A *low flow state* as a result of fluid protein and blood loss into the tissues are characteristic and must be aggressively treated to avoid additional shock-induced tissue damage. A crush type injury invariably results in a massive fluid loss into the injured tissue.

*Major vessel thrombosis* is well described, as is delayed rupture of large vessels with massive hemorrhage, even in the absence of surrounding tissue damage, indicating the low resistance to flow within vessels. Aneurysms occurring weeks to months after injury, although uncommon, must be anticipated with good follow-up measures. Treatment is specific to the disease process. *Cardiovascular problems* include:

- Cardiac arrhythmias
- Systemic hypertension
- Hypovolemic shock
- Vessel rupture or thrombosis
- Aneurysm formation

## Renal Injury

Renal failure is reported in 10% or more of injuries. Renal damage is caused by a multitude of processes, including:

- Myoglobin sludging in renal tubules
- Disseminated intravascular coagulation secondary to tissue damage
- Hypovolemic shock
- Direct current damage

Myoglobin and hemoglobin released from damaged muscle and red blood cells can precipitate in the renal tubules, producing an acute tubular necrosis picture. Myoglobin is colorless in circulating plasma, whereas free hemoglobin is, of course, pink to red. Both, however, will produce pink to red urine. Myoglobin precipitation is accentuated by an acid urine and decreased by an alkaline urine. Muscle necrosis also produces a tissue injury similar to a crush injury, with evidence of distant organ dysfunction. The kidney, i.e., glomerulus, is a well-known target organ with this type of process. The low flow state caused by hypovolemia will simply aggravate the injury. Direct renal vascular damage from the current can also result.

## Pulmonary Injury

The pulmonary abnormalities are the result of two processes:

- Central nervous system-induced hypoventilation
- Chest wall dysfunction

Impairment of respiratory center activity and severe central nervous system damage will lead to hypoventilation, which is frequently the cause of immediate death. Impairment of muscle activity in the chest wall caused by a chest burn, muscle damage, or second degree blunt traumatic injuries can markedly impair compliance. Injuries to the diaphragm are uncommon. Later pulmonary complications are comparable to those seen after thermal burn.

## Neurologic Injury

Both immediate and delayed neurologic abnormalities are common. Acute central nervous system dysfunction with coma, seizures, motor, and, to a lesser extent, sensory deficits are well described. Many of these abnormalities are permanent. In addition, a number of delayed injuries occur, including both peripheral neuropathies and cord damage with paralysis. The mechanisms believed to be responsible for the delayed injuries are *delayed vascular thrombosis leading to ischemia* and *progressive demyelinization from electrical current*. Because of the delayed nature of these injuries, the determination of functional impairment caused by electrical injury should be delayed for a year after the initial event.

## Abdominal Viscera

Hollow viscus damage is not common but certainly can occur. Many of the injuries appear to be vascular in origin, although local heat-induced damage to the intestine has been described. Peptic ulcers, cholecystitis, and gastrointestinal bleeding can be seen. It is difficult, however, to sort out whether these latter types of processes are due to a specific current injury or simply a manifestation of severe trauma or the resulting shock.

## Orthopedic Injury

Orthopedic injuries occur as a result of three processes:

> *Muscle spasm-induced fractures and dislocations*
> *Heat-induced local bone destruction*
> *Devascularization of bone*

The most common orthopedic injury occurs as a result of severe immediate muscle spasm, which is capable of producing long bone fractures and dislocation at major joints. Heat necrosis of local periosteum with subsequent production of nonviable bone and sequestrum formation is the next most common process. Devascularization of bone due to the same vascular injury affecting other tissues is less common.

## Ocular and Otic Injuries

Again, both immediate and delayed injuries are noted. Conjunctival and corneal burns as well as ruptured ear drums are well described early changes. Late changes (up to 1 year) include cataract formation, tinnitus, and decreased hearing.

## Hematologic Injury

Acute anemia due to hemolysis and blood loss in damaged muscle is a characteristic finding. Clotting abnormalities, in particular an initial consumptive coagulopathy, are also common.

## Infection

Infection in the areas of tissue necrosis and ischemia is a major problem beginning several days after injury, particularly if a skin burn is also present that will potentiate cross-contamination from wound to wound. Control of the wound is much more difficult than with the skin burn because topical antibiotics will not be able to reach subsurface pockets of infection.

## GENERAL TREATMENT PRINCIPLES

### Monitoring

The first principle of treatment is making the diagnosis of an electrical injury. *Any patient with an entrance and exit wound due to an electrical burn requires hospital admission.* These findings are pathognomonic of the passage of a significant amount of current. Since there is absolutely no way of ruling out deep injury on initial assessment, admission and observation are necessary (Table 15-3).

Cardiopulmonary monitoring and supportive care are clearly necessary given the high incidence of cardiac arrhythmias and pulmonary dysfunction. An initial urinalysis is essential not only to verify adequate renal perfusion, but also to check for myoglobinuria, which, if present, will require special management. Blood gases and acid-base balance are of particular importance in avoiding an acidosis that will accentuate pigment deposition in the kidney.

**Table 15-3**  Monitoring Patients After an Electrical Burn

| Systemic Changes | Local Changes |
|---|---|
| 1. Vital signs | 1. Doppler measurement of injured extremity blood flow |
| 2. Urine output | 2. Frequent assessment for evidence of nerve compression |
| 3. Urine myoglobin | 3. Frequent palpation of muscle compartments |
| 4. Serial hematocrits | |
| Consider | Consider |
| 1. Arterial line | Measurement of Compartment Pressures |
| 2. Pulmonary artery catheter in selected cases | |

Monitoring of peripheral perfusion and palpation of muscle compartments are of particular importance because of the concern of the development of compartment syndromes due to underlying muscle edema. Measurement of compartment pressures can also be performed (as described). Compartment pressure can be monitored using several types of available systems. The *Wick-type* catheter and the *solid state transducer* are two types commonly used. Placement of the catheter into the compartment is relatively safe, if not placed through overlying burn. The primary difficulty is the determination as to the reliability of the reading. Accurate leveling is necessary using the *Wick catheter*. The *solid state* system has the transducer in the catheter. Determination of the need for fasciotomy is based either on the absolute value of tissue pressure or the relationship of tissue pressure to blood pressure. *Indications for fasciotomy, escharotomy* are:

*Tissue pressure more than 40 mmHg*

*Tissue pressure within 30 mmHg of diastolic pressure*

Usually the number itself is not used as an absolute indication but is compared with any clinical evidence of nerve compression, i.e., tingling, increased pain, decreased sensation, or vessel compression. Thus, signs of increased pressure include:

Decreased peripheral pulse

Evidence of nerve compression

Onset of paresthesias

Decreased sensation or increased pain

Increased muscle turgor to palpation

Motor nerve dysfunction is more difficult to assess given the fact that muscle damage may be impossible to distinguish from nerve damage. Excessive tissue turgor is the single most useful sign of underlying muscle damage and the need for fasciotomy.

## Fluid Management

The same basic principles of fluid management apply as with a thermal burn alone. The primary resuscitation fluid is Ringer's lactate solution (or hypertonic lactated saline). There is no formula, however, to assist in management due to the unpredictable nature of the underlying tissue damage. In general, the fluid requirements per percent of burn are 1.5 to 2 times that of a skin burn alone given the nature of the added soft tissue injury. Colloid and blood are used more frequently during the early resuscitation period than after thermal burn alone due to red blood cell hemolysis and to the increased whole blood losses into the damaged muscle and other deep tissues. Excessive crystalloid may accentuate muscle edema and potentiate pressure necrosis even after fasciotomy, since this procedure does not totally eliminate the problem.

The *rate* of fluid administration is based on the amount necessary to maintain adequate perfusion using the same guidelines as for burn shock management. The exception is the presence of urine myoglobin or other evidence of early renal impairment. If the urine is red or reddish black, a massive myoglobin release from muscle has occurred and an increased washout of the tubular pigment is needed. A urine flow of 1 cc/kg/hr or more is needed until pigment load has decreased. Mannitol (12.5 g every 2 to 4 hours) is often required to maintain this level of output. In addition, sodium bicarbonate is often needed to maintain urine pH equal to or greater than 7 in order to minimize pigment precipitation. Loop diuretics may be needed beginning the next day to maintain a high urine flow if pigment persists. Thus, the treatment regimen is as follows:

1. Give mannitol 25 g bolus followed by 12.5 g every 2 to 4 hours in addition to fluids until pigment clears from urine
2. Add sodium bicarbonate to intravenous solution to maintain urine pH >7 but avoid increasing blood pH >7.5
3. Low-dose dopamine if excessive fluids required in addition to mannitol to maintain urine flow
4. Add loop diuretics after 18 to 24 hours to fluid infusion if pigment load persists

Furosemide increases tubular fluid flow and lowers renal vascular resistance. A similar approach at maintaining tubular patency is also initiated if evidence of nonpigment load renal dysfunction is noted from direct renal injury or that from disseminated intravascular coagulation or low flow state.

Fluid and osmotic agents are temporizing agents, however, and the injured muscle, if a large amount is present, must be removed very early to prevent renal shutdown. Subsequent fluid, electrolyte, nutritional support, and stress management follow the principles described for thermal burns.

## Infection Control

In general, infection control is obtained by wound debridement. *Tetanus prophylaxis is required* in view of the risks of deep tissue necrosis in a relatively anaerobic environment. Broad-spectrum antibiotics are not indicated as a prophylactic measure. However, perioperative antibiotics are indicated, as with management of skin burns. The principal organism of concern in the initial 2 to 3 days is *Staphylococcus aureus*. Coverage with a cephalosporin or methicillin is appropriate. Later, organisms such as *Pseudomonas aeruginosa*, which thrives in a low oxygen environment, will be the predominant organism. Topical antibiotics, such as silver sulfadiazine (Silvadene) and mafenide (Sulfamylon) can be used on the skin burns where an eschar is present. *General infection control measures include:*

Tetanus prophylaxis
No broad-spectrum prophylactic antibiotics
Use of perioperative antibiotics
Use of topical cream-based antibiotics—skin wound

## Escharotomy-Fasciotomy

In general, if there is a circumferential deep burn and any evidence of impaired distal perfusion, i.e., decreased pulses, an escharotomy is necessary. If there is also a concomitant electrical injury to underlying tissue and increasing compartment pressure, as evident from increased myoglobin, rigid muscle compartments, or nerve or vessel compression, i.e., tissue pressure (>35 to 40 mmHg), fasciotomy is indicated. Fasciotomy incisions are performed in the long axis of the limbs, as with the escharotomy. The fasciotomy incisions must split the investing fascia of all the involved compartments. The underlying muscle can then be inspected to determine viability. Electrocautery is often necessary with fasciotomy as opposed to escharotomy because fascial and muscle vessels will probably be patent. The fasciotomy defect exposing the viable but injured muscle must be covered preferably with a biologic or synthetic skin substitute to avoid desiccation. The escharotomy site and incisions through burn or nonviable tissue can be managed with topical antibiotics. It is not necessary and is actually disadvantageous to exposed muscle groups that are not clearly involved in a compartment syndrome. The exposure of muscle increases the risk of colonization and infection.

## Wound Management

The spectrum of injuries that can occur makes definitive comments on wound management difficult. In general, high voltage burns with large amounts of necrotic muscle must be treated aggressively with surgical debridement, including early amputation of nonviable extremities, to minimize subsequent organ dysfunction, infection, and eventual mortality. An early aggressive surgical approach also maximizes the salvage of marginal tissue, which is very susceptible to infection. If gross myoglobinuria is present for several hours or large exit sites or mummification of a large entrance wound, one can nearly guarantee that a large amount of dead muscle is present. *Evidence for severe muscle damage* include:

1. Large entrance site with mummification
2. Large exit sites: Tissue explosion
3. Gross myoglobinuria
4. Woody, hard nonfunctioning muscle by palpation

Early excision of obviously dead muscle is performed as soon as hemodynamic stability is obtained, preferably in the first 1 to 2 days. Also, the risks of renal failure increase as long as a large amount of dead and dying muscle is present. The *initial surgical treatment* is as follows:

1. Restore cardiopulmonary stability
2. Fasciotomies dictated by evidence of dead muscle or increasing pressure
3. Removal of dead muscle: Spare muscle with indeterminant viability
4. Early guillotine amputation of obviously nonsalvageable limbs (this can be lifesaving)
5. Use biologic dressings or moist, dilute antibiotic solutions (followed by dry, soft dressing with extremity elevation)
6. Perioperative systemic antibiotics against skin organisms, principally S. aureus
7. Reoperate in 24 to 48 hours

The goal of subsequent surgical procedures is to conserve remaining viable tissue while removing neighboring dead tissue. The uneven nature of the injury makes this approach difficult and very time consuming. Small scattered areas of injured muscle will be reabsorbed and replaced by fibrous tissue. Physiologic evidence of remaining infected dead tissue is often manifested by a high fever and tachycardia. The tissue along the bone is often the site of the necrosis.

Obviously dead muscle should be removed first. The extent of initial debridement is dictated by hemodynamic stability. Marginal muscle can be left in place for a second look in 24 to 48 hours. Further thrombosis of blood vessels should be anticipated. Serial debridements every 12 to 24 hours may be needed if the amount of dead tissue usually in multiple areas is more than that which can be safely removed at one time.

The wounds can be treated open using biologic dressings if available or dressings continually moistened with a dilute antibiotic solution (e.g., bacitracin, neomycin irrigant) to avoid wound desiccation. Surrounding skin burns can be treated with topical antibiotics. The *evidence for modest muscle damage* is:

1. Lack of severe tissue necrosis at entrance site
2. Small (punctate) exit sites
3. None-to-trace myoglobinuria
4. Absence of severe muscle swelling and dysfunction

## Managing Entrance and Exit Sites

Entrance and exit sites, although thermal burns, i.e., due to heat generation, are more complex than a standard skin burn. The problem is that devitalized tissue exists below the burn, especially at the exit site. Initial debridement to viable tissue should follow the same principles as with a thermal burn. However, it is best to use biologic or synthetic temporary skin substitutes initially. Further necrosis of tissues is expected. After 3 to 5 days, the temporary skin substitutes (or moist dressings) can be removed, any residual necrotic tissue debrided, and wound closure begun either with skin grafts or skin flaps. Tissue defects at the entrance and exit sites may eventually require soft tissue coverage by a tissue flap. Initial closure with skin grafts is often preferred, with the larger procedures to be performed later in a more stable patient.

## THERMAL BURNS TO THE SKIN

The heat generated by arcing (jumping) of a high-voltage current from a high-tension wire toward the patient will reach several thousand degrees because air has a high resistance. The heat will produce a flash skin burn comparable to that of any explosion of volatile substances. In addition, the intense heat frequently causes clothes to catch fire, leading to deep burns by this mechanism. It is easy to overlook an electrical burn in the presence of a large skin burn. The subsequent soft tissue edema and pain can be misinterpreted as due to the thermal injury rather than underlying damage. Thus, the two *mechanisms* are:

Heat generated by current arcing

Clothing catching fire

The treatment is essentially identical to that for any cutaneous burn alone except a higher urine output will be necessary if myoglobinuria is present. More fluid will be necessary and more initial cardiopulmonary support if an electrical burn is also present.

## BLUNT TRAUMA (FREE FALLS)

Well over one half of high voltage injuries occur to workers on towers and poles 20 or more feet above the ground. Free fall injuries therefore are the result. The nature and magnitude of the injury depend on:

1. Height of the fall
2. The impact surface (stopping distance)
3. Body mass
4. Body orientation on impact
5. Distribution of impact forces
6. Patient age, affecting tissue tolerance

A fall of 30 feet (two stories) generates an impact velocity of 30 mph.

$$KE = \tfrac{1}{2} \text{mass} \cdot V^2$$

where KE is kinetic energy and V is velocity (gravity constant of 35 ft/s$^2$ times height). Some of the kinetic energy generated during the fall is converted to potential energy, which is defined as mass times gravity times stopping distance. The greater the stopping distance the more kinetic energy is dissipated as potential energy. Fortunately, the surface near power poles is frequently dirt rather than concrete. The majority of kinetic energy is converted to mechanical energy, which is dissipated through the tissues, generating fractures and rupture of visceral organs. The injury patterns are given in Table 15-4.

Treatment is essentially the same as that for similar trauma in the absence of an electrical injury. Differences are primarily in the manner of treating fractures beneath burned skin or muscle damage where early fixation with hardware may not be as feasible. The *major treatment problem,* however, is *failure to recognize the existence of the blunt injury in the electrical burn patient.*

## LOW-VOLTAGE INJURY

The major injury produced is a cardiac arrhythmia, especially ventricular fibrillation. A wet skin surface markedly increases the amount of current passing through the body. Suffocation due to chest wall muscle tetany is less common because several minutes are required to produce this outcome and often some assistance is available to remove the patient from the source. The difficulty with the cardiac abnormality is the fact that only a small portion of the population is capable of rendering cardiopulmonary resuscitation

**Table 15-4** Injury Patterns (2 to 3 Stories: 30 to 45 Ft)

| Injuries | Incidence |
| --- | --- |
| Fracture of low extremity, ankle, foot | >40% |
| Fracture of vertebrae, thoracic, lumbosacral | 10–40% |
| Liver, spleen injury | >10% |

before the arrival of emergency personnel. The central nervous system abnormalities are usually the result of hypoxia from the cardiopulmonary arrest. It is good practice to observe patients for 24 hours in the hospital with cardiac monitoring to avoid missing a major myocardial injury. Fractures, as a result of tetany and muscle spasm from AC can also occur. Thus, the *most common injuries* are:

>Cardiopulmonary arrest
>Tetany-induced fractures

## PITFALLS IN MANAGEMENT

### Failure to Recognize Depth of Entrance and Exit Sites

Both entrance and exit wounds are extremely deep, extending well into the tissues beneath the skin. Excision of necrotic tissues is almost always necessary. Therefore, continued use of a topical antibiotic in hopes of primary healing only prolongs disability.

### Failure to Recognize the Potential Extent of Injury Along the Course of the Current

The electrical injury is usually far more extensive than is evident by the entrance and exit sites, which added together often make up a relatively small body surface "burn." The hidden injury can rapidly evolve into a complication, such as a compartment syndrome.

### Failure to Recognize Increased Compartment Pressure and Its Complications

One has to look actively for evidence of increasing compartment tissue pressure, nerve compression, etc., in order to initiate therapy, i.e., fasciotomy, in sufficient time to avoid significant damage.

### Failure to Recognize Increased Resuscitation Fluid Needs

The combined electrical and thermal burn requires 1.5 to 2 times the amount of fluid calculated for the skin burn alone due to the extensive losses into the subdermal tissues. Renal failure can develop rapidly if adequate renal blood flow is not maintained.

### Failure to Diagnose Blunt Traumatic Injuries on Admission

The electrical burn itself is often disfiguring and extensive. All attention becomes focused on the mummified extremities, etc. An organized initial assessment must be performed followed by a secondary survey, just as with any other trauma patient, to avoid missing major injuries.

## Failure to Be Aware of the Delayed Injury

Spontaneous hemorrhage and a late neuropathy or paraplegia or cataract can develop days to weeks after initial injury. Care providers must be aware of these potential problems in order to limit their morbidity and to inform the patient adequately.

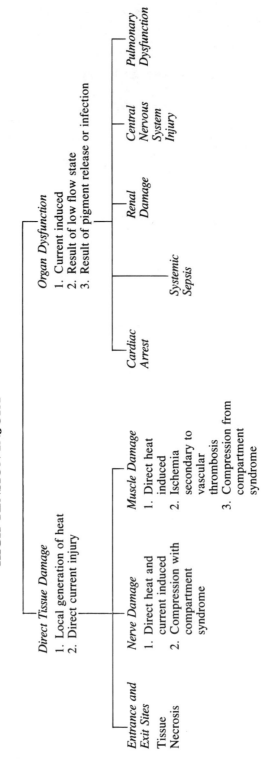

# SUMMARY OF INITIAL TREATMENT OF HIGH-TENSION INJURY

## Make the Diagnosis

1. Adequacy of airway, cardiopulmonary dysfunction
2. Consider possibility of muscle necrosis (look for exits)
3. Presence of blunt traumatic injuries
4. Size and depth of skin burn

### Fluid Treatment

1. Lactated Ringer's solution: add colloid and blood as necessary
2. Anticipate need for more than 4 cc/kg/% total body surface in first 24 hours
3. Maintain urine more than 1 cc/kg/hr with myoglobinuria (use mannitol 12.5 g bolus)
4. Maintain urine pH more than 7 (add sodium bicarbonate to intravenous fluids)

### Monitoring

1. Electrocardiography to control arrhythmias
2. Arterial, venous pressures (consider pulmonary artery catheter)
   a. To monitor adequate perfusion especially to injured central nervous system myocardium and kidneys
   b. To monitor blood gases, pH
3. Urine output, pH, Myoglobin
4. Serum electrolytes (especially $K^+$) myoglobin, clotting factors
5. Consider monitoring compartment pressures
6. Monitor flow to distal extremity (Doppler flow meter)
7. Monitor central and peripheral nerve function (watch for compression neuropathy)

## Wound Care

### Infection

1. Tetanus prophylaxis
2. No prophylactic systemic antibiotics
3. Topical antibiotics to areas of skin burn or necrosis
4. Debride as soon as stable

### Perfusion

1. Escharotomy, if distal pulses impaired in circumferential injury
2. Fasciotomy
   If evidence of vessel, nerve, muscle compression injury
   Interstitial pressure more than 35 to 40 mmHg

# 16

# Low Tension Oral Burns

## PATHOPHYSIOLOGY

Low-voltage electricity is the leading cause of electrical injury in children, especially 1 to 2 years old. Sucking an extension cord is responsible for more than half of the injuries, and biting on an electric cord accounts for about 30% (Color plate 17, page 318). The most common mechanism is the production of an electrical arc by the bared wires conducted by the childs saliva. Intense local heat is generated, producing severe local destruction of the mouth tissues. The local mouth burn is characteristically grayish-white in color and indented at the center due to tissue necrosis. Severe swelling then develops as venous thrombosis impedes blood return. The oral burn may involve the lip, tongue, or oval mucosa and underlying bone. The most frequent site is the lip, in particular the commissure area between upper and lower lips (Table 16-1). The edema of the lips may be intense, impairing control of saliva. The orbicularis oris muscle is frequently involved, further impairing control. Edema subsides over the next 5 to 10 days and local necrotic tissue begins to slough. Bleeding from the labial artery is a common occurrence (20%) during the period of slough (7 to 21 days) and should be anticipated. Granulation tissue then develops, followed by collagen deposition and wound remodeling. Local adhesions and microstomia may develop over a period of 3 to 5 months. Injury to the underlying bone will result in dental abnormalities over time.

To summarize, the pathophysiology consists of:

1. Local generation of high temperature from current in mouth
2. Intense local edema (5 to 10 days), impaired muscle function
3. Sloughing of necrotic tissue (1 to 3 week period) with bleeding from labial artery: common
4. Scar formation, adhesions, remodeling 3 to 5 months

## TREATMENT

Initial hospitalization is recommended to treat the local burn and observe for any current related injuries. Tetanus prophylaxis is necessary, but systemic antibiotics do not appear to be particularly beneficial. Local wound care with gentle washing followed three to four

**Table 16-1** Categorization of Electrical Burn to Lip

| | |
|---|---|
| Minor: | Less than one third of upper or lower lip involved sparing commissure |
| Moderate: | More than one third of lip involved sparing commissure or local commissure injury alone |
| Severe: | Loss of skin and muscle of more than one third of lip, including commissure |

times daily by local application of a petroleum-based antibiotic ointment. Tube feeding or via a syringe or straw is helpful to avoid any further local pressure. Occasionally, vessel ligation is required.

Since the extent of injury cannot be determined for several days, surgical debridement is delayed for about a week or longer. The present treatment of choice is the placement of a prosthetic intraoral splint after initial edema resolves (5 to 10 days). The splints, of which a variety of types exist, decreases the scar deformity of adhesion formation. Decreased scarring markedly decreases the need for later reconstruction of major cosmetic defects, which is required in about 80% of burns not splinted. The wound not splinted will heal by contraction. Splinting should continue for 6 to 12 months until the local scar relaxes, losing its contractile properties. Minor surgery can then be performed if needed on the residual defect.

## TREATMENT SUMMARY FOR ORAL BURNS

HOSPITAL ADMISSION
5 to 10 Days: Until Edema Resolves

*Infection Control*
1. Tetanus prophylaxis
2. Topical antibiotic ointment (four times daily)
3. No prophylactic systemic antibiotics

*Wound Care*
1. Minimize mouth trauma, use liquid feedings
2. Conservative wound debridement
3. Pressure control of local (labial artery) bleeding

*Cosmesis*
1. Use of intraoral splint (6 to 12 months)
2. Revision of remaining deformity after 1 year

# 17

# Lightning

## PATHOPHYSIOLOGY

Lightning is the result of an atmospheric electrical discharge occurring between a positive charge developing in an upper cloud level and a net negative charge at a lower cloud level. A lightning flash occurs when the potential difference between the layers exceeds the insulating properties of air. Air crossed by the lightning is rapidly heated and expands to develop a shock wave that decays to a sound wave perceived as thunder. The power of a lightning bolt is estimated at 10,000 to 20,000 amperes of current with more than 20 million volts of electromotive force. There are four mechanisms of injury: direct strike, flash discharge, ground current, and shock-wave.

A direct strike results when the person is outside and is the grounding site. Mortality rate is high, with head entry being quite common. A flash discharge is a more common injury as the lightning is deviated by another object. Injury is still severe, but not as great as a direct strike.

Ground currents can develop from the initial strike on the ground. A person standing may generate a sufficient potential difference between legs and ground that a current develops. Overall mortality rate from lightning injury is about 30%, with permanent sequelae involving two thirds of survivors.

The phenomenon of "flash-over" results when the lightning travels along the outside of the conductor, namely, the victim. The current vaporizes skin moisture and destroys clothing but spares the body tissues themselves. The shock wave produced by the heating and expansion of air produces tissue damange comparable to any large explosion. This form of tissue trauma is commonly overlooked in the patient.

## SPECIFIC PROBLEMS

### Cardiovascular Injury

The direct current of lightning produces myocardial depolarization and arrest. Subsequent respiratory arrest and hypoxia will make resuscitation efforts to restore a normal rhythm very difficult. Immediate resuscitation efforts are required. Intense vasoconstriction caused by the passage of current can lead to severe tissue ischemia. Treatment is supportive.

## Central Nervous System Injury

The central nervous system damage is due to either the electrical current or mechanical trauma. At least three fourths of patients with a lightning injury have at least a transient loss of consciousness. More than two thirds have a temporary paralysis of the upper or lower extremities, which resolves over hours to days. Permanent sequelae are common, especially those that result from an added anoxic injury from cardiorespiratory arrest. Treatment is supportive.

## Skin

Skin injuries vary from the burns seen with a high-voltage current to a superficial skin abnormality called "feathering" or "lightning prints." The latter process is characterized by linear fernlike erythematous skin markings that do not blanch. The markings are probably due to the "flash over" phenomenon as static electricity is transmitted along the superficial vasculature. They fade in several days. Recognition of this skin change in a comatose person can help make the diagnoses of a lightning injury. Treatment of the localized deep burns is the same as for other electrical burns with excision and wound closure when the wound has evolved.

## Musculoskeletal Injury

A typical high-tension injury with muscle necrosis can be seen with all the problems of a compartment syndrome, myoglobinuria, and renal failure. Treatment is the same as that outlined for high-tension injury.

## Eye

Cataracts are the most common intraocular injury caused by lightning. One type of cataract is traumatic in origin due to the initial concussion. The second type caused by the current itself is delayed in onset for several months. Lid lesions from a burn itself and conjuctivitis are also common. Treatment is based on the specific injuries produced.

## Ear

Ear injuries occur in more than 50% of lightning injuries, again due to both the concussion (ruptured tympanic membrane) and the current (direct nerve damage). Treatment is based on the specific injuries produced.

## Gastrointestinal Tract

Injuries are basically the same as seen in mechanical trauma and high-voltage electrical burns.

## GENERAL TREATMENT

Treatment is based on recognition, which is often the major problem after an unwitnessed lightning injury. The absence of a history or of evidence of flames or a fire often makes diagnosis difficult. Understanding of the magnitude of energy involved in the lightning injury will minimize the risk of missing major tissue damage, both the immediate and delayed type. The general treatment principles are the same as those given for a high-voltage electrical burn.

# SECTION 6
# Management of Burns in the Multiple Trauma Patient

# 18

# Management of Burns in the Multiple Trauma Patient

Management of the trauma patient is guided by well-defined principles of prioritization, as is the care of the burn patient. The surgeon providing the primary care to one of these two patient types is often not totally familiar with the management of the other patient type. This problem is particularly true of burns. The burn surgeon may be more familiar with general trauma care than the general surgeon or surgical subspecialist is in dealing with burns. The immediate course of action for the traumatic injury can be inappropriately disrupted by the concerns about what to do with the burn. However, the most dangerous situation is the unrecognized traumatic injury in the patient perceived to only have a burn injury. There are several reasons for this latter situation. First, there is usually an overwhelming desire to move the major burn patient out of the emergency room as soon as possible, either to the intensive care unit (ICU) or more appropriately to the nearest burn unit. This desire can lead to an inadequate workup before transfer. Second, once the patient arrives in an ICU or burn facility, the concern for other injuries is often diminished and a significant delay in the diagnosis can result.

The incidence of a combined injury is not well defined, but the problem is certainly not rare. There are five major injury categories in which a combined injury in the civilian population is most frequently seen: motor vehicle accidents, escape attempts from structural fires, explosions, aircraft accidents, and high-voltage electrical injuries.

In our experience, the most common cause is a motor vehicle accident followed by escape attempts from a fire. The first four causes are those at increased risk of the development of a smoke-inhalation injury. Smoke inhalation and its complications are major causes of the increased mortality seen in the combined injury. High-voltage electrical injuries are frequently associated with a fall.

## GENERAL PRINCIPLES OF MANAGEMENT

The initial approach to the combined trauma and burn injury should follow the same basic guidelines for trauma resuscitation, which include airway, breathing, circulation, and neurologic assessment.

## Airway

In the case of a compromised airway and a facial burn, the standard approach of naso- or oropharyngeal intubation with C-spine control is initiated. If there are clear indications for a surgical airway because of traumatic injuries, e.g., facial fractures, one should not hesitate to perform a cricothyrotomy even if a neck burn is present. Neck burn can then be excised and grafted within 24 to 48 hours when the patient is more stable, the cricothyrotomy can be removed, and a tracheostomy placed through the new skin graft, preferably a sheet graft.

Another important airway consideration relates to the trauma patient who has a patent airway and a facial burn that by itself does not require an immediate artificial airway. However, if a surgical procedure is planned, e.g., internal fixation of a fracture within the first 24 hours, it will be extremely difficult to place a tube at the time of the operation due to massive edema with considerable distortion of anatomic landmarks. This consideration needs to be made in the early resuscitation period (Table 18-1).

## Breathing

The same immediate concerns over adequate breathing that affect the trauma patient are present in the combined injury. Tension pneumothorax, open chest wound, and flail chest with underlying contusion remain major concerns with trauma. Management, even in the presence of a chest burn, should be the same. If a chest tube is required, it should be placed through nonburn tissue, if possible. However, a tube placed through burn has a minimal risk of infection if changed within the first 24 to 48 hours. As with the airway, deep burn in the area of the tube can be excised and grafted within 24 to 48 hours and a new tube placed through a graft. If an immediate thoracotomy is indicated, the incision site and surrounding burn can be excised and grafted and the wound closed in a standard fashion. The amount of excision depends on the stability of the patient. If skin grafting for some reason cannot be immediately performed, the local area preferably with a several inch border can be excised and the wound sealed with a skin substitute (synthetic, e.g.,

**Table 18-1** Airway Assessment

| Airway Patent But Inhalation Injury or Face Burn Present | Immediate Compromise Urgent Need for Airway |
|---|---|
| Place Artificial Airway<br>1. Prior to onset of airways edema<br>2. Prior to onset of anatomic distortion by edema, which can hamper placement<br>3. If surgical procedure is planned prior to adequate resolution of orofacial edema | Place Artificial Airway Following Standard Guidelines with C-Spine Control<br><br>Needs Surgical Airway and Burn Present<br>1. Perform cricothyrotomy through the burn<br>2. Excise and graft deep burn at 24 to 48 hours and convert to tracheostomy through graft<br>3. Cover superficial burn with skin substitute to seal wound around airway |

biobrane or biologic: cadaver skin, pigskin). The wound edges will be protected from bacterial colonization and will heal beneath the substitute in a normal fashion. When skin is available, preferably within a week, the substitute can be removed and a sheet of 1.5 to 1 meshed skin grafts applied. The early life-threatening problems that must be looked for are:

1. Tension pneumothorax
2. Open pneumothorax
3. Flail chest with contusion
4. Inhalation injury
5. Constricting chest wall burn

Since *Staphylococcus aureus* is commonly present on a burn, even in the early hours, we consider prophylactic antibiotics to be indicated. Coverage should be especially aimed at gram-positive organisms, in the first 24 to 48 hours until the burn wound can be excised and grafted.

## Circulation

There are two important considerations to be made in the combined injury in regards to initially *assessing* the circulation:

1. Recognition of the increased volume losses of a burn in a trauma patient
2. Recognition of blood loss from undiagnosed trauma in a burn patient

The first problem is recognizing the increased fluid requirements of a burn caused by the fluid shifts previously described. In addition, the burn alters red cells first by an initial heat injury, decreasing red cell life span, and second by a decreased production of erythropoietin. Occasionally, there is red cell hemolysis evident on admission. In any case, the decreasing hematocrit over the first several days after a major burn alone needs to be appreciated. A falling hematocrit does not necessarily mean ongoing blood loss in the combined injury.

Next, it is crucial to be able to recognize blood volume loss in the burn patient, when in excess of what is expected with the burn alone. This clue will greatly assist in the diagnosis of an unappreciated traumatic injury.

Once diagnosed, the initial management of the traumatic injury should not be dramatically altered by the presence of a burn. There are two important considerations regarding the *management* of the circulation:

1. Recognizing the differences and similarities for resuscitation endpoint for trauma and burns
2. Recognizing the differences in volume replacement for trauma versus burns:
    Rate of edema formation is directly proportional to fluid infusion rate.
    Replacement of blood and plasma loss with protein-free solution will markedly accentuate hypoproteinemia
    Access problems

The combined injury is best handled by initial isotonic crystalloid loading (2 to 3 L) to restore perfusion. This initial process can be followed by a continuous infusion of isotonic crystalloid at the estimated rate to correct for the burn loss along with replacement of blood products for blood loss guided by indicators of tissue perfusion and hematocrit. We believe that consideration should be given to replacement of plasma protein when serum albumin is less than 2.5 g/dl, given the fact that the burn losses will continue for several days. Low-dose dopamine is often very advantageous in maintaining renal perfusion and urine output. It is especially useful in the patient receiving a larger than predicted volume replacement in whom urine output is marginal but all other parameters indicate good perfusion. Since burn (inhalation injury) and trauma (lung contusion) as well as central nervous system injuries can be exaggerated with excess fluid, the resuscitation of the combined burn and trauma injury must be very carefully monitored.

## Disability (Neurologic)

Head injuries are a common occurrence in the trauma- and burn-injured patient given the nature of the type of accident that leads to both burns and trauma. As described with other traumatic injuries, one of the major difficulties is making the diagnosis. *Assessment* is impaired by the frequent occurrence of smoke inhalation and both hypoxia-induced and carbon monoxide-induced neurologic dysfunction. Hypoxia, carbon monoxide (and also cyanide) toxicity are global injuries and usually do not present with lateralizing signs. Severe global injury can lead to cerebral edema at 24 to 72 hours, with the potential of herniation. Traumatic brain injuries with epidural or subdural bleeding often develop lateralizing signs. The distinction between a traumatic and global injury can be better defined by a computed tomography (CT) scan. It is important to emphasize that one cannot assume that the neurologic problem is carbon monoxide in a burn patient if a history or evidence of trauma is present. Treatment of head trauma is based on first restoring systemic tissue oxygenation and perfusion, followed immediately by any surgery if indicated. Excessive brain edema as a result of overresuscitation or electrolyte abnormalities like hyponatremia should be avoided. However, it is also counterproductive to try to "dry out" a trauma patient with a burn in the early postinjury period, since ongoing burn losses will inevitably lead to brain hypoperfusion. Addition of an inotrope, dopamine, or dobutamine to supplement fluid resuscitation may help avoid complications of excessive fluid replacement.

Surgical indications in the presence of a burn are comparable to those without a burn. The complicating factors will be the difficulty of clinical assessment of head injury-induced neurologic dysfunction in the presence of carbon monoxide (or cyanide)-induced toxicity. The presence of a scalp burn should not preclude production of a surgical flap or pin placement for cervical traction. Potential scalp infection should be diminished by excision and grafting (first 24 to 48 hours) of the scalp burn in the area of the surgery. Insufficient data are currently available on this approach to document this concept; however, early wound closure would appear to be the most logical approach. Prophylactic antibiotics are indicated when an incision is placed through burn tissue.

A particular concern in the head injured-patient is avoiding hypervolemia in the postresuscitation period. Fluid will be mobilized from partial thickness burn edema beginning 48 to 72 hours after injury. Continued monitoring of filling pressures during this period will greatly assist in the diagnosis. Treatment is carefully administered diuretics. Low-dose dopamine can assist in the diuresis. Severe hyponatremia, again as a result of too much water in the presence of inappropriate antidiuretic hormone needs to be avoided. The continued evaporative water loss from the burn surface usually results in hypernatremia rather than hyponatremia.

## SPECIAL PROBLEMS

### Intra-Abdominal Injuries

*Assessment* of intra-abdominal injuries in the presence of burns can be a major problem because of the difficulty of interpreting physical findings, especially if a burn is present on the abdominal wall. Peritoneal lavage and CT scan should be used more liberally in this circumstance because interpretation of vital signs and pain will be extremely difficult. There is no contraindication for performing an initial lavage through burn if the area is appropriately prepared. The burn wound is not heavily colonized in the first hours after injury unless there is gross wound soilage. Cleaning the area in a similar fashion to that of procedure through nonburn skin should be effective. An open approach, i.e., a small incision carried down to the peritoneum, in a superficial burn should not present any major wound problem. A similar approach through a deep burn is best managed by excision and grafting of the incision area within 24 to 48 hours, i.e., before wound colonization. Subcutaneous tissue can be approximated with sutures and the skin incision and surrounding area will be covered with a skin graft. Peritoneal lavage, however, will not rule out retroperitoneal injuries and, since symptoms of pain will be difficult to assess, a computed tomography scan may be a more appopriate general early assessment. The evaluation of the pancreatic duodenal area is particularly important, since complications of post-traumatic pancreatitis several days later could readily be interpreted as burn wound sepsis or, if hyperamylasemia is present, burn-induced pancreatitis. Also, a modest hyperbilirubinemia, which could be a symptom of hepatobiliary trauma, is a common occurrence in the major burn patient when early severe hemolysis or an episode of shock is present. In addition, a decreasing hematocrit due to initial red blood cell injury and decreased red blood cell production are common findings in the postresuscitation period.

### Management

The indications for surgical management of intra-abdominal trauma in the presence of a burn is not different from that with trauma alone. The difficulties arise primarily from management of the surgical incision. The wound is, of course, at risk for infection and dehiscence. Dehiscence can result not only from infection but from inability to close all wound layers, as well as a result of postburn catabolism. Exploration through a midline incision remains the best approach for trauma, even if the incision is placed through burn. Several recent series indicate that the dehiscence rate of the abdominal incision in the burn patient when placed through burn is not increased compared with the multiple trauma patient if retention sutures are used, which encompass all layers. Stainless steel retentions appear to be the best. Early wound excision and grafting in the area of the incision should decrease the potential of infection in the local wound. However, no prospective studies on this problem have been performed. If the deep skin burn is not excised and grafted immediately, the skin incision should not be closed primarily. A skin substitute may be of particular benefit in sealing the wound until skin grafting can be performed. A diverting colostomy should be placed through nonburn skin if at all possible. If not, the area should be excised and grafted as soon as possible.

## Orthopedic Injuries

### Fractures

The most common traumatic injury associated with burns is a fracture. The burn produces problems both in assessment and treatment. Diagnosis is often hampered by the fact that burn edema and the burn eschar can disguise the clinical evidence of both pain and local swelling. Hemodynamic instability in excess of that expected for a burn alone indicates that a traumatic injury is present unless proved otherwise. Considerable blood loss can occur in a fracture site. Fracture dislocations are particularly common in the high-voltage electrical injury patient from both the tetany produced by the current itself and the frequent fall from a utility pole. Once the diagnosis is considered, standard radiographs can define the problem. Although correct assessment simply requires a high index of suspicion, treatment can be considerably complicated by the presence of a burn in the area of the fracture. Bone healing appears to be normal in burn patients if infection and other wound complications can be avoided. The standard recommendations before the advent of early excision and grafting was to avoid internal fixation because of the high risk of infection with a plate present beneath an overlying infected wound. Skeletal traction for a number of weeks was utilized until the overlying wound was healed. However, this immobility results in a high risk of long-term disability due to joint stiffness and overlying wound contractures. Plaster casts placed over a burn are discouraged because of inability to treat the wound.

The current recommended approach is to use a combination of external and internal fixation for those fractures requiring reduction and immobilization. The determining factors include: (1) The necessity for reduction and immobilization of the fracture; (2) the stability of the patient, allowing for an operative approach; (3) access to the burn for wound care; and (4) ability to institute aggressive physical therapy. External fixation is most appropriate for open fractures or massively contaminated wounds and wounds in which immobilization of the joints adjacent to the fracture do not markedly interfere with patient mobility. External fixation requires minimal anesthesia and can be performed in the early resuscitation period. This approach is particularly useful for the unstable pelvic fracture in the hemodynamically unstable patient. Internal fixation is ideal once the patient is hemodynamically stable, i.e., after 24 to 48 hours. Excision and grafting of deep burn in the area of the incision is ideal, to avoid a subsequent wound infection. A combination of external and internal fixation may be required. Pin sites through burn need to be treated with topical antibiotics until the wound is excised and closed. Temporary skin substitutes can be used on superficial burns. Systemic antibiotics (first choice is a first generation cephalosporin) are indicated until the wound is closed.

## Compartment Syndrome

The combination of a deep burn and an underlying fracture or soft tissue hematoma increases the risk of a compartment syndrome or decreased blood flow, especially to the distal extremity. The deeply burned skin leads to subdermal edema, which cannot be compensated for by skin elasticity because the covering eschar is very inelastic. This process alone can lead to impaired distal perfusion. An underlying fracture with tissue edema and hematoma formation will magnify the problem. Assessment of symptoms of pain, paresthesias, distal pallor, and also clinical assessment of pulses will be hampered by the local burn wound. A Doppler flowmeter will assist in detecting the adequacy of distal blood flow but may not accurately detect a compartment syndrome, especially if the problem is confined to one compartment. Measurement of compartment pressures is indicated with severe fractures or underlying muscle damage, just as it would be with a fracture alone. This procedure will require penetrating burn tissue with a needle to measure tissue pressure. The complications of this procedure are minimal compared with compression damage to the neurovascular bundle. The treatment of impaired perfusion as a result of the overlying burn is an escharotomy. The treatment for subfascial edema and hematoma formation is fasciotomy.

## SUMMARY OF INTRA-ABDOMINAL INJURIES

*Management*
1. Indications for surgery on traumatic injuries not changed with burn
2. Midline (or transverse incision) preferred to paramedian incision
3. Close wound with through and through retention sutures, anticipating delayed healing
4. Leave skin incision through burn open
    Can excise and graft area early to remove burn
    Can cover open incision with skin substitute temporarily awaiting excision and grafting

*Assessment*
1. Recognition of risks of missing a traumatic injury
    Early systemic findings can be due to burn alone
    Decrease in hematocrit, increase in bilirubin can be due to burn alone
    Late symptoms of intra-abdominal inflammation from missed diagnosis can be masked by burn infection
2. Liberal use of peritoneal lavage or computed tomography scan (the latter will also help define retroperitoneal injuries)

# SUMMARY OF BREATHING PROBLEMS

*Immediately Impaired*

### Need for Thoracotomy with Chest Burn
1. Place on perioperative antibiotics (first generation cephalosporin)
2. Excise and graft deep burn around incision and cover either temporarily with a skin substitute or permanently with skin grafts if the patient is sufficiently stable

### Burn Related
1. Look for evidence or history of smoke inhalation
2. Look for constricting chest wall burn and perform necessary escharotomy

### Trauma Related
1. Look for airway problem, pneumothorax, flail chest with contusion
2. Place chest tube if needed, preferably through nonburn tissue
3. If tube through or close to burn:
   Place on short courses of antibiotics (first generation cephalosporin)
   Excise and graft deep burn at tube site and surrounding area in 24 to 48 hours and change tube site
   Cover superficial burn around tube site with skin substitute (biobrane, cadaver skin, pigskin) to seal wound and minimize colonization

# SUMMARY OF CIRCULATORY CHANGES

## Management

### Replace Estimated Burn Losses
1. Use constant infusion
2. Add plasma proteins if also losing whole blood
3. Preserve some intravenous access sites for the long haul
4. Prefer nonburn intravenous sites

### Replace Estimated Trauma Loss
1. Use bolus (2 to 3 L) of crystalloid to restore perfusion
2. Replace ongoing blood loss with blood products, including protein if burn is of large size

### Monitoring Endpoint
1. Recognize difficulty of "filling the tank" in the presence of a large burn
2. Recognize intense catechol and antidiuretic hormone release after burn
3. Consider use of low-dose dopamine in addition to adequate fluids

## Assessment

### Recognize Increased Losses from Burn in Trauma Patient
1. First 24 hours 4 cc/kg/% total body surface being plasma
2. After 24 hours: evaporation losses cc/hr = $(25 + \%burn) \times m^2$ total body surface
3. Increased burn-induced red blood cell destruction
4. Decreased red blood cell production in burn

### Recognize Blood Loss in Burn Patient
1. Decreasing red cell mass in absence of hemolysis

255

# SUMMARY OF NEUROLOGIC DYSFUNCTION

*Management*

1. Restore and maintain adequate cerebral perfusion
   Fluids
   Consider addition of inotrope
2. Surgical indications same as for trauma alone
   Consider early excision and grafting of surgical site if deep burn
   Consider skin substitute to seal superficial burn
   Perioperative antibiotics, especially covering *S. aureus*
3. Watch for late (2 to 4 days) hypervolemia due to mobilization of burn edema

*Assessment (Differential Diagnosis)*

Head Injury
1. Often focal signs
2. Do not assume dysfunction secondary to carbon monoxide toxicity if evidence of trauma
3. Need computed tomography to define injury

Hypoxia, Carbon Monoxide, Cyanide Toxicity
1. Usually global, not localized
2. May have semilucid interval with carbon monoxide

# SUMMARY OF FRACTURES

*Management*

1. Watch for compartment syndrome or distal perfusion abnormalities
   Burn tissue inelasticity plus edema
   Underlying fracture with hematoma
   Difficult pain assessment
2. Assess by Doppler and tissue pressure
3. Perform escharotomy or fasciotomy when indicated

1. Avoid casts over burn
2. Avoid prolonged immobilization of joints in burn area
3. External and internal fixation techniques are treatment of choice
   Decision based on patient hemodynamic stability
   Excise and graft burn area near operative area

*Assessment*

1. Need high index of suspicion
2. Local pain and deformity can be masked by burn eschar and edema

# SECTION 7
# Reference Section

This section contains information useful for the cardiopulmonary and metabolic support required for the burn patient, in particular the critically ill patient, including respiratory function, hemodynamics and perfusion, nutritional support, and topical antibiotics

# 19

# Respiratory Function

## MONITORING RESPIRATORY FUNCTION

Respiratory monitoring can be divided into two major categories: the adequacy and efficiency of oxygen exchange and the adequacy of respiratory mechanics and ventilatory reserve.

### Defining Ventilation-Perfusion Mismatch

Even in the normal lung, there is some ventilation-perfusion (V/Q) mismatch because there is relatively more ventilation to the upper lobes of the lung and relatively more perfusion to the lower lobes. This mismatch can be magnified by ventilatory abnormalities, such as bronchoconstriction, alveolar collapse or flooding (pulmonary edema), or perfusion abnormalities, such as vascular occlusion or hypoperfusion from hypovolemia. When an area of the lung with no ventilation is perfused, no oxygenation occurs. This is known as a "shunt," and the amount of total pulmonary blood flow that perfuses nonventilated areas is known as the *shunt fraction* ($Q_S/Q_T$). A true shunt does not respond to administration of oxygen because the excess oxygen cannot reach the perfusing blood through a nonventilated area. An area of the lung that is ventilated but not perfused is referred to as *dead space*. The ratio of the portion of tidal volume ($V_T$) that is dead space ($V_D$) is calculated as $V_D/V_T$. Most V/Q mismatch is not the result of a total lack of ventilation or perfusion to an area, and therefore some response to exogenous administration of oxygen is usually seen.

### Defining Adequacy of Oxygen Exchange

#### Arterial Oxygen Tension

This parameter measures the amount of oxygen dissolved in plasma and determines the percent saturation of hemoglobin, the major factor in blood oxygen content. Arterial oxygen tension ($PaO_2$) will be affected by pulmonary processes impairing oxygen exchange, i.e., impaired diffusion, increased shunt, V/Q mismatch. In addition, $PaO_2$ will be affected by the venous oxygen tension ($PvO_2$), especially in the presence of an increased shunt. Hypercapnia will affect $PaO_2$, especially when breathing room air (fractional inspired oxygen [$FiO_2$] is 0.2):

$$P_AO_2 = (P_B - P_{H_2O}) \times FiO_2 - \frac{PaCO_2}{0.8}$$

where $PAO_2$ is alveolar oxygen tension, $P_B$ is barometric pressure, and $PaCO_2$ is carbon dioxide tension.

## Alveolar-Arterial Oxygen Gradient

This parameter is a more sensitive measure of an impairment to oxygen exchange from lung to blood.

Although measurable at any given $FiO_2$, it is commonly determined with the patient inhaling 100% oxygen ($FiO_2 = 1.0$) for 20 minutes. When the patient is breathing $FiO_2$ of 1.0, the $PO_2$ is the same in all ventilated alveoli. The normal gradient is less than 50 mmHg on 100% oxygen (less than 30 mmHg on room air). It must be noted that the calculation of the alveolar-arterial oxygen gradient ($A$-$aDO_2$) at $FiO_2 = 1.0$ may cause absorption atelectasis, which can then further increase the shunt.

## Pulmonary Shunt

The percent of pulmonary shunt ($Q_S/Q_T$, i.e., the right-to-left shunt) is defined as that portion of the cardiac output ($Q_T$) (pulmonary blood flow) that is perfusing unventilated alveoli ($Q_S$).

In the normal person, $Q_S/Q_T$ is in the range of 3 to 5%. The $Q_S/Q_T$ can be measured with the patient either on 100% oxygen or on a lesser oxygen concentration. When breathing 100% oxygen, the calculation of the $Q_S/Q_T$ is simplified (because the calculation of the $P(A-a)O_2$, which is required in the shunt equation, is simplified). The calculation is:

$$Q_S/Q_T = \frac{CcO_2 - CaO_2}{CcO_2 - CvO_2}$$

where $Q$ = total pulmonary blood flow, $CaO_2$ = oxygen content of arterial blood, $CvO_2$ = oxygen content of mixed venous blood, $CcO_2$ = oxygen content of pulmonary capillary blood. The calculation of $CcO_2$, however, requires one to assume that this would be the oxygen content that arterial blood would have if fully equilibrated with alveolar air, because of the inaccessibility of pulmonary capillary blood for direct measurement.

The *causes of pulmonary shunt* are:

1. Alveolar consolidation or edema
2. Anatomic right to left shunts
3. Alveolar collapse, atelectasis

## Monitoring Respiratory Mechanics

### Physiologic Dead Space

Dead space is that portion of the tidal volume not exchanging with pulmonary blood. A portion of this is *anatomic*, e.g., trachea, large airways (150 ml in adults). The remainder of the measured $V_D/V_T$ is called *alveolar dead space*, which is made up of nonperfused ventilated alveoli, e.g., from embolic occlusion. The normal $V_D/V_T$ is 0.2 to 0.4. $V_D/V_T$ = anatomic plus alveolar dead space:

$$V_D/V_T = \frac{PaCO_2 - P_ECO_2}{PaCO_2}$$

where $V_D/V_T$ = dead space; $PaCO_2$ = arterial carbon dioxide tension; $P_ECO_2$ = mean expired carbon dioxide tension.

The $V_D/V_T$ will vary with changes in either anatomic or alveolar dead space or tidal volume. However, the measured $V_D/V_T$ does not differentiate anatomic from alveolar dead space. The *causes of increased $V_D/V_T$* are:

1. Vascular obstruction, e.g., embolus
2. Hypovolemia impairing lung perfusion
3. Increased airway pressure impairing perfusion
4. Decreased $V_T$ with constant $V_D$

In the presence of refractory atelectasis, a portion of this redistributed blood flow will go to atelectatic areas. As a result, both $V_D/V_T$ and $Q_S/Q_T$ will be increased.

## Inspiratory Force

Inspiratory force is measured as the maximum pressure below atmospheric pressure that a patient can exert during a period of 5 to 10 seconds against a completely occluded airway. This measurement is not dependent on the cooperation of the patient and is particularly useful with unconscious or anesthetized patients. The normal value for inspiratory force is $-75$ to $-100$ cm $H_2O$. A force of more than $-25$ cm $H_2O$ is usually required to generate a vital capacity of 15 ml/kg.

## Vital Capacity

Vital capacity is defined as the lung volume after a maximal inspiration preceded by a maximal expiration. Normal vital capacity is 65 to 75 ml/kg. A vital capacity of less than 15 ml/kg reflects severe lung dysfunction and inadequate lung inflation and is an indication for mechanical ventilatory assistance.

## Functional Residual Capacity

Functional residual capacity (FRC) is defined as the gas remaining in the lung after a normal expiration that maintains the alveoli patent. Total collapse during expiration would, of course, result in a marked impairment in gas exchange. Patients with pulmonary insufficiency have a decreased FRC leading to atelectasis. It has been observed that positive end-expiratory pressure (PEEP) increases FRC.

## Dynamic Compliance

Dynamic compliance ($C_{DYN}$) is the term reflecting lung expansibility during air flow. $C_{DYN}$ is obtained during inspiration at the peak impedance to lung expansion, namely, at the peak inspiratory pressure. Tidal volume is the volume change. The pressure change is calculated as peak inspiratory pressure minus atmospheric or 0 unless continuous positive airway pressure (CPAP) is present

$$C_{DYN} = \text{tidal volume/peak inspiratory pressure} - \text{PEEP}$$

It is a reflection of not only lung expansibility but resistance to flow of air. The resistance includes the ventilator, the airways, and chest wall.

## Static Lung Compliance

Static lung compliance ($C_{STAT}$) is a measure of the recoil properties of lung and chest wall or the ability of the system to stay inflated and end inspiration. $C_{STAT}$ is measured at no flow, at the end of inspiration. The $V_T$ is held in the lung at the end of inspiration and pressure measured. On a ventilator, this is obtained by using an end-inspiratory pause or plateau, the pressure now measured at no air flow is called the *plateau pressure*:

$$C_{STAT} = \text{tidal volume/plateau pressure} - \text{PEEP}$$

Decreased $C_{STAT}$ can reflect a tendency toward alveolar collapse, such as surfactant denaturation or alveolar edema. A stiff chest wall will also decrease $C_{STAT}$.

## Work of Breathing

Work of breathing is an important parameter in ventilation. Normally, less than 5% of total oxygen consumption ($VO_2$) is used for the work of breathing. An increase in dead space, or shunt, or decrease in compliance can markedly increase the work load. If the increased oxygen demands cannot be met or muscle fatigue occurs, respiratory distress will occur.

## Minute Ventilation

Minute ventilation ($\overset{\circ}{V}$) is defined as total air movement through the lungs per unit time. The value of $\overset{\circ}{V}$ includes both alveolar and dead space ventilation:

$$\overset{\circ}{V} = \text{tidal volume} \times \text{rate}$$

## Alveolar Ventilation

Alveolar minute ventilation ($\overset{\circ}{V}_A$) refers to that portion of V that is actually responsible for gas exchange. $PaCO_2$ is linearly related to $\overset{\circ}{V}_A$ with the value of $PaCO_2$ changing inversely with changes in $\overset{\circ}{V}_A$:

$$\overset{\circ}{V}_A = \overset{\circ}{V} - (\overset{\circ}{V} \times V_D/V_T)$$

The stimuli for maintaining adequate $\overset{\circ}{V}$ are the $PaO_2$ in peripheral chemoreceptors (carotid body and aortic arch) and the pH of the central chemoreceptors in the brainstem. The pH is altered by dissolved carbon dioxide, which rapidly crosses the blood-brain barrier, whereas plasma buffers such as $HCO^-_3$ cannot cross. Small changes in carbon dioxide therefore produce significant changes in pH. A decrease in pH (increase in carbon dioxide) is a strong stimulus to increase ventilation, whereas an increase in pH will decrease the ventilatory drive. A decrease in $PaO_2$ initiates a similar increase in $\overset{\circ}{V}$ via the carotid body.

*Arterial Carbon Dioxide Tension*

The normal value of $PaCO_2$ is 39 to 42 mmHg with the normal value in mixed venous blood being 41 to 50 mmHg. The alveolar (end-expiratory) $PCO_2$ should be numerically close to $PaCO_2$, assuming reasonable uniformity of ventilation. Increase in carbon dioxide production in the absence of a compensatory increase in $\mathring{V}_A$ will result in an increase in $PaCo_2$.

## DIAGNOSING RESPIRATORY DYSFUNCTION

## Defining Respiratory Dysfunction

A significant impairment in any of the following functions will eventually result in respiratory insufficiency: adequacy of lungs as gas exchanger, adequacy of work of breathing, and adequacy of alveolar ventilation.

*Adequacy of Lung as a Gas Exchanger*

It has been empirically established that a *shunt, greater than 20%* or a $V_D/V_T$, *greater than 0.6,* is incompatible with adequate spontaneous ventilation. Shunt can be directly measured if a pulmonary artery catheter is present or can be estimated from values of $PaO_2$ and $FiO_2$, the latter approach being satisfactory in most clinical situations.

*Adequacy of Work of Breathing*

The maximum inspiratory effort, i.e., ability to generate negative intrapleural pressure of at least $-25$ cm $H_2O$ and the ability to generate a vital capacity of at least 10 ml/kg body weight are predictors. However, these values only reflect the ability of the patient's breathing capacity over a very short period while *endurance* also needs to be assessed by determining the changes in lung function with time. An increasing respiratory rate and chest wall retraction are indicators of excessive respiratory work.

*Adequacy of Alveolar Ventilation*

Alveolar hypoventilation or a decrease in $\mathring{V}_A$ could be considered to be a specific form of V/Q mismatch caused by a mechanical or central nervous system impairment to alveolar ventilation. Insufficient alveolar ventilation will result in both hypoxia and hypercapnia because neither gas will be exchanged (Table 19-3). Exogenous administration of oxygen may maintain sufficient content of oxygen in the alveolus even during hypoventilation to maintain reasonable oxygen exchange. Hypoxia will therefore be a late finding in this case. The $PACO_2$, however, will increase relatively rapidly and in direct proportion to the decrease in alveolar ventilation. The $PaCO_2$ will increase (respiratory acidosis) and correspond to the end-inspiratory $PACO_2$ of that alveolus. A halving of alveolar ventilation will result in a doubling of $PaCO_2$, and vice versa.

*Total minute ventilation* may be normal but *alveolar ventilation* can be decreased if $V_D/V_T$ is increased above the normal 0.3 to 0.4. This can even occur in the absence of lung parenchymal injury. With shallow breathing, the anatomic dead space (100 to 150 ml) becomes a larger fraction of a decreased tidal volume. Patency subsequently decreases

Table 19-1  Standard Measurements of Respiratory Function

| Parameters of Gas Exchange | Acronym | Measurement | Normal Values |
|---|---|---|---|
| Partial pressure $O_2$ arterial blood | $PaO_2$ | Direct | Varies with age<br>80-95 mmHg (room air) |
| Partial pressure $CO_2$ in arterial blood | $PaCO_2$ | Direct | 40 mmHg |
| Partial pressure $O_2$ mixed venous blood | $PvO_2$ | Direct | Varies with $VO_2$<br>35-40 mmHg |
| Partial pressure $CO_2$ | $PvCO_2$ | Direct | 41-51 mmHg |
| Alveolar oxygen tension | $PAO_2$ | $(P_B - P_{H2O}) \times FiO_2 - \dfrac{PaCO_2}{0.8}$ | Depends on $P_B$ and $FiO_2$<br>95-110 room air<br>630-670 $FiO_2$ 1.0 |
| Alveolar-arterial $O_2$ gradient | $A\text{-}aDO_2$ | $P_AO_2 - P_aO_2$ | 25-50 mmHg at $FiO_2$ 1.0 |
| Percent arterial oxyhemoglobin saturation | $SaO_2$ | Direct | Varies with $PaO_2$<br>by oximeter 97% (room air) |
| Percent venous oxyhemoglobin saturation | $SvO_2$ | Direct | Varies with $VO_2$<br>by oximeter 75% (room air) |
| Right to left shunt | $Q_S/Q_T$ | $\dfrac{CcO_2 - CaO_2}{CcO_2 - CvO_2}$ | 5-8% |
| Respiratory mechanics | | | |
| Tidal volume | $V_T$ | Direct | 4-5 ml/kg |
| Vital capacity | $V_C$ | Direct | 65-75 ml/kg |
| Functional residual capacity | FRC | Direct | 2000-2600 ml |
| Inspiratory force | IF | Direct | $-75$ to $-100$ cm $H_2O$ |
| Dead space to tidal volume | $V_D/V_T$ | $\dfrac{PaCO_2 - P_ECO_2 \text{ (exp } PCO_2)}{PaCO_2}$ | 0.2-0.3 |
| Effective dynamic | $C_{DYN}$ | $\dfrac{\text{(Peak inspiratory pressure} - \text{PEEP)}}{V_T}$ | Mechanical ventilation<br>60-80 ml/cm $H_2O$ |
| Static compliance | $C_{STAT}$ | $\dfrac{\text{(Plateau pressure} - \text{PEEP)}}{V_T}$ | Mechanical ventilation<br>80-100 ml/cm $H_2O$ |
| Total minute ventilation | $\dot{V}_T$ | $V_T \times$ rate | 4-6 L/min |
| Alveolar ventilation | $\dot{V}_A$ | $\dot{V}_T - \dot{V}_D$ | 3-5 L/min |
| Dead space ventilation | $\dot{V}_D$ | $\dot{V}_T \times V_D/V_T$ | 1-2 L/min |

Table 19-2  Causes of Decreased Compliance

|  | Dynamic Compliance ($C_{DYN}$)<br>(Airway or Parenchymal) | Static Compliance ($C_{STAT}$)<br>(Parenchymal) |
|---|---|---|
| Lung | Bronchospasm, or airway obstruction | Pneumothorax |
|  | Pneumothorax | Surfactant impairment |
|  | Stiff lung parenchyma, e.g. fibrosis, ARDS* | Atelectasis, edema, pneumonia, ARDS |
| Chest | Noncompliant chest wall, edema, muscle spasm, rib fractures | Same |

*ARDS: Adult respiratory distress syndrome.

in the absence of an adequate tidal volume. Airways collapse and atelectasis results if FRC decreases below closing volume.

## Treatment

The primary treatment is to remove increased carbon dioxide by increasing alveolar ventilation, often by mechanical assist. The initiating cause must be corrected at the same time to avoid returning to a state of hypoventilation. Correction of an impaired respiratory drive is usually the easiest to accomplish, since most drug-related hypoventilation in surgery patients is narcotic induced. Correction of increased dead space must focus on the cause, i.e., obstruction of vessels or low output (either absolute, i.e., shock, or relative from positive pressure breathing). Increasing blood volume and cardiac output and

Table 19-3  Causes of Hypercapnia

Extrapulmonary
    Impaired ventilatory response to carbon dioxide
        Central nervous system depressant drugs; head trauma
        Starvation, hypothyroidism
    Increased carbon dioxide production
        Increased temperature 6-10% per degree centigrade
        Increased muscle activity: shivering, seizures
        Increased respiratory quotient from excess carbohydrate calories
Pulmonary
    Airway obstruction
    Impaired chest wall motion
        Chest wall trauma, instability
        Chest wall pain, splinting
        Neuromuscular disorders
    Increased dead space ventilation
        Shallow breathing
        Pulmonary emboli
        Low cardiac output
        Positive-pressure ventilation

decreasing mean airway pressure are useful maneuvers to control increasing dead space ventilation.

Increased carbon dioxide production is controlled by controlling increasing temperature and increased muscle activity, e.g., shivering or seizure activity will markedly increase carbon dioxide production. Excessive carbohydrate calories will increase the respiratory quotient, which can exceed 1.0, thereby generating very large amounts of excess carbon dioxide. Respiratory acidosis should not be treated with sodium bicarbonate unless the pH is less than 7.2 or unless there are severe complications of the acidosis, e.g., cardiac arrhythmias, hyperkalemia. Since there is no base deficit with respiratory acidosis, the addition of base will result in an alkalosis once alveolar ventilation is restored. In addition, the bicarbonate load will increase total carbon dioxide. Overcorrection of the impairment in alveolar ventilation should also be avoided because an alkalotic state has its own set of complications.

## TREATING RESPIRATORY DYSFUNCTION

### Endotracheal Intubation

There are four indications for controlling the airway by endotracheal intubation (rule of 4 P's): patency of the airway: restoration, protection (from aspiration), pulmonary toilet (=inadequate cough), positive pressure applied to the airway (mechanical ventilation with or without PEEP, CPAP with spontaneous breathing). *Each* of these items in itself is an *absolute* indication for intubation.

*Patency of the airway* relates to current and anticipated problems of the adequacy of the airway. Direct injury from trauma or burns resulting in mucosa edema or external compression by edema or hemorrhage are examples.

*Protection,* in particular from aspiration, relates to the status of the awake state as well as the structural integrity of the larynx and the ability of the epiglottis to protect the airway when necessary.

*Pulmonary toilet* relates to the ability to clear secretions to avoid airway obstruction, atelectasis, and infection. An inadequate cough would necessitate a more direct access to the airways for suctioning. Patients with an adequate cough but with voluminous secretions, e.g., inhalation injury, may also require intubation to avoid fatigue from increased work.

*Positive-pressure breathing* is indicated when the criteria for adequacy of spontaneous ventilation are not met: the larger the diameter of the tube, the less resistance to airflow through the tube.

### Mechanical Ventilation

*Definition*

Mechanical ventilation is largely defined as *positive-pressure ventilation*. The necessary increase in *mean airway pressure* can also produce complications. A potential disruption of the normal V/Q matching seen with spontaneous ventilation can occur with lung overexpansion leading to regional hypoperfusion. Cardiac output and oxygen delivery can be impaired by both a decrease in venous return and an increase in pulmonary vascular

**Table 19-4** Nonpulmonary Side Effects

Cardiac
1. Impairment of preload due to decrease in venous return
2. Increase in right ventricle and a decrease in left ventricle size due to right to left septal shift
3. Support of the failing ventricle by the surrounding positive pressure and by reduction of preload and afterload

Renal
1. Decrease in renal blood flow comparable to overall decrease in cardiac output
2. Redistribution of blood flow from cortical to medullary areas decreasing filtration rate and urine output. The flow shift is believed to be due to increased renal vein pressure
3. Increase antidiuretic hormone due to increased intrathoracic pressure and a neural reflex initiated by the pressure-distorted atrial wall
4. Increase in plasma renin activity

---

resistance, both the result of the transmission of positive airway pressure to the mediastinal structures and the pulmonary vasculature. The *more compliant the lung or the less compliant the chest wall, the greater will be the transmission of the positive airway pressure to the mediastinum*. The concomitant decrease in cardiac output can, in large part, be overcome by volume loading.

## Adjusting the Ventilator

*Tidal volume* with positive pressure is usually set at 10 to 12 ml/kg body weight, which is considerably increased over the 5 to 6 ml/kg seen with spontaneous ventilation. This

**Table 19-5** Guidelines for the Institution and Discontinuation of Mechanical Ventilatory Support in Patients with Pulmonary Insufficiency

| Parameter | Normal Range | Indication for Ventilatory Assistance |
|---|---|---|
| Mechanics | | |
| Respiratory rate | 12–20 | >35 |
| Vital capacity (ml/kg body wt)* | 65–75 | <15 |
| Inspiratory force (cm $H_2O$) | >−75 | <−25 |
| Compliance (L/cm $H_2O$) | 0.1 | 0.02 |
| Oxygenation | | |
| $PaO_2$ (mmHg) | >75 (room air) | <70 |
| $P(A-a)O_2$ ($FiO_2 = 1.0$) (mmHg) | 25–50 | 450 |
| Shunt $Q_S/Q_T$ | 5% | >20% |
| Ventilation | | |
| $PaCO_2$ (mm Hg) | 35–45 | 55† |
| $V_D/V_T$ | 0.2–0.3 | 0.60 |

*Use ideal body weight.
†Exception is chronic lung disease.

allows for a slower rate, which in turn decreases mean airway pressure. In addition, the sense of dyspnea created by stiff lungs is diminished and anxiety is decreased. The higher tidal volume also decreases atelectasis and in turn the shunt fraction. A portion of the set tidal volume (3 to 8 ml/cm $H_2O$ air pressure) is lost in the circuit through *compression loss* as tubing distends with positive pressure. This loss must be anticipated and corrected, if necessary, by either decreasing airway pressure or increasing tidal volume.

*Respiratory rate* should be set to meet ventilatory needs, usually beginning with 10 to 12 breaths/min.

*Inspiratory to expiratory ratio* is usually set at 1:2. Patients with severe airways disease may require a longer relative expiratory time to avoid air trapping and hyperinflation with subsequent breaths.

*Inspired oxygen concentration* is set to allow for at least 90% saturation of hemoglobin, i.e., $PaO_2$ of 60 mm/Hg or higher. An $FiO_2$ of 0.5 or less is preferred if possible to diminish the potential of oxygen toxicity.

## Use of Positive End-Expiratory Pressure and Continuous Positive Airway Pressure

PEEP has been demonstrated to be useful in the management of acute respiratory failure by returning FRC toward normal, thereby decreasing atelectasis and shunt. In addition, PEEP has been shown to be able to increase lung compliance by recruiting additional areas of the lung for ventilation. PEEP can therefore improve oxygenation by decreasing shunt and improve ventilatory mechanics by increasing compliance. The addition of positive pressure during inspiration and expiration to the spontaneously breathing patient is known as CPAP. The addition of some PEEP to all mechanical ventilation modes is common practice in order to improve arterial oxygen tension. PEEP can improve lung mechanics by alveolar recruitment, but mechanics can also be impaired if lung hyperinflation occurs because the latter will accentuate a V/Q mismatch. PEEP is also not indicated when there is already regional hyperinflation, such as with emphysema.

The major disadvantages of PEEP and CPAP are the increase in mean airway pressure-induced complications. PEEP of 10 cm $H_2O$ or less usually does not lead to major impairments in cardiac output (Table 19-6).

## Acute Respiratory Decompensation on Mechanical Ventilation ("Fighting the Ventilator")

The term "fighting the ventilator" is frequently applied to the situation in which the patient is clearly struggling to maintain ventilation.

Troubleshooting should begin with *disconnecting* the patient from the ventilator and Ambu *bagging* with 100% oxygen. Easy ventilation with the Ambu bag and patient stabilization would suggest a ventilator problem. Decreased sensitivity of the machine to patient initiation of a ventilatory cycle could occur, as could a number of other mechanical problems. Ambu bagging, however, usually results in an increased $V_T$, which can also be responsible for the patient's improvement. Patients with stiff lungs frequently are dyspneic despite adequate gas exchange. This appears to be due to activation of the J receptors in the lung from increased interstitial fluid. Often increasing the $V_T$ will correct this subjective feeling. Dead space can be added to the system if this maneuver also leads to hyperventilation and hypocapnia.

Difficult bagging on ventilator disconnect strongly suggests a problem with the tube

**Table 19-6** Positive End-Expiratory Pressure

---
Advantages
1. Increases functional residual capacity
2. Recruits additional lung units, improving compliance
3. Reduces pulmonary shunt fraction
4. Allows for a decrease in $FiO_2$
5. Can decrease preload in congestive heart failure

Disadvantages
1. Increases mean airway pressure leading to reduced venous return
2. Can increase $V_D/V_T$ by impairing perfusion to hyperexpanded lung
3. Can increase pulmonary vascular resistance and right heart dysfunction
4. Altered renal blood flow with increase in antidiuretic hormone release
5. Barotrauma caused by increased pressure

Primary indications
1. Treat hypoxemia when patient already on $FiO_2$ of 0.5 or greater and with bilateral diffuse pulmonary infiltrates
2. Treat a shunt of 20% or greater in patient with diffuse disease
3. To maintain FRC after airways injury, such as smoke inhalation
---

or the lung chest wall complex. Endotracheal tube narrowing from inspissated secretions or malposition of the tube must be rapidly diagnosed and treated. Blood gases, chest examination, and chest radiographs should be ordered. A suction catheter should be passed to check for narrowing or blockage. Checking the marking of the tube at the orifice entrance compared with its prior position will assist with the malposition issue. Tube replacement should be performed if the problem cannot be rapidly corrected.

Easy passage of the catheter and deterioration suggest a pneumothorax, which can be diagnosed clinically in many cases and a chest tube placed. Lack of tube obstruction in the absence of a pneumothorax suggests increased oxygen demands, as seen with sepsis, or impaired oxygen delivery, as seen in the case of heart failure, or an acute pulmonary injury, as occurs with pulmonary emboli, or acid aspiration.

The patient may need to be paralyzed in order to allow for effective mechanical ventilation if "fighting" persists after other treatable causes have been eliminated. A list of nondepolarizing agents is presented in Table 19-7.

## Weaning from the Ventilator: Weaning Criteria

Withdrawal of mechanical ventilatory support is the term referred to as "weaning." The timing of the initiation of weaning is crucial. A premature attempt will result in a weaning failure as well as increase patient anxiety for a second attempt. If weaning is started too late, one runs the risk of an iatrogenic dependence on the ventilator occurring as well as a ventilator or positive-pressure–induced complication. Certain criteria must be present before weaning is instituted. The patient must be hemodynamically stable. An adequate cardiac output and oxygen delivery to the respiratory muscles must be present as well as sufficient reserve to allow a further increase in work. Thus, for *decision-making*, the *criteria for weaning* are:

1. Stable clinical condition
2. Adequate oxygen delivery
3. Control of sepsis

**Table 19-7** Paralyzing Nondepolarizing Agents

| Drug | Intravenous Dosage | Properties | Side Effects |
|---|---|---|---|
| Pancuronium (Pavulon) | Initial 0.06–0.1 mg/kg with rate of injection not significant<br>Followed every 30–60 minutes by 0.01–0.10 mg/kg | Dose-dependent muscle paralysis<br>Onset of action in 2–3 minutes with short half-life of 2 hours<br>Eliminated by kidneys and liver | Some histamine release<br>Has sympathetic stimulation that can increase heart rate and blood pressure<br>Decreased clearance with liver or kidney disease |
| Metocurine (Metubine) | Initial 0.2–0.4 mg/kg given over 30–60 seconds<br>Followed every 30–90 minutes by 0.02–0.1 mg/kg | Dose-dependent muscle paralysis<br>Onset of action 1–3 minutes with longer half-life of 4 hours<br>Eliminated by kidney, not liver | Histamine release more than pancuronium<br>No sympathetic effect; therefore less effect on heart rate<br>Hypotension and vasodilation can occur if given too rapidly<br>Decreased clearance with kidney disease |
| Atracurium | Initial 0.25–0.5 mg/kg<br>Later doses to effect | Dose-dependent muscle paralysis<br>Minimal sympathetic effect<br>Nonspecific metabolism; therefore no active metabolite buildup with liver or renal failure<br>Half-life 20–35 minutes | Mild hypotension, vasodilation |
| Vecuronium | Initial 0.05–0.12 mg/kg<br>Later doses to effect | Dose-dependent muscle paralysis<br>No sympathetic effect<br>Half-life 25–50 minutes<br>Metabolites excreted by kidney | Less of a problem with renal failure than is metocurine |

*Patient assessment for weaning* is as follows:

1. Is the state of consciousness adequate? Are drugs being given that depress respiratory drive or muscle activity?
2. Adequacy of lung function: Is the shunt less than 20%, $V_D/V_T$ less than 0.6, inspiratory force more than $-20$ cm $H_2O$, vital capacity more than 10 ml/kg body weight, and respiratory rate less than 30.
3. Appropriate acid-base balance: Is base excess (BE) within $-5$ to $+5$ mEq/L. Large base deficit, i.e., pH less than 7.32, may produce too strong a respiratory drive, and weaning may fail. Large BE leads to carbon dioxide retention (physiologic compensation) with production of a small $V_T$, leading to a weaning failure. *Arterial pH is a more reliable index for weaning than $PCO_2$*. In patients with chronic lung disease and chronic carbon dioxide retention, patients are prepared for weaning by setting $PaCO_2$ at the preoperative value.
4. Adequacy of oxygen delivery: Since $VO_2$ will increase as a result of the increased respiratory work, the status of cardiac output and blood hemoglobin will be very important determinants of the success of weaning.
5. Are significant electrolyte disturbances corrected? Alterations in potassium, calcium, and magnesium can cause muscle weakness.

**Weaning Techniques.** There are two standard techniques for gradual removal from ventilatory support: use of a T-piece and intermittent mandatory ventilation (IMV).

With the *use of the T-piece with complete ventilator disconnect,* the patient breathes spontaneously through the endotracheal tube and high-flow oxygen system for set periods of time, dictated by early evidence of fatigue. Continuous positive pressure of 5 to 10 cm $H_2O$ can be used with this technique if weaning will require several days or if FRC is sufficiently decreased and shunt increased with ventilator disconnect.

With *IMV,* the patient is more gradually removed from the ventilator, with a gradual decrease in the rate of mechanical ventilation, there being no sudden large changes.

Since the IMV weaning process is more gradual, weaning can be started earlier, i.e., before even a small period of total spontaneous ventilation is possible. Again, CPAP or PEEP can be used with this approach.

## Endotracheal Extubation

The patient's status must be such that *all* the P's will be corrected with return to spontaneous ventilation:

*Patency:* Is the edema or external compression sufficiently resolved? May require laryngoscopy to determine.

*Protection:* Is mental status and gag reflex adequate? Is vomiting likely?

*Pulmonary toilet:* Is mental status, adequacy of cough, cooperation adequate?

*Positive pressure* to the airway: See *criteria* for weaning from mechanical ventilation. If weaning is possible but one or more of the other P's are present, weaning should be undertaken and the patient left intubated.

# 20

# Hemodynamics and Perfusion

## HEMODYNAMIC MONITORING

The role of hemodynamic monitoring is to assess the adequacy of tissue perfusion. This is reflected in measurements of vascular pressures, blood flow, and adequacy of cardiac activity. The primary factor being assessed is the adequacy of tissue oxygenation.

### Pressure Measurements

Vascular pressures are used to reflect the status of blood volume. Remember: *Pressure equals flow times resistance.* A change in either parameter will alter the value.

*Arterial pressure* measurements obtained continuously by an indwelling catheter are frequently desirable. It must be remembered that arterial pressure is a poor reflection of blood volume and blood flow in view of the smooth muscle activity of the arterioles, which can increase systemic vascular resistance (SVR). The catheter should be removed if there is any evidence of impaired perfusion to the extremity distal to the catheter. Thrombotic complications increase markedly after 3 days of artery cannulation.

*Central venous pressure* (CVP) can be used indirectly to reflect blood volume if one recognizes its limitations. In the healthy heart, right ventricular filling pressure will correlate with left ventricular filling pressure, and therefore CVP will correspond to the adequacy of preload and cardiac output. With an impairment of the right heart function alone as, e.g., pulmonary hypertension, or tricuspid insufficiency, or with more severe left heart than right heart disease, the CVP will not correlate with left heart function. The most valuable information is the change in the CVP with a maneuver such as volume loading rather than the absolute value of CVP.

*Pulmonary artery pressure* (PAP) is monitored through a Swan-Ganz catheter. Acute increases in PAP reflect a number of disease processes. Thus, the *causes of pulmonary hypertension* are:

1. Increased left atrial pressure
2. Increased pulmonary vascular tone
3. Pulmonary vascular obstruction (emboli)
4. Hypoxia-induced vasoconstriction
5. Positive-pressure ventilation

Blood sampled from the pulmonary artery is true mixed venous blood and allows calculation of the arteriovenous oxygen content difference. This can then be used in the measurement of shunt ($Q_S/Q_T$). PAP monitoring is indicated when this information is necessary for adequate patient care decisions. Because the pulmonary circulation is a low-pressure system, the zero point is very important. Complications are similar to those for a CVP catheter. In addition pulmonary hemorrhage from vessel rupture with balloon inflation, as well as lung infarction from prolonged maintenance in the wedge position, has been well described. The balloon must not be left in the wedge position beyond the time necessary for obtaining the pressure measurements.

*The pulmonary artery end-diastolic pressure* (PADP) is a good reflection of left atrial pressure, provided that pulmonary arterial resistance is not greatly elevated. In the absence of increased PVR and abnormal left ventricular function, the PADP will closely approximate the pulmonary artery wedge pressure (PAWP), mean left atrial pressure, and left ventricular end-diastolic pressure (LVEDP).

*Pulmonary artery wedge pressure.* Because there are no valves between the left atrium and pulmonary arteries, the inflation of the balloon on the Swan-Ganz catheter occludes proximal flow, and the pressure obtained is a back pressure from the left atrium. The PAWP correlates well with mean left atrial pressure (LAP) and reflects *pulmonary capillary hydrostatic pressure*. In addition, in the absence of mitral valvular disease, PAWP will closely approximate LVEDP. Monitoring of *capillary hydrostatic pressure* is important, since a significant *increase* will lead to pulmonary congestion and possibly *edema*. At a PAWP above 25 mmHg, there is usually radiographic evidence of pulmonary congestion, hilar engorgement, etc. When PAWP exceeds 30 mmHg, pulmonary edema is often present.

Equating *wedge pressure* with *LAP* assumes an open circuit from the catheter tip to the left atrium. This is not the case if the cannulated vessel is not patent or if the catheter is located in lung zones, where alveolar pressure is greater than arterial pressure (zone I) or venous pressure (zones I and II). In this case PAWP is really reflecting airway pressure. In zone III, (dependent portion of the lung) where both arterial and venous pressures exceed alveolar pressure, there is continuous flow, and PAWP correlates with LAP. Most of the lung enters zone III when the patient is supine, and most pulmonary-artery catheters will preferentially float into zone III. *It has been shown that if the tip of the catheter is at or below the left atrium, then the conditions in zone III exist even if positive end-expiratory pressure (PEEP) values are as high as 30 cm of water,* assuming no embolic obstruction. A cross-table lateral film will confirm the location of the catheter tip relative to the left atrium. If the tip is above the atrium, the catheter should be repositioned. A damped tracing, balloon overinflation, and wide pressure changes with respiration can alter the reliability of the measurement.

The *complications of a pulmonary artery catheter* are:

1. Arrythmia during placement (both atrial and ventricular)
2. Bundle branch block (usually right and usually temporary)
3. Thrombosis of catheter resulting in emboli from tip and false readings
4. Pulmonary infarction usually caused by prolonged catheter wedge
5. Pulmonary artery rupture (balloon overinflation, distal catheter migration)
6. Catheter knotting

7. Infectious complications
8. Complications during placement, e.g., bleeding, pneumothorax

## Flow Measurements

### Cardiac Output

Thermodilution is an application of the indicator-dilution principle and its application in the pulmonary artery flow-directed Swan-Ganz catheter avoids the necessity for separate catheters for injection and sampling. The solution may be iced or at room temperature, with the key value being a reliable injectate temperature. Although the technique is relatively simple and allows simple calculation of cardiac output if a computer is used, there are some possible sources of error, e.g., the injectate may be allowed to rewarm above the temperature recorded by the machine thermometer before injection, or errors are induced if the catheter is against the arterial wall in a wedged position or if the solution is injected too slowly. Normalizing cardiac output to body surface area termed "cardiac index" is the optimal way of expressing this term.

### Preload

Preload is the volume in the ventricle just before systole, i.e., the end-diastolic volume (EDV) distending the ventricular muscle fibers. The increase in fiber length increases the power of contraction. The EDV is a function of ventricular compliance and transmural ventricular filling pressure. Preload is very difficult to measure directly and is usually inferred by the measure of CVP and PAWP.

### Afterload

This term defines the resistance against which each ventricle contracts or the tension that the ventricular muscle must generate to reject the stroke volume. Afterload is a function of EDV and transmural ejection pressure. It closely corresponds to the degree of vascular resistance. As afterload increases, the work of ventricle ejection increases. If afterload decreases, the ventricle can empty more effectively and increase blood flow.

### Systemic Vascular Resistance

This parameter is largely responsible for the left ventricle afterload. An inappropriate increase in SVR can depress cardiac output by requiring increased heart work and myocardial oxygen consumption, whereas a decrease in SVR by vasodilation will decrease work and increase cardiac output.

### Pulmonary Vascular Resistance

This parameter cannot only greater affect right ventricular function but the left ventricle as well due to the increased distensibility of the right heart. A shift of the ventricular septum from right to left can result from increased afterload-induced right ventricular distention.

## Contractility

This parameter reflects the capacity of the myocardium to function as a pump and is described in terms of heart work per stroke. Depressed contractility defines a state of reduced heart work at a constant preload.

## Monitoring Perfusion and Tissue Oxygenation

The endpoint in determining the adequacy of cardiovascular function is maintenance of sufficient oxygen in the cell. *Oxygen delivery (transport)* is the major function of the circulation.

### Oxygen Demand

This is the amount of oxygen necessary to satisfy the metabolic requirements of the cell and is the sum of the oxygen required by all tissues in the body. It is determined by the metabolic rate and is modified by factors such as temperature, metabolic activity, and activity level or work.

### Oxygen Content

This term refers to the amount of oxygen present in blood, usually measured as milliliters of oxygen per 100 ml:

$CaO_2$ = (Hgb [g/dl] × $SaO_2$ × 1.34) + [0.003 × $PaO_2$ (mmHg)].

where $CaO_2$ = arterial oxygen content, Hgb = hemoglobin, $SaO_2$ = arterial oxygen saturation, $PaO_2$ = arterial oxygen tension. Almost all the oxygen delivered to tissues is carried as oxyhemoglobin. Each gram of hemoglobin carries about 1.34 ml oxygen per 100 ml, whereas serum carries only 0.003 ml oxygen per 100 ml/mmHg $PaO_2$ as dissolved oxygen. With a normal hemoglobin level of 15 g/dl, each 100 ml of blood carries about 20.1 ml oxygen as oxyhemoglobin and 0.3 ml dissolved, for a total of 20.4 ml/100 ml.

### Oxygen Delivery (Transport)

The amount of oxygen delivered to the tissues is determined by cardiac output, hemoglobin concentration, and arterial hemoglobin $SaO_2$. In the presence of an impairment in adequate oxygen transport, one should keep the hemoglobin level at or above 10 g/dl. Once the lung provides an adequate $PO_2$ to saturate an adequate amount of hemoglobin, then oxygen delivery is dependent on an adequate cardiac output:

Oxygen delivery = $CaO_2$ × cardiac output (L/min) × 10 = ml $O_2$/100 ml

Cardiac output can triple in the normal host to meet increased oxygen demands.

### Oxygen Extraction

This term defines the difference between the *oxygen content* in ml/100 ml (volume %) of blood $CaO_2$ and mixed venous ($CvO_2$) blood. Under normal conditions with normal hemoglobin, cardiac output and oxygen saturation, 4 to 5.5 vol% of oxygen are extracted from arterial blood (hemoglobin 14 and $SaO_2$ 97%), mixed venous hemoglobin saturation ($SvO_2$) being about 75% and $PvO_2$ about 40 mmHg. With increased oxygen demands, increased oxygen extraction from blood can occur. It is believed that the critical range, below which some tissue hypoxia occurs, is a $PvO_2$ of 25–30 mmHg or an $SvO_2$ of 40 to 55%. Beyond this point, the heart has no reserve for further oxygen extraction and will rely on increased blood flow for the needed oxygen. If systemic blood flow is shunted from less critical organs, such as the gut, these tissues will become hypoxemic even though the central blood $PvO_2$, measuring the sum total of all the tissue oxygen extraction, is normal. An increasing lactic acidosis may then be evident.

## Percent Oxygen Saturation of Hemoglobin

The percent of oxygen saturation of hemoglobin in arterial and venous blood is a major factor in the oxygen delivery, oxygen extraction, and tissue oxygen utilization. A value of $SaO_2$ by itself does not reflect the adequacy of blood oxygen content if, e.g., anemia is present. In general, at the normal $PaO_2$ of 90 to 100 mmHg (at sea level, breathing room air) the $SaO_2$ is approximately 97%. As long as the $PaO_2$ is kept above 60 mmHg, the $SaO_2$ will be at least 90%. Increasing the $PaO_2$ above 100 mmHg will have little effect on the $SaO_2$ because the oxygen saturation cannot exceed 100%. On the venous end of the curve, when the value of $PvO_2$ is around 40 mmHg, the situation is quite different. In this range of $Pvo_2$, a small change in $PO_2$ has a significant effect on the venous saturation ($SvO_2$). A decrease of $PvO_2$ from 40 to 35 mmHg will cause the $SvO_2$ to decrease from 75 to 65%. The $P_{50}$ is the oxygen tension at which 50% of the hemoglobin is saturated with oxygen. At a pH of 7.4 and temperature = 37°C, the $P_{50}$ is 26 ± 2 mmHg.

## Oxygen Consumption

This parameter is a measure of the amount of oxygen utilized by the body:

$VO_2$ = cardiac output ($CaO_2 - C_VO_2$)

where $VO_2$ = rate of oxygen consumption, $C_VO_2$ = mixed venous oxygen content. The normal range is 120 to 160 ml/min/m². When insufficient oxygen is available, aerobic metabolism is diminished and instead of pyruvate entering the Krebs cycle, pyruvate is converted to lactate, i.e., lactic acid. Normal arterial *lactate* is less than 2 mM/L. The magnitude of lactic acidosis usually corresponds to the severity of the perfusion deficit (see "Acid-Base Balance"). Inadequate $VO_2$ can result from a decrease in cardiac output, anemia, or hypovolemia or a maldistribution of blood flow, as in sepsis. In a burn-injured or postshock man, $VO_2$ increases from 50 to 100% above normal because injured tissue not only requires more oxygen for repair but stimulates the development of a hypermetabolic state:

$\overset{\circ}{V}O_2$ Increased: Hypermetabolism, temperature, trauma, sepsis anxiety, stress, increased work

$\overset{\circ}{V}O_2$ decreased: Hypothermia, anesthesia, shock sedation, inactivity

## Arterial Lactate Concentration

The measurement of arterial lactate concentration is a very useful monitor of the magnitude of perfusion failure. Lactic acidosis is due to both increased lactate production

**Table 20-1** Hemodynamic Monitoring

| Parameters | Acronym | Formula | Normal Values |
|---|---|---|---|
| **Pressure** | | | |
| Mean arterial pressure | MAP | Direct measurement | 80–100 mmHg |
| Central venous pressure | CVP | Direct measurement | 1–10 cm $H_2O$ |
| Mean pulmonary artery pressure | MPAP | Direct measurement | 11–15 mmHg |
| Pulmonary artery wedge pressure | PAWP | Direct measurement | 8–12 mmHg |
| **Flow-related** | | | |
| Cardiac index | CI | Direct measurement | 2.8–3.6 l/min/$m^2$ |
| Stroke index | SI | CI/HR* | 30–50 ml/min/$m^2$ |
| Mean transit time | MTT | Direct measurement | 12–18 s |
| Left ventricular stroke work | LVSW | SI $\times$ (MAP-PAWP) $\times$ 0.014 | 44–68 g·M/$m^2$ |
| Right ventricular stroke work | RVSW | SI $\times$ (MAP-CVP) $\times$ 0.014 | 7–12 g·M/$m^2$ |
| **Resistance** | | | |
| Systemic vascular resistance | SVR | $\dfrac{80(\text{MAP-CVP})}{\text{CI}}$ | 1700–2600 $\dfrac{\text{dyne·sec}}{cm^5 \cdot m^2}$ |
| Pulmonary vascular resistance | PVR | $\dfrac{80(\text{MPAP-PAWP})}{\text{CI}}$ | 150–300 $\dfrac{\text{dyne.sec}}{cm^5 \cdot m^2}$ |
| **Tissue oxygenation** | | | |
| Arterial oxygen content | $CaO_2$ | Hgb* $\times$ $SaO_2$ $\times$ 1.34 + (0.003 $\times$ $PaO_2$) | 19–20 ml/100 ml |
| Mixed venous oxygen content | $C_vO_2$ | Hgb $\times$ $S_vO_2$ $\times$ 1.34 + (0.003 $\times$ $PaO_2$) | 14–15 ml/100 ml |
| Arteriovenous oxygen content difference | C(a-v)$O_2$ | $CaO_2 - C_vO_2$ | 4–5.5 ml/100 ml |
| Oxygen delivery | $O_2$ deliv | $CaO_2 \times$ CI $\times$ 10 | 520–720 ml/min/$m^2$ |
| Oxygen consumption | $VO_2$ | C(a-v)$O_2 \times$ CI $\times$ 10 | 120–160 ml/min/$m^2$ |
| % oxygen extraction | $O_2$ ext | $\dfrac{(CaO_2 - C_vO_2)}{CaO_2}$ | 22–30% |
| Arterial pH | pH | Direct measurement | 7.36–7.44 |
| Carbon dioxide production | $VCO_2$ | Direct measurement | 100–140 ml/min/$m^2$ |

*Hgb: hemoglobin; HR: heart rate.

Table 20-2  Adrenergic Receptors

| Receptor | Location and Stimulation | Physiologic Response |
|---|---|---|
| Alpha$_1$ | Receptor on the effector cell<br>Stimulation: vasoconstriction, intestinal relaxation, pupil dilatation | Increase in vascular resistance<br>Increasing pressure and afterload |
| Beta$_1$ | Receptor predominately in myocardium<br>Stimulation: increase in rate and contractility | Increased cardiac output<br>Increased heart oxygen consumption |
| Beta$_2$ | Receptor in respiratory and vascular smooth muscle<br>Stimulation: broncho- and vasodilation | Decreases airway and vascular resistance |
| Dopaminergic | Receptor in central and peripheral nervous system<br>Stimulation: renal and mesenteric vasodilation, suppression of aldosterone secretion with increase in renal sodium excretion | Increase in renal and mesenteric blood flow |

and impaired clearance by the hypoperfused liver. *Normal lactate* equals 0.5 to 1.9 mM/L.

## PHARMACOLOGIC SUPPORT

### Adrenergic Receptors

The sympathetic nervous system and its mediators, the catecholamines, modulate tissue perfusion and oxygen delivery by their effects on myocardial *inotropic* and *chronotropic* activity and on vasomotor tone. There are two major categories of response to catecholamines, indicating two major receptor populations known as alpha and beta. A third receptor, less well-distributed, is known as the dopaminergic receptor. Compounds that initiate the receptor response are known as agonists, and blockers are called antagonists. The specific physiologic effects of the various receptors are listed in Table 20-2.

### Receptor Agonists

A number of pharmacologic agents to be described can be used to produce a specifically desired physiologic effect based on these agents' mode of activity on the various adrenergic receptors (Table 20-3). Other agents, in particular the vasodilators used for reduction of afterload, have a direct smooth muscle effect not related to the adrenergic receptors. The $\beta_1$ agonist in heart muscle and alpha agonist in vascular smooth muscle enhance calcium influx into the muscle cell via the calcium channels. The $\beta_2$ agonist vasodilation appears to be the result of stimulation of the $Na^+$, $K^+$-ATPase system, thereby decreasing the intracellular calcium.

## ACID-BASE BALANCE

### Defining an Acid-Base Disturbance

Normal arterial pH is between 7.37 and 7.43. If the pH is less than 7.37, the patient has an acidosis. If the pH is greater than 7.43, the patient has an alkalosis. The normal arterial

**Table 20-3** Effect of Pharmacologic Agents on Adrenergic Receptors

|  | Inotropic $\beta_1$ | Chronotropic $\beta_1$ | Vasoconstrictor $\alpha$ | Vasodilation $\beta_2$ |
|---|---|---|---|---|
| Isoproterenol | +++ | +++ | 0 | +++ |
| Dobutamine | +++ | 0-+ | 0-+ | +-++ |
| Dopamine | +++ | + | 0-+++ | +† |
| Epinephrine | +++ | +++ | +++ | ++ |
| Norepinephrine | ++ | ++ | +++ | 0 |

*Effects are dose dependent
†Dilates renal and splanchnic bed via dopaminergic effect at doses less than 5 µg/kg/min.

Table 20-4  Actions and Doses of Vasoactive Drugs (inotropic agents)

| Drug | Actions | Indications | Dose |
|---|---|---|---|
| Digoxin | Inhibits $Na^+$, $K^+$-ATPase, thereby allowing influx of intracellular calcium. Increases force and velocity of contraction. Decreases atrioventricular conduction. Toxicity will lead to heart block with ventricular arrythmias | To improve contractility when immediate inotropic support is not needed. To control ventricular rate with atrial tachyarrythmias | 0.125–0.25 mg daily maintenance. Rapid digitalization 0.5 mg initially and 0.25 mg every 2 hours (up to 2 mg) |
| Dopamine | An endogenous precursor of norepinephrine that has α and β and specific dopamine receptor effects. Less increase in myocardial oxygen consumption than isoproterenol or norepinephrine. *Low-dose effect* is a renal and mesenteric vasodilatation. *Moderate dose effect* mimics a β agonist without a peripheral vasoconstriction. *High-dose effect* is that of both an α and β agonist, which includes peripheral vasoconstriction. Tachyarrythmias can occur at this dose | *Low dose*: increase renal blood flow improving urine output<br>*Moderate dose*: improves cardiac output but avoids increasing afterload<br>*High dose*: maximize inotropic action | Low <5 µg/kg/min<br><br>Moderate 5–10 µg/kg/min<br><br>High >15 µg/kg/min. Tachyphylaxis develops |

| Drug | Description | Clinical Use | Dose |
|---|---|---|---|
| Dobutamine | A synthetic dopamine analogue acting directly on $\beta_1$ receptors, thereby maximizing inotropic action with less increase in heart rate. Has some $\beta_2$, with little $\alpha$ receptor activity. Arrhythmias are the main complication | May be preferred to dopamine when an inotropic action is desired with no $\alpha$ stimulation. Useful when filling pressures increased | 2–10 $\mu$g/kg/min. Tachyphylaxis develops |
| Epinephrine | In low doses, a $\beta$ effect is seen while an $\alpha$ adrenergic effect is noted with higher doses. Exhibits both inotropic and chronotropic effects | Low doses ($\beta_1$) to increase cardiac output and decrease SVR. Bronchodilation. High doses increase afterload and blood pressure by increasing SVR. | Begin 0.02 $\mu$g/kg/min Low-moderate, 1–15 $\mu$g/min High, >20 $\mu$g/min. Less tachyphylaxis |
| Nitroprusside | Vasodilator, primarily arteriolar. Some venodilation, increasing venous capacitance. Rapid onset of action. Can result in severe hypotension. Can result in cyanide toxicity if use is prolonged. Can impair hypoxic pulmonary vasoconstriction, increasing shunt fraction | Reduction of afterload to improve cardiac performance. Some preload reduction. A hypotensive agent to treat severe hypertension | 0.5–8 $\mu$g/kg/min intravenously. Protect infusion from light. Prepare new infusion every 4 hours |
| Nitroglycerin | Primarily a venodilator increasing venous capacitance. Less reduction in blood pressure. Also may dilate coronary arteries directly, improving myocardial blood flow. Can impair hypoxic pulmonary vasoconstriction, increasing pulmonary shunt | Reduction of preload and afterload. Treatment of angina | 10–400 $\mu$g/min intravenously 2% ointment 0.5–2 inches every 6 hours |

carbon dioxide tension ($PaCO_2$) is between 37 and 43 mmHg. If the $PaCO_2$ is greater than 37 mmHg, there is a respiratory acidosis. If the $PaCO_2$ is less than 37 mmHg, there is a respiratory alkalosis. The normal bicarbonate (measured as carbon dioxide content) is between 22 and 28 mEq/L. If the bicarbonate (carbon dioxide content) is less than 22 mEq/L, there is a metabolic acidosis. If the bicarbonate is greater than 28 mEq/L, there is a metabolic alkalosis.

## Primary Versus Secondary Disturbances

It is useful and necessary to distinguish between primary and secondary disturbances in acid-base balance. *A primary disturbance* is the cause of the shift of the pH away from normal. *A secondary disturbance* is initiated to move the pH toward normal and represents the attempt of the body to compensate for the primary disturbance. *A mixed acid-base disturbance* exists when there is more than one simultaneous primary acid-base disturbance. When two primary disturbances, i.e., respiratory and metabolic acidosis tend to move the pH in the same direction, it is usually not difficult to diagnose the presence of these disturbances. However, when the disturbances are such that they tend to move the pH in opposite directions, then it may be difficult to distinguish the lesser primary disturbance from normal compensatory mechanisms. Compensatory (secondary) disturbances do not return the pH to normal, so the value of the pH will determine what the primary disturbance is, i.e., an acidosis or alkalosis.

## Compensatory Mechanisms

There are two mechanisms of compensation: (1) An immediate compensation by the *lungs* as carbon dioxide ($CO_2$) is removed or retained, restoring the normal $HCO_3^-/H_2CO_3$ ratio; and (2) a slower compensation by the *kidneys* through retention of bicarbonate or increased secretion of acid salts.

Chemoreceptors in the brainstem respond to even the slightest changes in arterial $PaCO_2$, to alter the rate and depth of breathing. The $H^+$ concentration in cerebrospinal fluid is the regulator. Carbon dioxide, but not buffers, can cross the blood-brain barrier. With the low buffer content, $H^+$ content changes of cerebrospinal fluid are quite large with changes in carbon dioxide. The normal $HCO_3^-/H_2CO_3$ ratio is restored. Conversely, if $PaCO_2$ because of, for example, hyperventilation, $H^+$ content decreases and chemoreceptor activity decreases (Table 20-5).

The maximum excretion of acid by the kidney is $3 \times 10^{-5}$ mol/L or a pH of urine of 4 to 5. The primary pathway for $H^+$ excretion depends on the balance between filtration and absorption of $HCO_3^-$. The $HCO_3^-$ is primarily delivered to the renal tubule as the $Na^+$ salt. As the *$Na^+$ and $HCO_3^-$ are resorbed*, $H^+$ is excreted by the renal tubule on a one to one equivalent basis. Another mechanism is the release of ammonia ($NH_3$) by the tubules, which then combines with $H^+$ to result in *$NH_4^+$ production* and urinary removal. *Potassium* reabsorption occurs as an active process in the loop of Henle. Sodium reabsorption is exchanged for $H^+$ secretion in the distal tubule via aldosterone. A high plasma $K^+$ results in a decrease in $H^+$ secretion and *alkaline urine*. A low plasma $K^+$ results in $K^+$ resorption, $H^+$ secretion, and an *acid urine*, even in the presence of an alkalotic state.

Table 20-5  Results of Acid-Base Disturbances

| | Acute (Uncompensated) | | | Chronic (Partial Compensation) | | |
|---|---|---|---|---|---|---|
| | pH | $PaCO_2$ | $HCO_3^-$ | pH | $PaCO_2$ | $HCO_3^-$ |
| Respiratory acidosis | Decrease | Increase | Normal | Decrease | Increase | Increase |
| Respiratory alkalosis | Increase | Decrease | Normal | Increase | Decrease | Decrease |
| Metabolic acidosis | Decrease | Normal | Decrease | Decrease | Decrease | Decrease |
| Metabolic alkalosis | Increase | Normal | Increase | Increase | Increase | Increase |

## Base Excess (Deficit)

Base excess is a term devised for the clinical assessment and treatment of acid-base disorders and refers to the milliequivalence of acid or base needed to titrate 1 L of blood to a pH of 7.4 at 37°C with a $PCO_2$ of 40 mmHg. A normal value would be zero ($0 \pm 2$ mEq/L). A positive number indicates an alkalotic state and a negative number, an acidotic state. Base excess is only changed by *nonvolatile acids* and therefore is a measure of the *nonrespiratory (metabolic)* acid-base disorders.

## Anion Gap

Changes in the content of strong cations and anions, e.g., from electrolyte disorders, can result in alterations in acid-base balance reflected in changes in base excess. Also, the addition of other nonvolatile acids, e.g., lactate, ketoacids, or sulfate and phosphate from decreased renal clearance, will also cause a base deficit. Determination of the anion gap helps distinguish these two processes:

Anion gap = $Na^+ - (Cl^- + HCO_3^-)$     Normal = $12 \pm 2$ mEq/L

or

$Na^+ + K^+ - (Cl^- + HCO_3^-)$     Normal = $16 \pm 2$ mEq/L

This concept is basically the same as measuring the strong electrolyte difference with the addition of $HCO_3^-$ as an anion.

A normal or low *anion gap* with a metabolic acid-base disorder indicates an electrolyte abnormality.

An increased *anion gap* with metabolic acidosis indicates the presence of another source of acids, e.g., lactic acidosis, ketoacidosis, uremia, and salicylate poisoning.

Plasma proteins, in particular albumin, are circulating buffers making up part of the normal anion gap. A decrease in proteins decreases the anion gap by *3 for each 1 g/dl* decrease in albumin. This change must be considered when assessing the presence of additional nonvolatile acids because an increase in acids could be masked by a decrease in proteins.

## Primary Respiratory Acidosis

An increased $PCO_2$ would tend to elevate the $H^+$, resulting in the condition of *respiratory acidosis*. The normal arterial $PCO_2$ ranges from 35 to 45 mmHg. A respiratory acidosis is present if $PCO_2$ is greater than 45 mmHg and pH is decreased. The pH decreases by 0.3 for an acute doubling of $PCO_2$ before any renal compensation. Plasma $HCO^-_3$ will increase 1 mEq for every 10 mmHg increase in $PaCO_2$.

The most common causes of hypoventilation in the surgical patient are drug related, i.e., either central nervous system depression from narcotics, sedations, anesthesia, or impaired respiratory muscle function from paralytic agents not completely reversed or potentiated by other agents (lidocaine, aminoglycosides, etc.). A decreased sensitivity of the central nervous system chemoreceptors can also be seen in the semistarvation state and in endocrine abnormalities, such as hypothyroidism.

Causes of mechanical impairment to ventilation include airway obstruction, impaired chest wall stability (fractures), pain-induced chest wall splinting, pneumothorax, and any impairment in neuromuscular function.

Processes that increase dead space ventilation will also lead to increased carbon dioxide. Acute increases in dead space will significantly increase total ventilatory requirements and can lead to severe hypoventilation. Work of breathing will be substantially increased. The most common causes of increased dead space are: (1) pulmonary embolus; (2) decreased cardiac output; and (3) adult respiratory distress syndrome, (ARDS), especially with positive-pressure ventilation where nondependent lung is preferably ventilated while perfusion is increased in dependent lung. Increased carbon dioxide production can rapidly lead to respiratory acidosis, especially in the patient with marginal respiratory reserves who cannot generate a compensatory increase in alveolar ventilation ($\mathring{V}_A$). A process that increases metabolic rate will increase carbon dioxide production, e.g., increased temperature, increased muscle activity, especially uncontrolled activity (shivering, seizures). Excess carbohydrate calories will increase the respiratory quotient, exceeding 1, thereby leading to a marked inappropriate increase in production. Treatment is increasing alveolar minute ventilation.

## Primary Respiratory Alkalosis

This process, caused by excess lung removal of carbon dioxide, is diagnosed when the arterial $PCO_2$ is less than 37 mmHg and the pH is greater than 7.43. Since $PaCO_2$ and $HCO^-_3$ are in equilibrium, a decrease in $HCO^-_3$ of 2 to 3 mEq/L is expected for every 10 mmHg decrease in $PaCO_2$. An acute decrease in $PCO_2$ of 10 mmHg from normal will cause pH to increase by 0.1 U. There are three primary physiologic causes for an increase in alveolar ventilation. The most common cause in the setting of the intensive care unit is in response to arterial hypoxemia. Central nervous system dysfunction is also a common cause. Processes such as anxiety and pain will increase respiratory rate, as will direct central nervous system process, such as trauma or infection. Endotoxin and other products released in sepsis can lead to hyperventilation. Metabolic acidosis will result in direct stimulation of hypothalamic receptors to increase $\mathring{V}_A$. A common iatrogenic cause is increased carbon dioxide removal with mechanical ventilation. High tidal volume and PEEP necessary to decrease shunt can cause a respiratory alkalosis. Thus, the *causes of hyperventilation* are:

    Hypoxia-induced increased minute ventilation

    Excessive mechanical ventilation

    Increased respiratory drive: due to pain, sepsis endotoxin, liver failure, etc.

The treatment is decreasing alveolar ventilation either by decreasing respiratory drive and by decreasing tidal volume or rate of mechanical ventilation, or both.

## Primary Metabolic Acidosis

A primary metabolic acidosis is the result of an excess of nonvolatile acids relative to buffer. This process is diagnosed when the pH is less than 7.37 and the bicarbonate (carbon dioxide content) is less than 22 mEq/L. The $PaCO_2$ should decrease by 1 to 1.5

times the decrease in plasma $HCO^-_3$ concentration. Metabolic acidosis is the result of one of two abnormalities or a combination of both.

## Increased Anion Gap

An increase in $H^+$ production due to an increase in *nonvolatile* acid production will lead to an increase in the number of anions relative to cations and will result in an acid excess or *base deficit*. The primary problem, in this form of acidosis, is the underlying disease process producing the increased acid. Increased lactic acid production as a result of anaerobic glycolysis will produce an increased anion gap acidosis. Measurement of serum lactate will help differentiate this process from other causes. Normal lactate is less than 2 mMol/L. Increased ketoacids (ketones) due to uncontrolled diabetes, malnutrition, or toxins will result in a base deficit and an acidosis. Renal dysfunction leading to increased plasma anions of sulfate and phosphate is the third major cause.

Anion gap = $Na^+ - (CL^- + HCO^-_3)$ normal = $12 \pm 2$ mEq/L

In summary, an *increased anion gap* results from:

1. Lactic acidosis
2. Ketoacidosis
   Diabetes
   Starvation
   Toxins
3. Renal Dysfunction

**Normal Anion Gap.** An imbalance of electrolytes will result in an excess of $H^+$ relative to available base. An increase in $Cl^-$ anion due to excess $Cl^-$ intake (e.g., saline loading) or a decrease in $HCO^-_3$ (gastrointestinal, renal losses) will produce a metabolic acidosis without the addition of nonelectrolyte anions; i.e., normal gap. Gastrointestinal losses from diarrhea and fistulas are the most common form of $HCO^-_3$ loss. Inability of the kidney to conserve $HCO^-_3$ is seen with hereditary or acquired renal tubular acidosis. The acquired form is due to, e.g., amphotericin. An alkaline urine in the presence of a metabolic acidosis is characteristically seen. A low $Na^+$ content in the distal tubule impairs the potential for $H^+$ exchange and renal compensation.

In summary, a *normal anion gap* results from

1. Administration of excess $Cl^-$ relative to $Na^+$ and $HCO^-_3$, e.g., saline loading
2. Loss of excess $HCO^-_3$ relative to $Cl^-$, diarrhea, bowel fistula
3. Renal wasting of $HCO^-_3$, renal tubular acidosis, carbonic anhydrase inhibition
4. Dilutional acidosis from extracellular space expansion
5. Sodium depletion leading to impaired renal $H^+$ excretion

The treatment of metabolic acidosis should be aimed at correcting the underlying disorder. This correction is particularly important in an increased anion gap acidosis. Administration of $HCO^-_3$ will temporarily eliminate the acidemia but will have no effect on and actually disguise the severity of the causative disorder. Lactic acidosis must be corrected by restoration of perfusion. Ketosis, depending on the cause, is corrected with insulin for diabetes or nutrition for starvation. Remember that β-hydroxybutyrate, the reduced form and often predominant ketone, is not measured with standard ketone analysis. Often a $K^+$ deficiency is also present. Diagnosis of a large $K^+$ deficit is evident from a normal serum $K^+$ in an acidemic state. $K^+$ replacement will be an important component of therapy and must be considered severe life-threatening hypokalemia. $HCO^-_3$ is given if pH is less than 7.2 or severe acidemia symptoms are present. Since the $HCO^-_3$ distribution space is the extracellular fluid, calculation of base requirements is based on 25% of ideal body weight. Renal dysfunction must be improved or controlled in cases of renal-induced metabolic acidosis.

Normal anion gap metabolic acidosis is treated by correcting or at least replacing the increased $HCO^-_3$ losses, usually gastrointestinal or renal in origin. Iatrogenic hyperchloremia induced by excessive saline administration must also be controlled. Adequate total body $Na^+$ must be present to avoid hypovolemia. In cases of severe hyperchloremia, $Cl^-$ wasting in the kidney can be accomplished using a loop diuretic.

## Primary Metabolic Alkalosis

Primary metabolic alkalosis is diagnosed when the pH is greater than 7.43 and the serum bicarbonate is greater than 28 mEq/L. The $PaCO_2$ will also increase with the increase in $HCO^-_3$.

The cause of the alkalemia is due to a decrease in plasma $Cl^-$ relative to $Na^+$ and $HCO^-_3$ or other base. The result is a *base excess*. There are two general forms of hypochloremic alkalosis. The first category is *chloride-responsive alkalosis*, where replacement of $Cl^-$ losses correct the problem. Losses of $Cl^-$ are due usually to upper gastrointestinal losses, e.g., nasogastric suction or renal losses, usually as a result of use of loop diuretics. Volume contraction will result in an extracellular fluid concentration of body buffer of which $HCO^-_3$ is the most prominent. Urinary chloride is usually less than 10 mEq/L because $Cl^-$ resorption (in loop of Henle) is maximal. Excess base administration also fits in this category. Massive resuscitation with Ringer's lactate solution can commonly result in an alkalotic state. The second category is *chloride-resistant alkalosis*. These disease states are characterized by a urine chloride greater than 20 mEq/L. Severe $K^+$ depletion is the most common form. $Cl^-$ resorption is impaired in the ascending loop and $H^+$ excretion is increased in the distal tubule as inadequate $K^+$ is available for $Na^+$ exchange.

Treatment is based on correcting the underlying disorder producing the alkalotic state. Restoration of extracellular fluid volume using solutions containing sodium chloride is the primary treatment. Isotonic saline extracellular fluid expansion increases the distribution space for $HCO^-_3$ and decreases aldosterone release, thereby decreasing $H^+$ losses in the kidney. Potassium replacement is crucial, since $Cl^-$ losses in the kidney will persist until adequate $K^+$ is available for $Cl^-$ reabsorption. In addition, less $H^+$ will be excreted in the distal tubule. Spironolactone can be added to the volume regimen if increased aldosterone levels are to persist. Excessive base infusion, usually in the form of sodium lactate or acetate should be controlled. Continued use of $HCO^-_3$ to correct increased anion gap acidotic states should also be controlled to minimize the inevitable base excess that will result.

Table 20-6  Acid-Base Disorder

| Primary Disorder | Defect | Common Causes | Compensation | Treatment |
|---|---|---|---|---|
| Respiratory acidosis | Carbon dioxide retention (hypoventilation) | Central nervous system depression Airway, lung Impairment | Renal excretion of acid salts $HCO_3^-$ retention $Cl^-$ shift into red blood cells | Restoration of adequate ventilation Control excess carbon dioxide production |
| Respiratory alkalosis | Hyperventilation | Central nervous system excitation. Excess ventilator support | Renal excretion of $Na^+$, $K^+$, $HCO_3^-$. Absorption of $H^+$, $Cl^-$ Lactate release from red blood cells | Correction of hyperventilation |
| Metabolic acidosis | Excess loss of base Increased nonvolatile acids | Excess $Cl^-$ to $Na^+$ Increase $HCO_3^-$ loss lactic, ketoacidosis Uremia Dilutional acidosis | Respiratory alkalosis Renal excretion $H^+$, $Cl^-$ Resorption $K^+$, $HCO_3^-$ | Increase $Na^+$ load Correct underlying process waste $Cl^-$ Give $HCO_3^-$ for pH < 7.2 Restore buffers, Proteins, hemoglobin |
| Metabolic alkalosis | Excess loss of $Cl^-$, $K^+$ Increase $HCO_3^-$ | Gastrointestinal losses of $Cl^-$ Excess intake $HCO_3^-$ Diuretics Hypokalemia Extracellular fluid volume contraction | Respiratory acidosis may be hypoxia Renal excretion, $HCO_3^-$, $K^+$ Absorption, $H^+$, $Cl^-$ | Increase $Cl^-$ content $K^+$ replacement Acetazolamide to waste $HCO_3^-$ Vigorous volume replacement Occasional 0.1 N hydrochloric acid needed |

If more rapid correction of the alkalotic state is required, a carbonic anhydrase inhibitor such as acetazolamide can be used to increase urine $HCO_3^-$ losses. Rarely, i.e., in extreme cases, is hydrochloric acid infusion required. Indications are usually a pH more than 7.6 and $HCO_3^-$ more than 40 mEq/L. Dosage, as with $HCO_3^-$, is based on an extracellular fluid distribution space, i.e., 25% of total body weight. Half of the calculated acid deficit (base excess) is given as 0.1 N hydrochloric acid in 2 to 4 hours, with remaining over the next 24 hours.

# 21
# Nutritional Support

## PARENTERAL NUTRITIONAL SUPPORT

### Central Vein Hyperalimentation

### Central Parenteral Nutrition

*Indications*

1. Nonfunctioning gastrointestinal tract.
2. Hypermetabolic state.
3. Provide adequate calories, protein.
4. Fluid restriction.
5. Renal or hepatic dysfunction.

*Nutritional Composition*

The nutritional composition can be adjusted to needs. A standard central vein solution is recommended. Table 21-1 lists the contents of each standard liter bag.

*Major Considerations*

1. Sufficient nonprotein calories need to be provided to spare protein from being used as calories.
2. Fat emulsions can be given to increase the total caloric intake.
3. Lack of gastrointestinal feeding results in gastrointestinal tract mucosal atrophy and altered permeability.
4. Central venous lines risk infection and must be managed with strict aseptic technique.

### Peripheral Parenteral Nutrition

*Indications*

1. No safe central line access.
2. Nonfunctioning gastrointestinal tract.
3. Supplementation of gastrointestinal feedings.

## Table 21-1  Sample Contents of Liter of Central Vein Solution*

| | | | | | |
|---|---|---|---|---|---|
| Crystalline amino acids | | (5%) | Protein | = | 50 g |
| Dextrose | | (25%) | Dextrose | = | 250 g |
| Sodium | 30 | mEq | Nitrogen | = | 8.4 g |
| Potassium | 30 | mEq | Calories/N | = | 126 |
| Magnesium | 5 | mEq | Total calories | = | 1060 |
| Calcium | 4.7 | mEq | mOsm | = | 1970 |
| Phosphate | 15 | mM | | | |
| Acetate | 73 | mEq | | | |
| Chloride | 28 | mEq | | | |

*All components can be varied.

    4. Calories to minimize or prevent weight loss.
    5. For the patient who can tolerate a large fluid volume (at least 2500 ml/day).

## *Nutritional Composition*

The contents of a liter bag of a standard peripheral vein solution are listed in Table 21-2.

## *Major Considerations*

1. Sufficient nonprotein calories need to be provided to spare protein from being used for calories.
2. Fat emulsion can be given mixed with peripheral parenteral nutrition to increase the total calories and also to decrease osmolarity.
3. An osmolarity value over 650 results in an increased risk of phlebitis in peripheral veins.
4. Lack of gastrointestinal feeding can substantially alter the gastrointestinal tract mucosa, leading to a decrease in absorptive surface and increased permeability.

Suggested additives for parenteral solutions are given in Table 21-3.
The weekly intake of vitamin K should be 10 mg (contraindicated in patients receiving warfarin). Insulin should be added to the nutritional solution for the treatment of

## Table 21-2  Sample Contents of Liter of Peripheral Vein Solution*

| | | | | | |
|---|---|---|---|---|---|
| Crystalline amino acids | | (2.5%) | Protein | = | 25 g |
| Dextrose | | (5%) | Dextrose | = | 50 g |
| Sodium | 30 | mEq | Nitrogen | = | 4.2 g |
| Potassium | 30 | mEq | Calories/N | = | 65 |
| Magnesium | 5 | mEq | Total calories | = | 275 |
| Calcium | 4.7 | mEq | mOsm | = | 655 |
| Phosphate | 5 | mM | | | |
| Acetate | 52 | mEq | | | |
| Chloride | 18 | mEq | | | |

*All components can be varied.

**Table 21-3** Additives to Parenteral Solutions

| Vitamins (Given Daily) | | Trace Elements | |
|---|---|---|---|
| Thiamine | 3 mg | Zinc | 5.0 mg |
| Riboflavin | 3.6 mg | Copper | 1.0 mg |
| Vitamin $B_6$ | 4 mg | Manganese | 0.5 mg |
| Niacin | 40 mg | Chromium | 10 mg |
| Dexpanthenol | 15 mg | | |
| Biotin | 60 µg | | |
| Ascorbic acid | 500 mg | | |
| Folate | 400 µg* | | |
| Vitamin $B_{12}$ | 5 µg | | |
| Vitamin A | 3300 IU | | |
| Vitamin D | 200 IU | | |
| Vitamin E | 10 IU | | |

*Contraindicated in patients receiving methotrexate.

sustained hyperglycemia (more than 200 mg/dl). Less than 10 U of insulin per liter is not effective.

## Fat Emulsions

Intralipid is a sterile fat emulsion containing soybean oil, egg yolk, phospholipids, glycerin, and water. It provides a source of calories and essential fatty acids. A 20% intralipid solution provides 1000 kcal/500 ml.

### Major Considerations

1. The fat must be sufficiently cleared from the plasma to justify continuing administration. A plasma triglyceride level exceeding 250 mg/dl indicates inadequate clearance and the rate of fat emulsion should be decreased.
2. Patients receiving peripheral parenteral nutrition should receive fat emulsion daily to provide adequate nonprotein calories.
3. Fat emulsion should not provide more than 50% of the total calories. The amount given should not exceed 2.5 g/kg body weight per day.
4. Fat emulsion is contraindicated in patients with egg allergies.

Table 21-4 lists the disease states in which fat intolerance may be a problem.

### Administration

1. Fat may be administered through peripheral or central access catheters.
2. Fat may be administered via a triple mix solution (that is, dextrose, amino acids, and fat) in one bag as long as glass bottles are not used.

Table 21-4  Disease States Related to Fat Intolerance*

| | |
|---|---|
| Liver disease | Lipid metabolism abnormalities |
| Pancreatitis | Coagulopathies |
| Pulmonary disease | Pregnancy |

*If the triglyceride levels are normal before administration and not excessively elevated with infusion, fat emulsions can be used.

## Branched Chain Amino Acid Rich Solutions

Branched chain amino acids (valine, leucine, isoleucine) are the only amino acids that do not need to be metabolized by the liver as a source of energy via gluconeogenesis. Branched chain amino acids can be used directly by tissues for protein synthesis and energy production. Their oxidation yields energy without the conversion to glucose. Normally only about 6% of the total energy comes from branched chain amino acids. This percentage increases markedly (up to 30%) in patients with sepsis or liver failure due to decreased glucose utilization.

### Potential Benefits of Branched Chain Amino Acid Solutions

1. As an energy source if carbohydrate or fat calories are not adequate.
2. To help increase the impaired hepatic protein synthesis seen with liver dysfunction.
3. To help decrease muscle breakdown and the resulting increase in potentially toxic aromatic amino acids, which cannot be cleared by the injured liver.
4. As an energy source in multiorgan system failure when carbohydrate utilization is impaired.

Table 21-5 provides a summary of complications and their management in patients receiving parenteral nutrition.

## ENTERAL NUTRITIONAL SUPPORT

Since enteral feeding promotes more efficient utilization of nutrients and better preservation of intestinal integrity than does parenteral feeding, the gut is the preferred route for nutritional support. In addition, enteral feeding is safer and more economical. Adequate intestinal function must be present. However, sufficient gastrointestinal function is frequently available in the critically ill patient to at least allow some enteral feeding, which will help minimize gut mucosal atrophy and may provide sufficient calories so that peripheral rather than central vein alimentation is sufficient for the remainder of the calories.

If impaired gastrointestinal function is present, correctable causes should be sought and eliminated. If only a gastric atony is present, a tube can be placed through the pylorus endoscopically or by other maneuvers or a feeding jejunostomy placed, preferably at the

Table 21-5  Complications of Parenteral Nutritional Support

| Problem | Possible Concerns | Solution |
|---|---|---|
| **Glucose** | | |
| Hyperglycemia, glycosuria, osmotic diuresis, hyperosmolar nonketonic dehydration, coma | Excessive total dose or rate of infusion of glucose; inadequate endogenous insulin; increased glucocorticoids; sepsis | Reduce amount of glucose infused; increase insulin; administer a portion of calories as fat emulsion |
| Ketoacidosis in diabetes mellitus | Inadequate endogenous insulin response; inadequate exogenous insulin therapy | Give insulin; reduce glucose input |
| Postinfusion (rebound) hypoglycemia | Persistence of endogenous insulin production secondary to prolonged stimulation of islet cells by high carbohydrate infusion | Administer 5 to 10% glucose |
| **Fat** | | |
| Pyrogenic reaction | Fat emulsion, other solutions | Exclude other causes of fever |
| Altered coagulation | Hyperlipidemia | Restudy after fat has cleared from blood |
| Hypertriglyceridemia | Rapid infusion, decreased clearance | Decrease rate of infusion; allow clearance before blood tests |
| Impaired liver function | May be due to fat emulsion or to an underlying disease process | Exclude other causes of hepatic dysfunction |
| Cyanosis | Altered pulmonary diffusion capacity | Discontinue fat infusion |
| Essential fatty acid deficiency | Inadequate essential fatty acid administration | Administer essential fatty acids in the form of one 500 ml bottle of 20% fat emulsion every week |

| | | |
|---|---|---|
| Amino acids | | |
| Hyperchloremic metabolic acidosis | Excessive chloride and monohydrochloride content of crystalline amino acid solutions | Administer sodium and potassium as acetate salts |
| Prerenal azotemia | Excessive amino acid infusion with inadequate calorie administration | Reduce amino acid intake; increase glucose calories |
| Miscellaneous | | |
| Hypokalemia | Potassium intake inadequate relative to increased requirements for protein anabolism; diuresis | Increase $K^+$ administration |
| Hyperkalemia | Excessive potassium administration, especially in metabolic acidosis; renal failure | Decrease $K^+$ administration |
| Hypomagnesemia | Inadequate magnesium administration, relative to increased requirements for protein anabolism and glucose metabolism | Increase $Mg^+$ administration |
| Hypophosphatemia | Inadequate phosphorus administration; redistribution of serum phosphorus into cells, bone, or both | Administer phosphorus (20 mEq potassium dihydrogen phosphate/1000 intravenous calories) |
| Anemia | Iron deficiency; folic acid deficiency; vitamin $B_{12}$ deficiency; copper deficiency; other deficiencies | Alter nutrient administration |
| Bleeding | Vitamin K deficiency | Alter nutrient administration |
| Hypervitaminosis A | Excessive vitamin A administration | Alter nutrient administration |
| Elevations in SGOT, SGPT, and serum alkaline phosphatase levels | Enzyme induction secondary to amino acid imbalance or to excessive deposition of glycogen, fat, or both in liver | Reevaluate status of patient<br>Consider alteration in substrate profile |

time of any initial intra-abdominal procedures. Thus, the *common correctable causes of ileus* are:

> Hypoalbuminemia (value less than 2.5 g/dl)
> Narcotic use
> Electrolyte abnormalities
> Increased fat in diet

Although oral consumption of a diet is the easiest approach, this is usually inadequate in the sick patient and therefore tube feeding is necessary. Small feeding tubes, once confirmed in proper position, are utilized. Constant infusion is better tolerated than bolus feeding. The initial route and strength (tonicity) of the feedings is dependent on the length of time the gut has not been used. Mucosal atrophy begins after several days of nothing by mouth status and therefore the absorptive surface is diminished. In addition deficiencies in mucosal enzymes, such as lactase, may be present that alter the type of initial solution used. The *guidelines for tube feeding* are:

1. Place patient in sitting position (at least 45°) during feeding
2. Begin slow continuous infusion 30 cc/hr
3. Check for amount of residuals if feeding into stomach every several hours
4. If residuals more than 100 ml, decrease or temporarily terminate feeding
5. Increase rate as tolerated every 12 hours up to 150 to 200 ml/hr
6. Begin with hypoosmolar solution gradually increasing osmolarity to isoosmolar; (hyperosmolar solutions are less well tolerated and are reserved for patients with fluid restriction)
7. Type of tube feeding, i.e., nutrient-mix is dictated by same criteria as for parenteral feeding

The major complication of tube feeding is diarrhea, and the cause and treatment are given in Table 21-6. Mechanical, gastrointestinal, and metabolic complications are given in Table 21-7.

## Types of Tube Feeding

There are a large variety of tube feeding solutions available with nutrient mixes to meet a number of different clinical disease states (Table 21-8). In general, most are somewhat hyperosmolar and free water may need to be added to allow for gastrointestinal tolerance. Most also have a calorie to nitrogen ratio above 150:1. Several high protein solutions are now available that approach the 100:1 to 150:1 ratio. Protein supplement can be provided as protein powder or given intravenously to meet protein needs.

Solutions are also available for the patient with organ dysfunction, in particular renal and hepatic failure. The concepts of these nutrient mixes are identical to those described for parenteral feedings.

**Table 21-6** Major Complication of Tube Feeding: Diarrhea

| Cause | Treatment |
|---|---|
| Osmolarity too high | Dilute: Use of opiates |
| Rate too high | Decrease: Use of opiates |
| Lactose intolerance | Lactose-free diet |
| Fat malabsorption | Use medium-chain triglycerides |
| Bacterial contamination of feeding solution | Stop feedings until enteritis resolves |

**Table 21-7** Complications of Tube Feeding

| | Treatment |
|---|---|
| Mechanical | |
|   Nasopharyngeal irritation | Topical anesthetics |
|   Sinusitis | Decongestants |
|   Mucosal erosions; bleeding | Ice water lavage, remove or reposition tube |
|   Aspiration | Discontinue tube feeding until airway protected |
| Gastrointestinal | |
|   Cramping and distention | Reduce rate; if lactase deficient, put on lactose-free diet |
|   Vomiting and diarrhea | Reduce rate, concentration, change formula, antidiarrhea agents |
| Metabolic | |
|   Hyperosmolarity | Add more free water: Decrease feeding |
|   Hyperglycemia | Give insulin: Reduce carbohydrate |
|   Hepatic encephalopathy | Decrease protein content |
|   Renal failure | Decrease: $Mg^+$, $K^+$, $PO_4^-$ Use essential amino acids |
|   Cardiac failure | Decrease $Na^+$ and fluid |

Table 21-8  Examples of Enteral Products Available*

| Enteral Product Name | CHO+ (g) | PRO+ (g) | FAT (g) | NA+ mEq | K+ MEq | Kcals/cc | Osmol | Cal/N Ratio | Comments |
|---|---|---|---|---|---|---|---|---|---|
| Lactose free | 145 | 37 | 39 | 24 | 26 | 1.1 | 300 | 180:1 | Standard tube feeding, isotonic. Not recommended for oral feeding |
| Ensure | 145 | 37 | 37 | 32 | 32 | 1.0 | 460 | 180:1 | High protein content, both oral and tube feeding |
| Ensure Plus | 200 | 55 | 53 | 50 | 60 | 1.5 | 600 | 170:1 | High protein, high calorie feeding for volume restricted patients. Used for oral and tube feeding |
| Isocal | 132 | 34 | 44 | 23 | 34 | 1.0 | 300 | 200:1 | |
| Sustacal | 140 | 61 | 23 | 40 | 53 | 1.0 | 600 | 100:1 | |
| Chemically defined | | | | | | | | | |
| Vital HN | 188 | 42 | 11 | 20 | 34 | 1.0 | 450 | 150:1 | Minimal fecal residue. Low fat, partially digested protein. Used for patients with poor absorption or digestion |
| Vivonex | 226 | 20 | 2 | 37 | 30 | 1.0 | 525 | 300:1 | |

*Nutrient Analysis per 1000 ml

# 22
# Topical Antibiotics

## TOPICAL AGENTS

### Silver Sulfadiazine (Silvadene) 1% Cream

*Actions*

The active agents are the sulfa component and a slow release of silver from the cream base. This agent is the most commonly used topical antibiotic for major burns, in large part because of its low toxicity. The agent has moderate tissue penetration properties and causes rehydration and softening of the eschar. The antibacterial properties last for 12 to 24 hours, depending on the amount applied and wound contact. It is effective against a wide range of gram-positive and gram-negative organisms and fungi, including *Staphylococcus aureus,* Pseudomonas, and *Candida albicans*. Bacterial resistance will develop with continued use and with the more virulent hospital strains. Its action can be inhibited by pus or body fluids.

*Complications*

Pain is usually minimal on application. Skin allergy is uncommon. A transient leukopenia believed to be due either to eschar sequestration or bone marrow suppression is seen, which resolves after several days even with continued use. Some retardation of wound healing is seen.

*Effect on Wound*

Generally produces wound maceration and increased exudate, increasing eschar separation. The characteristic yellow slimy appearance of the agent after contact with the wound can be misinterpreted as being a grossly infected wound. Appears to increase the growth of hypertrophic granulation tissue when applied to the granulating wound. Epithelialization is retarded.

*Use*

Apply in a thin layer 1 to 2 mm thick directly to the burn. Although dressings are not mandatory, application of a layer of fine mesh gauze improves antibiotic contact and assists in wound debridement. The old cream and loose eschar are removed with dressing changes.

## Indications

It is the first choice as a prophylactic agent for controlling infection in deep burn and heavily contaminated superficial burns.

## Less Useful

It is less useful in small superficial epithelializing burns, especially to face, or in a clean granulating wound.

## Not Indicated

It is not indicated for placement on fresh skin grafts because of macerating effect or excised wounds (in cream base form), or when the patient has a sulfur allergy.

# Mafenide (Sulfamylon) 8.5% Cream

## Actions

Although the active ingredient is a sulfa compound, this agent is not a true sulfonamide chemically. The antibacterial spectrum is similar to silver sulfadiazine, but better coverage of *Pseudomonas aeruginosa* and anaerobes and better eschar penetration makes this agent more effective for the burn with a thick eschar, heavily colonized. Antibacterial action is not inhibited by pus or secretions. Bacterial resistance can develop. The agent should be applied every 12 to 18 hours, although some antibacterial action will persist in the eschar for up to 72 hours.

## Complications

Pain is significant on application, producing a burning sensation lasting 10 to 15 minutes, most prevalent with its use on a partial thickness burn. It is a carbonic anhydrase inhibitor, which therefore leads to increased $HCO^-_3$ wasting, metabolic acidosis, secondary respiratory alkalosis with tachypnea. The degree of metabolic acidosis is proportional to the surface area covered and age, particularly prevalent in the very young and elderly. Some impairment in wound healing is noted.

## Effect on Wound

Less maceration than silver sulfadiazine is noted. Eschar separation, in fact, is usually delayed due to decrease in bacterial content. Local impairment in wound healing and surrounding skin reaction seen in 5 to 10%.

## Use

Apply in a thin layer 1 mm thick directly to the wound. Dressings can be applied over the wound but are not necessary for antibacterial action. Eschar separation is delayed so that a more aggressive mechanical debridement will be necessary.

*Indicated*

It is the first choice for small deep *infected* wound. Can be used to impede eschar separation, e.g., on back, buttocks. Useful on deep burn when bacterial resistance to silver sulfadiazine develops.

*Less Useful*

It is less useful for uninfected partial thickness burn because of pain, toxicity.

*Not Indicated*

It is not indicated for most uninfected burns, for large body burns due to toxicity, in the patient with sulfa allergy, for clean, excised wounds, or for use on new grafts.

## Povidone-Iodine 1% Ointment

The active agent is the iodophor present in a viscous petroleum base (not water soluble). Iodine is a very effective antimicrobial that is leached from the base in several hours; therefore several applications (two to three times daily) is usually required with an active infection. Effective against most gram-positive and gram-negative organisms and fungi (less effective against Pseudomonas than mafenide). Eschar penetration is only moderate. Antimicrobial resistance will develop with continued use.

*Complications*

Pain on application is common. Iodine toxicity can occur but is very uncommon. Toxicity is more likely in the presence of renal dysfunction. Some impairment in wound healing is noted.

*Effect on Wound*

Less maceration than the preceding cream-based agents. Eschar actually appears to remain firm and dry, delaying separation. Some local wound toxicity, less than mafenide. Less tendency toward development of hypertrophic granulation tissue but produces wound hyperemia, probably due to irritant effect.

*Use*

Apply in a thin layer several times a day. Use of a layer of fine mesh gauze improves wound contact and antibacterial action.

*Indicated*

It is used as a substitute for silver sulfadiazine in a partial thickness burn. It is also indicated for use on granulation tissue after eschar separation for the treatment of wound bacteria that have developed resistance to other creams, for yeast or fungal wound colonization or infection, as long as eschar is not too thick, for burns in the perineum or buttocks where maceration is disadvantageous, and for small open areas between healed or grafted areas where maceration should be avoided.

*Not Indicated*

It is not indicated for superfical burns because pain is significant and healing can be retarded.

## Gentamicin (Cream, Ointment) 0.1%

The active agent is present in either a water-soluble cream or petroleum base ointment.

*Actions*

The antibacterial spectrum is primarily gram negative. Fungi, yeast, and anaerobes are not covered. At least two applications daily are needed. Eschar penetration is moderate.

*Complications*

Oto- and nephrotoxicity occur if excessive amounts are used. Selection for fungi will occur with prolonged use.

*Use*

Apply twice a day in a thin layer onto wound surface.

*Effect on Wound*

It does not produce as much exudate and maceration as silver sulfadiazine or mafenide, and it has less drying effect than povidone-iodine. Yeast (fungal) overgrowth can occur.

*Indicated*

It is used for wounds colonized with gram-negative organisms resistant to other more standard agents, for small superficial burns at risk for gram-negative infection, e.g., ear or perineal burns, and for small open areas on skin grafts or healing wounds.

*Not Indicated*

It is not indicated for large surface areas because of potential toxicity, or as a first choice agent.

## Bacitracin Ointment

The active agent is present in a petroleum base.

*Actions*

The antibacterial spectrum is predominately gram positive. Frequent applications are needed. Eschar penetration is limited.

*Complications*

It is nephrotoxic if absorbed in large amounts, e.g., use on extensive partial thickness burns. It has less retardation of wound healing than silver sulfadiazine. Yeast overgrowth can occur.

*Effect on Wound*

Maceration occurs less than with silver sulfadiazine.

*Indicated*

It is used for superficial burns, especially on the face, where usual infecting agent in first week is *S. aureus,* and for small open areas on reepithelialized burns or skin grafts.

*Not Indicated*

It is not indicated for deep second or third degree burns, or burns colonized with gram-negative organisms or yeast.

## Nitrofurazone (Furacin) Ointment or Cream

Active agent is in water-soluble cream or petrolatum ointment.

*Actions*

Agent is effective against *S. aureus* and some gram-negative organisms. Usually, it is not a good agent for *Pseudomonas*. Eschar penetration is limited.

*Complications*

It is nephrotoxic if large amounts used. Selection for yeast, fungi can result. Pain occurs on application.

*Effect on Wound*

Exudate production is minimal. Maceration is not usually seen.

*Use*

Apply twice daily to wound surface.

*Indications*

It is used for the treatment of resistant gram-positive or gram-negative organisms.

*Not Indicated*

It is not indicated as a first choice agent, or for burns with a thick eschar.

Table 22-1 Standard Topical Antibiotic Creams and Ointments

| | Silver Sulfadiazine | Mafenide Cream | Gentamycin Cream or Ointment | Povidone-Iodine Ointment | Bacitracin Ointment | Nystatin Cream | Nitrofurazone Ointment |
|---|---|---|---|---|---|---|---|
| Antimicrobial Spectrum | Good gr−,* Fair gr+ Fair fungi | Excellent gr− Good fungi Fair gr+ | Mostly gr− No fungi | Good gr−, gr+, and fungi | Mostly gr+ No fungi | Fungi | Good gr+ Some gr− |
| Eschar penetration | Good | Excellent | Good | Fair | Fair | Fair | Fair |
| Local tissue toxicity | Low | Some | Low | Some | Low | Low | Low |
| Systemic toxicity | Low transient marrow suppressor | High† metabolic acidosis | Low† ototoxicity and renal | Low† Iodine toxicity | Low† Renal | Low | Low† Renal |
| Pain | Rare | Yes 5–10% | Rare | Yes | No | No | Yes |
| Skin allergy | Rare | | Rare | Rare | Rare | Rare | Rare |

*gr−: gram-negative; gr+: gram positive
†All agents if used in excess amounts will lead to significant systemic toxicity

# Index

Acidosis
  anion gap, 286, 287
  lactate, 34, 194, 196, 197, 276
  types, 87, 88, 279–286, 288
Acute respiratory failure
  definition, 75
  diagnosis, 263–265
Adrenergic
  activity, 27, 95
  receptors, 95, 278, 279
Adult respiratory distress syndrome, 77–79, 159–164
Age, 46
Airways
  edema, 8, 9, 71, 72
  infection, 74–77
Alkalosis, 284, 287
Anemia, 86, 169
Anesthesia, 80, 81, 119–121, 185, 188
Antibiotics
  systemic, 57, 199, 200, 232
  topical, 57, 116, 117, 232, 301–307

Bacteria, *see* Infection
Behavior changes, 212, 213
Biobrane, 59, 60, 130
Blood gas, 19, 34, 39, 94, 259
Blunt trauma and burns
  airway, 248
  breathing, 248, 249
  circulation, 249, 250
  intra-abdominal, 251, 252
  neurologic, 250, 251
  orthopedic, 252, 253
Bronchoconstriction, 12, 13, 14, 17
Bronchodilators, 15
Burn area
  abdomen, 137

  axilla, 138
  back, 143
  breast, 138
  buttocks, 149
  chest, 17, 18, 22, 73, 83, 137
  eyes, 61
  face, 9, 60
  foot, 61, 141
  hand, 61, 141
  lower extremity, 62
  neck, 9, 138
  perineum, 62, 144
  upper extremity, 141
Burn
  categorization, 52, 66, 67
  depth, 44, 45, 102, 103
  size, 47, 48
  survival, 48
Burn center, 66
Burn wound
  cleaning, 55, 56, 65
  debridement, 55, 65, 113–117, 185, 201
  second degree, 44, 52, 65, 102, 105, 113–115, 179–180, 183, 191
  third degree, 45, 52, 65, 103, 105, 113–115, 135–137, 180, 181, 184, 191
  zone of ischemia, 46

Donor sites, 130–132
Dressing, burn
  antibiotic, 57, 116, 117, 301–307
  biologic, 58, 59
  synthetic, 58, 59, 133
  techniques, 58, 59, 113–117

Edema
  airway, 8, 9, 72

305

Edema (Cont.)
  burn, 25, 26, 85
  nonburn, 27, 85
Electrical burns, high voltage
  complications, 226–230, 238
  debridement, 233, 234
  etiology, 224–228
  fluids, 231
  monitoring, 230, 231
  treatment, 231–236
Endotracheal intubation
  indications, 7, 10, 16, 266
  size, 20
Entrance site, 226
Escharotomy, 19, 62, 64
Evaporative loss, 85, 91, 105, 169
Excisional therapy
  fascial, 122, 130, 188
  indications, 119, 135–137, 145, 233
  tangential, 122–127, 188
Exercise, 213, 214, 220

Facial burns, 9, 60
Fasciotomy, 233
Fat emulsions, 297, 293
Feeding, see Nutrition
Fiberoptic bronchoscopy, 9, 12, 16
Fluid loss
  evaporative, 85, 91
  initial burn, 25–28
Fluid replacement
  evaporation, 85, 91, 105
  initial burn, 30
  operating room, 91, 120, 121
  protein infusion, 91, 239
Fluid types, 29–33
Full thickness burn, 44, 45

Grafting
  bleeding, 131, 187, 188
  dressing, 131–134, 188
  donor sites, 130–132, 188
  procedure, 130–133, 186–188

Hand
  burns, 141
  heat loss, 50, 51, 120, 212
  hematologic changes, 28, 29, 36, 86
  hemodynamic monitoring, 27, 28, 33–36, 98, 122, 230, 231, 272–277
  hypercapnia, 265, 266

hyperkalemia, 88
hypermetabolism, 88, 170–173, 196
hypernatremia, 88
hyperthermia, 88
Hypoproteinemia, 26, 78, 85, 94, 296
Hypothermia, 35, 50
heterotopic calcification, 211
rehabilitation, 208–220

Immunologic response, 105, 106, 151–153, 193
Infection
  biopsy diagnosis, 110
  burn, 56, 57, 105, 106, 108, 110, 111, 185
  control, 111–113, 150
  pneumonia, 76, 77, 149–156
  sepsis, 193
  tracheobronchitis, 72, 76, 77, 151–153
Inflammation
  lung, 77–79
  wound, 101
Inhalation injury
  airway response, 3–17, 71, 72, 74–77, 151–153
  carbon monoxide, 5–7, 19
Inotropic support, 37, 95, 96, 201, 279, 280
Intravenous access, 32, 92, 93

Laryngoscopy, 12, 16
Lightning, 242–244
Low voltage injury, 235, 236, 240–242
Lung defenses, 151–153, 155
Lung changes
  burn alone, 16, 17
  inhalation, see Inhalation injury
  power failure, 156–158, 166

Mafenide, 302
Mannitol, 231
Mechanical ventilation, 13, 74, 266–269
Mediators, 17, 25, 80, 171, 172, 202
Metabolic changes, 88, 170–173
Mortality, 48

Nutrition
  assessment, 89, 173, 174, 177, 202
  enteral, 293, 297–300
  parenteral, 290–294

Operating room
  environment, 119–122, 192
  transport, 119, 120

Oral burn electrical, 240–242
Osmotic pressure, 26, 89, 92
Oxygen delivery, 28
Oxygen consumption,
        88, 93, 154, 178, 193,
        199, 276

Pain treatment, 55
Paralyzing agents, 270
Permeability
  burn tissue, 25, 26, 85
  lung, 79, 80
Pharmacologic support, 37, 95, 96, 279, 280
Physical therapy
  exercise, 213, 214, 220
  splinting, 215, 216
Pneumonia, 76, 77, 149–153, 165
Positioning, 215, 216, 220
Positive end expiratory pressure,
  13, 74, 163, 185, 199, 268, 269
Pressure garments, 217, 218
Pseudomonas, 111, 232
Psychosocial support, 218
Pulmonary edema
  high pressure, 77–79
  low pressure (ARDS), 79–81

Rehabilitation, 207–222
Renal injury, 228
Rotating bed, 76

Scar tissue, 182, 184, 210
Scar management, 184, 217, 218

Sepsis
  burn, 200
  causes, 198
  definition, 193, 194
  hyperdynamic, 194, 195
  hypodynamic, 194, 195
  metabolic response, 196, 197
Shunt pulmonary, 260
Silver sulfadiazine, 301
Skin anatomy, 42
Skin grafts, *see* Grafting
Skin substitutes, 59, 60, 130
Smoke inhalation, *see* Inhalation
Splints, 215, 216
Staphylococcus aureus, 109, 111, 181, 232
Surgical excision, *see* Excisional therapy

Topical antibiotics, 57, 116, 117, 232, 301–307
Transfer, 66, 67
Trauma and burns
  airway assessment, 248
  chest injuries, 249
  intra-abdominal, 251
  neurological, 250
  orthopedic, 252
Tube feeding
  complications, 297, 298
  technique, 293, 296, 297

Ventilation monitoring, 261–263
Ventilation-perfusion, 259, 260
Ventilators, 268, 269
Vitamins, 175, 292

Wound Healing, 103, 106, 181–183

# Color Plates

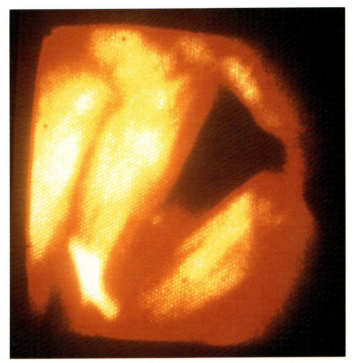

**Color plate 1.** Erythema and edema of the larynx 18 hours after burn as seen through a fiberoptic bronchoscope.

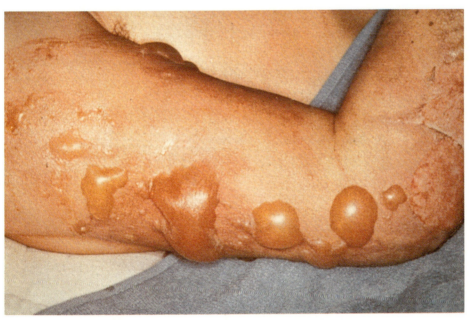

**Color plate 2.** A typical superficial second degree burn is shown with blister formation.

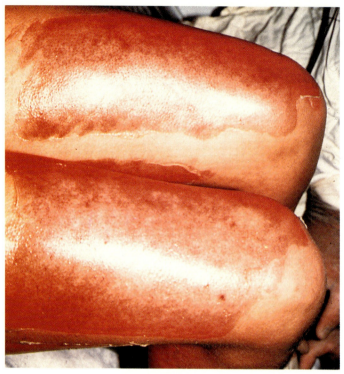

**Color plate 3.** A deep dermal burn, produced by flames, is shown. The red appearance with deeper whitish areas is typical.

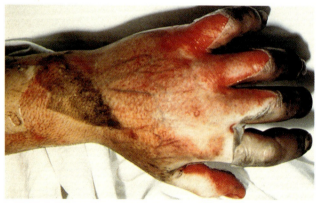

**Color plate 4.** A full-thickness burn of the hand is shown that actually extends below dermis into subdermal tissues.

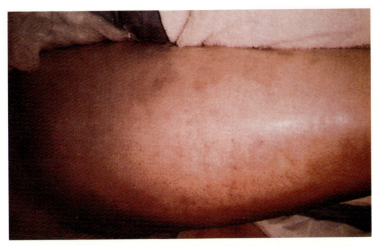

**Color plate 5.** A typical indeterminate burn is shown where a distinction between very deep dermal versus full thickness cannot be made at this time.

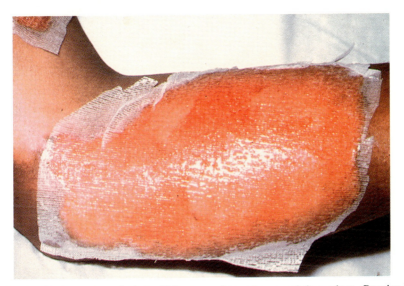

**Color plate 6.** Synthetic skin substitute, biobrane, used to cover second degree burn. Dressing is well adhered.

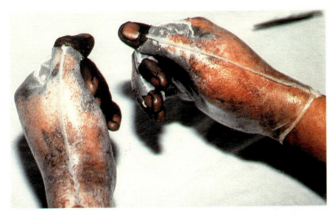

**Color plate 7.** Biobrane gloves applied to superficial second degree burn to the hands.

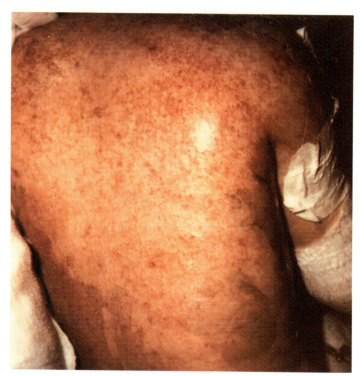

**Color plate 8.** A, Mid-deep second degree burn to back, 1 day after silver sulfadiazine treatment.

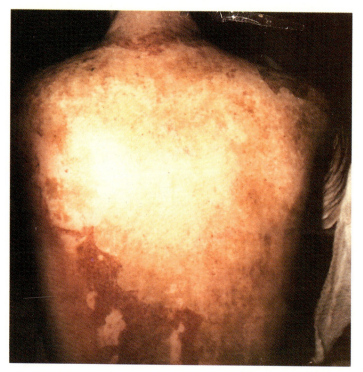

**Color plate 8.** B, Same burn 5 days later. Note thin yellow eschar, which is peeling away from the edges. Wound looks deeper because of superficial exudate, but it healed in 16 days.

Color Plates   315

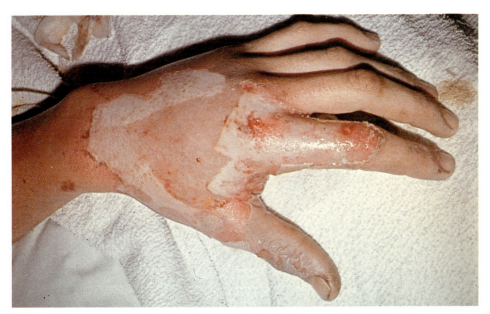

**Color plate 9.**  A deep dermal hand burn is shown, which is ideally treated with early tangential excision and grafting.

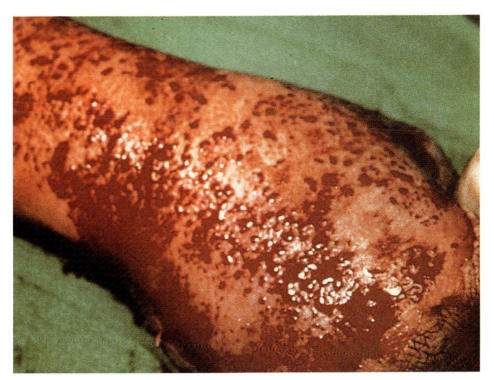

**Color plate 10.**  Brisk punctate bleeding from adequately excised hand burn is shown.

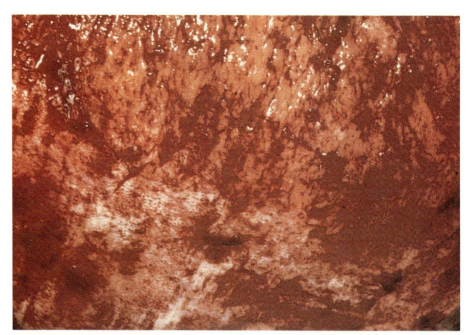

**Color plate 11.** Tangential excision endpoint for full-thickness burn is shown. Fat is light yellow in color and shiny. Surrounding areas have some remaining viable dermis.

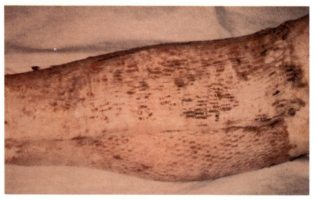

**Color plate 12.** Meshed skin graft. Note exposed fascia between mesh, which needs to be kept moist.

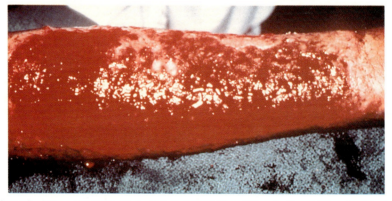

**Color plate 13.** Clean granulation tissue bed on full-thickness injury is shown. The wound is painful and bleeds easily when manipulated. Very gentle cleaning is required.

*Color Plates* **317**

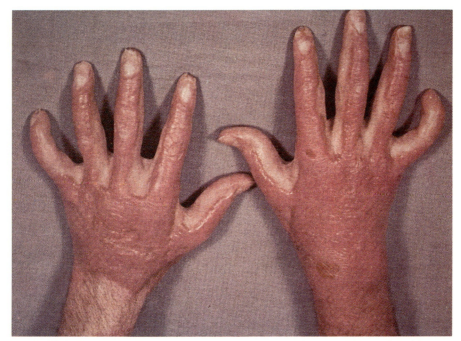

**Color plate 14.** Hypertrophic scarring.

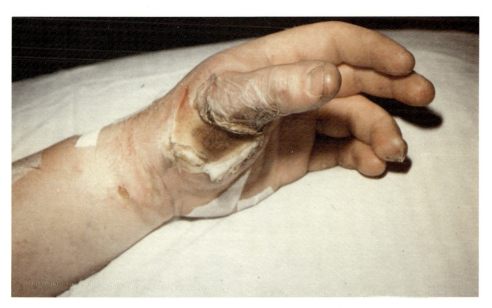

**Color plate 15.** Typical entrance site of a high voltage injury is shown on a hand. Note desiccation of tissue at entrance site.

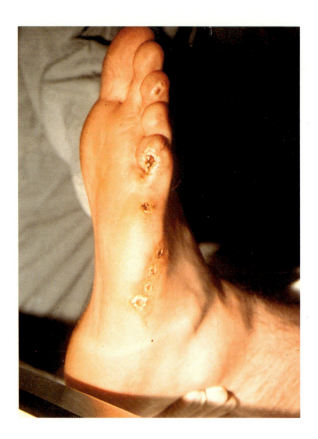

**Color plate 16.** Typical exit sites on foot where current exits from body. Areas are often small, round, and punctate, appearing quite innocuous.

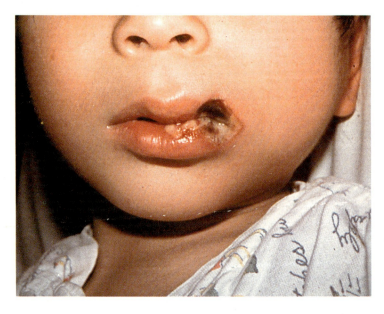

**Color plate 17.** Typical oral burn from biting on an electrical cord. Note tissue necrosis at corner of mouth.